Anxiety Disorders
SOURCEBOOK

First Edition

First Edition

Anxiety Disorders
SOURCEBOOK

Basic Consumer Health Information about Mental Health Disorders and Associated Myths and Facts, Types of Anxiety Disorders, Including General Anxiety Disorder, Obsessive-Compulsive Disorder, Posttraumatic Stress Disorder, Panic Disorder, Social Anxiety Disorder, Specific Phobia, Separation Anxiety, Illness Anxiety Disorder, Somatic Symptom Disorder, and More

Along with Information about Causes, Risk Factors, Treatment Options, Including Medications, Psychotherapy, and Complementary and Alternative Medications, Financial Assistance, Tips for Caregivers, a Glossary of Related Terms, and a Directory of Resources for More Information

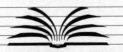

OMNIGRAPHICS

615 Griswold, Ste. 901, Detroit, MI 48226

Bibliographic Note
Because this page cannot legibly accommodate all the copyright notices, the Bibliographic
Note portion of the Preface constitutes an extension of the copyright notice.

* * *

OMNIGRAPHICS
Siva Ganesh Maharaja, *Managing Editor*
***

Copyright © 2018 Omnigraphics

ISBN 978-0-7808-1587-2
E-ISBN 978-0-7808-1588-9

Library of Congress Cataloging-in-Publication Data

Names: Omnigraphics, Inc., issuing body.

Title: Anxiety disorders sourcebook: basic consumer health information about
mental health disorders and associated myths and facts, types of anxiety
disorders, including general anxiety disorder, obsessive-compulsive disorder,
posttraumatic stress disorder, panic disorder, social anxiety disorder, specific
phobia, separation anxiety, illness anxiety disorder, somatic symptom disorder,
and more; along with information about causes, risk factors, treatment options,
including medications, psychotherapy, and complementary and alternative
medications, financial assistance, tips for caregivers, a glossary of related terms,
and a directory of resources for more information.

Description: First edition. | Detroit, MI: Omnigraphics, [2018] | Series: Health
reference series | Includes bibliographical references and index.

Identifiers: LCCN 2017036996 (print) | LCCN 2017039335 (ebook) | ISBN
9780780815889 (eBook) | ISBN 9780780815872 (hardcover: alk. paper)

Subjects: LCSH: Anxiety disorders--Popular works.

Classification: LCC RC531 (ebook) | LCC RC531.A6137 2018 (print) | DDC
616.85/22--dc23

LC record available at https://lccn.loc.gov/2017036996

Table of Contents

Part II: Types of Anxiety Disorders

Part IV: Anxiety and Other Chronic Illnesses

Part V: Managing Stress and Everyday Anxiety

Part VI: Looking Ahead

Preface

About This Book

According to the Office on Women's Health (OWH), nearly 40 million American adults suffer some form of anxiety. Concerns over finances, work, family, and the future are common sources of anxiety. In many cases individuals cope with such stressors and lead a healthy life. However, for others, worry becomes uncontrollable, taking a profound physical and mental toll. Prolonged anxiety can also lead to severe conditions such as heart disease and diabetes, and may also make an individual more vulnerable to substance abuse.

Anxiety Disorders Sourcebook, First Edition provides insight into the various ways people experience anxiety and its various types of disorders, including general anxiety disorder, obsessive-compulsive disorder, posttraumatic stress disorder (PTSD), and panic disorder. It provides information about chronic illnesses linked to anxiety and ways to overcome them. It also discusses anxiety in specific populations such as pregnant women, children, older adults, and the LGBT community. The book explains various treatment therapies such as psychotherapy, cognitive processing therapy, and complementary and alternative therapies for the anxiety disorders. Suggestions for coping with anxiety disorders are also included. The book concludes with a glossary of related terms and a directory of mental health organizations for people with anxiety disorders and other mental health concerns.

How to Use This Book

This book is divided into parts and chapters. Parts focus on broad areas of interest. Chapters are devoted to single topics within a part.

Part I: Introduction to Mental Health Disorders and Anxiety begins with an overview of mental health and mental health disorders. It dispels common myths and provides facts about mental health. It discusses anxiety disorders in general and provides statistical information on anxiety disorders in the United States, and its incidence in specific populations.

Part II: Types of Anxiety Disorders gives an overview of anxiety disorders and the signs, symptoms, diagnosis, and treatment-related aspects of the most common types of anxiety-related mental health disorders including agoraphobia, general anxiety disorder, obsessive-compulsive disorder, panic disorder, posttraumatic stress disorder, selective mutism, separation anxiety disorder, social anxiety disorder, somatic symptom disorder, specific phobia, and test anxiety.

Part III: Causes, Risk Factors, and Treatment for Anxiety Disorders highlights genetic, biological, environmental, and situational factors that can predispose a person to developing anxiety. The impact of smoking and bullying on anxiety is included. Therapies for alleviating anxiety disorders such as antianxiety medications, cognitive behavioral therapy and complementary approaches including abdominal breathing, chamomile capsules, meditation, mindfulness, relaxation therapy, and yoga have been highlighted. Technological frontiers in the treatment of mental health disorders are also discussed.

Part IV: Anxiety and Other Chronic Illnesses discusses the signs, symptoms, diagnosis, and treatment of chronic illnesses and conditions often linked to anxiety, such as attention deficit hyperactive disorder (ADHD), bipolar disorder, body dysmorphic disorder (BDD), borderline personality disorder, cancer, depression, eating disorders, erectile dysfunction, fibromyalgia, human immunodeficiency virus/acquired immunodeficiency syndrome (HIV/AIDS), irritable bowel syndrome (IBS), sleep disorders, and substance abuse.

Part V: Managing Stress and Everyday Anxiety describes how one can manage and cope with the symptoms of anxiety. It discusses on how exercise and animal companionship help in managing stress and other anxiety-related disorders. It also talks about developing resilience and coping with emotions related to anxiety.

Part VI: Looking Ahead highlights ways individuals with anxiety disorders can lead productive lives. It discusses about coping strategies for maintaining emotional wellness in people who have anxiety. It provides details about financial assistance and help available for people with anxiety disorders. Mental health issues among caregivers and coping strategies are also covered. The part concludes with clinical trials available for people with anxiety disorders and with a glance on the latest ongoing research.

Part VII: Additional Help and Information provides a glossary of terms related to anxiety disorders and directories of mental health resources and organizations for people with anxiety disorders and other mental concerns.

Bibliographic Note

This volume contains documents and excerpts from publications issued by the following government agencies: Centers for Disease Control and Prevention (CDC); Centers for Medicare and Medicaid Services (CMS); *Eunice Kennedy Shriver* National Institute of Child Health and Human Development (NICHD); Federal Emergency Management Agency (FEMA); National Cancer Institute (NCI); National Center for Complementary and Integrative Health (NCCIH); National Institute of Diabetes and Digestive and Kidney Diseases (NIDDK); National Institute of Mental Health (NIMH); National Institute on Aging (NIA); National Institute on Drug Abuse (NIDA); National Institutes of Health (NIH); National Institutes of Health (NIH); National Park Service (NPS); *NIH News in Health*; Office on Women's Health (OWH); Substance Abuse and Mental Health Services Administration (SAMHSA); U.S. Department of Health and Human Services (HHS); U.S. Department of Veterans Affairs (VA); and U.S. Public Health Service Commissioned Corps.

It may also contain original material produced by Omnigraphics and reviewed by medical consultants.

About the Health Reference Series

The *Health Reference Series* is designed to provide basic medical information for patients, families, caregivers, and the general public. Each volume takes a particular topic and provides comprehensive coverage. This is especially important for people who may be dealing with a newly diagnosed disease or a chronic disorder in themselves or in a family member. People looking for preventive guidance, information about disease warning signs, medical statistics, and risk factors for health problems will also find answers to their questions in the *Health Reference Series*. The *Series*, however, is not intended to serve as a tool for diagnosing illness, in prescribing treatments, or as a substitute for the physician/patient relationship. All people concerned about medical symptoms or the possibility of disease are encouraged to seek professional care from an appropriate healthcare provider.

A Note about Spelling and Style

Health Reference Series editors use *Stedman's Medical Dictionary* as an authority for questions related to the spelling of medical terms and the *Chicago Manual of Style* for questions related to grammatical structures, punctuation, and other editorial concerns. Consistent adherence is not always possible, however, because the individual volumes within the *Series* include many documents from a wide variety of different producers, and the editor's primary goal is to present material from each source as accurately as is possible. This sometimes means that information in different chapters or sections may follow other guidelines and alternate spelling authorities. For example, occasionally a copyright holder may require that eponymous terms be shown in possessive forms (Crohn's disease vs. Crohn disease) or that British spelling norms be retained (leukaemia vs. leukemia).

Medical Review

Omnigraphics contracts with a team of qualified, senior medical professionals who serve as medical consultants for the *Health Reference Series*. As necessary, medical consultants review reprinted and originally written material for currency and accuracy. Citations including the phrase, "Reviewed (month, year)" indicate material reviewed by this team. Medical consultation services are provided to the *Health Reference Series* editors by:

Dr. Vijayalakshmi, MBBS, DGO, MD
Dr. Senthil Selvan, MBBS, DCH, MD
Dr. K. Sivanandham, MBBS, DCH, MS (Research), PhD

Our Advisory Board

We would like to thank the following board members for providing initial guidance on the development of this series:

- Dr. Lynda Baker, Associate Professor of Library and Information Science, Wayne State University, Detroit, MI

- Nancy Bulgarelli, William Beaumont Hospital Library, Royal Oak, MI

- Karen Imarisio, Bloomfield Township Public Library, Bloomfield Township, MI

- Karen Morgan, Mardigian Library, University of Michigan-Dearborn, Dearborn, MI

- Rosemary Orlando, St. Clair Shores Public Library, St. Clair Shores, MI

Health Reference Series *Update Policy*

The inaugural book in the *Health Reference Series* was the first edition of *Cancer Sourcebook* published in 1989. Since then, the *Series* has been enthusiastically received by librarians and in the medical community. In order to maintain the standard of providing high-quality health information for the layperson the editorial staff at Omnigraphics felt it was necessary to implement a policy of updating volumes when warranted.

Medical researchers have been making tremendous strides, and it is the purpose of the *Health Reference Series* to stay current with the most recent advances. Each decision to update a volume is made on an individual basis. Some of the considerations include how much new information is available and the feedback we receive from people who use the books. If there is a topic you would like to see added to the update list, or an area of medical concern you feel has not been adequately addressed, please write to:

Managing Editor
Health Reference Series
Omnigraphics
615 Griswold, Ste. 901
Detroit, MI 48226

Part One

Introduction to Mental Health Disorders and Anxiety

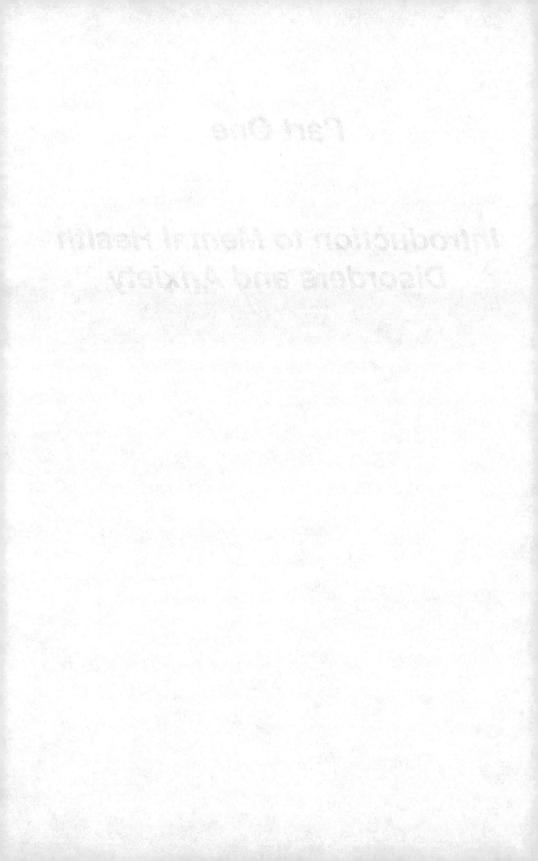

Chapter 1

Introduction to Mental Health Disorders

Chapter Contents

Section 1.1

What Is Mental Health?

This section contains text excerpted from the following
sources: Text in this section begins with excerpts from
"Mental Health," MedlinePlus, National Institutes of Health (NIH),
April 2, 2015; Text under the heading "Facts about Mental Health
Disorders" is excerpted from "Mental Disorders," Substance Abuse
and Mental Health Services Administration (SAMHSA),
October 27, 2015.

Mental health includes our emotional, psychological, and social
wellbeing. It affects how we think, feel and act as we cope with life.
It also helps determine how we handle stress, relate to others, and
make choices. Mental health is important at every stage of life, from
childhood and adolescence through adulthood.

Mental illnesses are serious disorders which can affect your thinking, mood, and behavior. There are many causes of mental disorders.
Your genes and family history may play a role. Your life experiences,
such as stress or a history of abuse, may also matter. Biological factors can also be part of the cause. Mental disorders are common, but
treatments are available.

Facts about Mental Health Disorders

The following are descriptions of the most common categories of
mental illness in the United States.

Anxiety Disorders

Anxiety disorders are characterized by excessive fear or anxiety
that is difficult to control and negatively and substantially impacts
daily functioning. Fear refers to the emotional response to a real or
perceived threat while anxiety is the anticipation of a future threat.
These disorders can range from specific fears (called phobias), such
as the fear of flying or public speaking, to more generalized feelings
of worry and tension. Anxiety disorders typically develop in childhood
and persist to adulthood. Specific anxiety disorders include generalized

4

anxiety disorder (GAD), panic disorder, separation anxiety disorder, and social anxiety disorder (social phobia).

National prevalence data indicate that nearly 40 million people in the United States (18%) experience an anxiety disorder in any given year. According to Substance Abuse and Mental Health Services Administration's (SAMHSA) report, *Behavioral Health, United States–2012*, lifetime phobias and generalized anxiety disorders are the most prevalent among adolescents between the ages of 13 and 18 and have the earliest median age of first onset, around age 6. Phobias and generalized anxiety usually first appear around age 11, and they are the most prevalent anxiety disorders in adults.

Evidence suggests that many anxiety disorders may be caused by a combination of genetics, biology, and environmental factors. Adverse childhood experiences may also contribute to risk for developing anxiety disorders.

Attention Deficit Hyperactivity Disorder (ADHD)

ADHD is defined by a persistent pattern of inattention (for example, difficulty keeping focus) and/or hyperactivity-impulsivity (for example, difficulty controlling behavior, excessive and inappropriate motor activity). Children with ADHD have difficulty performing well in school, interacting with other children, and following through on tasks. Adults with ADHD are often extremely distractible and have significant difficulties with organization. There are three subtypes of the disorder:

- Predominantly hyperactive/impulsive

- Predominantly inattentive

- Combined hyperactive/inattentive

ADHD is one of the more common mental disorders diagnosed among children. Data from the 2011 National Health Interview Survey (NHIS) indicate that parents of 8.4 percent of children aged 3 to 17 years had been informed that their child had ADHD. For youth ages 13 to 18, the prevalence rate is 9 percent. The disorder occurs four times as often among boys than girls. It is estimated that the prevalence of ADHD among adults is 2.5 percent.

Current research suggests that ADHD has a high degree of heritability, however, the exact gene or constellation of genes that give rise to the disorder are not known. Environmental risk factors may include low birth weight, smoking and alcohol use during pregnancy, exposure to lead, and history of child maltreatment.

The three overarching features of ADHD include inattention, hyperactivity, and impulsivity. Inattentive children may have trouble paying close attention to details, make careless mistakes in schoolwork, are easily distracted, have difficulty following through on tasks, such as homework assignments, or quickly become bored with a task. Hyperactivity may be defined by fidgeting or squirming, excessive talking, running about, or difficulty sitting still. Finally, impulsive children may be impatient, may blurt out answers to questions prematurely, have trouble waiting their turn, may frequently interrupt conversations, or intrude on others' activities.

Bipolar and Related Disorders

People with bipolar and related disorders experience atypical, dramatic swings in mood, and activity levels that go from periods of feeling intensely happy, irritable, and impulsive to periods of intense sadness and feelings of hopelessness. Individuals with this disorder experience discrete mood episodes, characterized as either a:

- **Manic episode**—abnormally elevated, expansive, or irritable mood accompanied by increased energy or activity that substantially impairs functioning

- **Hypomanic episode**—similar to a manic episode, however not severe enough to cause serious social or occupational problems

- **Major depressive episode**—persistent depressed mood or loss of interest or pleasure

- **Mixed state**—includes symptoms of both a manic episode and a major depressive episode

People exhibiting these symptoms are most frequently identified as having one of two types of bipolar disorders: bipolar I disorder or bipolar II disorder. The bipolar I diagnosis is used when there has been at least one manic episode in a person's life. The bipolar II diagnosis is used when there has been a more regular occurrence of depressive episodes along with a hypomanic episode, but not a full-blown manic episode. Cyclothymic disorder, or cyclothymia, is a diagnosis used for a mild form of bipolar disorder.

The combined prevalence of bipolar I disorder, bipolar II disorder and cyclothymia is estimated at 2.6 percent of the U.S. adult population and 11.2 percent for 13 to 18-year-old.

A family history of bipolar disorder is the strongest risk factor for the condition, and the level of risk increases with the degree of kinship.

As mentioned previously, bipolar disorders are characterized by manic and depressive episodes. In children, manic episodes may present as an excessively silly or joyful mood that is unusual for the child or an uncharacteristically irritable temperament and are accompanied by unusual behavioral changes, such as decreased need for sleep, risk-seeking behavior, and distractibility. Depressive episodes may present as a persistent, sad mood, feelings of worthlessness or guilt, and loss of interest in previously enjoyable activities. Behavioral changes associated with depressive episodes may include fatigue or loss of energy, gaining or losing a significant amount of weight, complaining about pain, or suicidal thoughts or plans.

Depressive Disorders (Including Major Depressive Disorder)

Depressive disorders are among the most common mental health disorders in the United States. They are characterized by a sad, hopeless, empty, or irritable mood, and somatic and cognitive changes that significantly interfere with daily life. Major depressive disorder (MDD) is defined as having a depressed mood for most of the day and a marked loss of interest or pleasure, among other symptoms present nearly every day for at least a two-week period. In children and adolescents, MDD may manifest as an irritable rather than a sad disposition. Suicidal thoughts or plans can occur during an episode of major depression, which can require immediate attention (to be connected to a skilled, trained counselor at a local crisis center, people can call National Suicide Prevention Hotline: 800-272-TALK (800-272-8255) anytime 24/7.

Based on the 2014 National Survey on Drug Use and Health (NSDUH) data, 6.6 percent of adults aged 18 or older had a major depressive episode (MDE) in 2014, which was defined by the 4th edition of the *Diagnostic and Statistical Manual of Mental Disorders* (DSM-IV). The NSDUH data also show that the prevalence of MDE among adolescents aged 12 to 17 was 11.4 percent in 2014, while female youths were about three times as likely as male youths to experience a MDE.

MDD is thought to have many possible causes, including genetic, biological, and environmental factors. Adverse childhood experiences and stressful life experiences are known to contribute to risk for MDD. In addition, those with closely related family members (for

7

example, parents or siblings) who are diagnosed with the disorder are at increased risk.

A diagnosis for MDD at a minimum requires that symptoms of depressed mood (for example, feelings of sadness, emptiness, hopelessness) and loss of interest or pleasure in activities are present. Additional symptoms may include significant weight loss or gain, insomnia or hypersomnia, feelings of restlessness, lethargy, feelings of worthlessness or excessive guilt, distractibility, and recurrent thoughts of death, including suicidal ideation. Symptoms must be present for at least two-weeks and cause significant impairment or dysfunction in daily life.

Disruptive, Impulse Control, and Conduct Disorders

This class of disorders is characterized by problems with self-control of emotions or behaviors that violate the rights of others and/or bring a person into conflict with societal norms or authority figures. Oppositional defiant disorder and conduct disorder are the most prominent of this class of disorders in children.

Oppositional Defiant Disorder

Children with oppositional defiant disorder (ODD) display a frequent and persistent pattern of angry or irritable mood, argumentative/defiant behavior, or vindictiveness. Symptoms are typically first seen in the preschool years, and often precede the development of conduct disorder.

The average prevalence of ODD is estimated at 3.3 percent, and occurs more often in boys than girls.

Children who experienced harsh, inconsistent, or neglectful child-rearing practices are at increased risk for developing ODD.

Symptoms of ODD include angry/irritable mood, argumentative/defiant behavior, or vindictiveness. A child with an angry/irritable mood may often lose their temper, be frequently resentful, or easily annoyed. Argumentative or defiant children are frequently combative with authority figures or adults and often refuse to comply with rules. They may also deliberately annoy others or blame others for their mistakes or misbehavior. These symptoms must be evident for at least six months and observed when interacting with at least one individual who is not a sibling.

Conduct Disorder

Occurring in children and teens, conduct disorder is a persistent pattern of disruptive and violent behaviors that violate the basic rights of others or age-appropriate social norms or rules, and causes significant impairment in the child or family's daily life.

An estimated 8.5 percent of children and youth meet criteria for conduct disorder at some point in their life. Prevalence increases from childhood to adolescence and is more common among males than females.

Conduct disorder may be preceded by temperamental risk factors, such as behavioral difficulties in infancy and below-average intelligence. Similar to ODD, environmental risk factors may include harsh or inconsistent child-rearing practices and/or child maltreatment. Parental criminality, frequent changes of caregivers, large family size, familial psychopathology, and early institutional living may also contribute to risk for developing the disorder. Community-level risk factors may include neighborhood exposure to violence, peer rejection, and association with a delinquent peer group. Children with a parent or sibling with conduct disorder or other behavioral health disorders (for example, ADHD, schizophrenia, severe alcohol use disorder) are more likely to develop the condition. Children with conduct disorder often present with other disorders as well, including ADHD, learning disorders, and depression.

The primary symptoms of conduct disorder include aggression to people and animals (for example, bullying or causing physical harm), destruction of property (for example, fire-setting), deceitfulness or theft (for example, breaking and entering), and serious violations of rules (for example, truancy, elopement). Symptoms must be present for 12 months and fall into one of three subtypes depending on the age at onset (childhood, adolescent, or unspecified).

Obsessive-Compulsive and Related Disorders

Obsessive-compulsive disorder (OCD) is defined by the presence of persistent thoughts, urges, or images that are intrusive and unwanted (obsessions), or repetitive and ritualistic behaviors that a person feels are necessary in order to control obsessions (compulsions). OCD tends to begin in childhood or adolescence, with most individuals being diagnosed by the age of 19.

In the United States, the 12-month prevalence rate of OCD is estimated at 1.2 percent or nearly 2.2 million American adults.

The causes of OCD are largely unknown, however there is some evidence that it runs in families and is associated with environmental risk factors, such as child maltreatment or traumatic childhood events.

Prerequisites for OCD include the presence of obsessions, compulsions, or both. Obsessions may include persistent thoughts (for example, of contamination), images (for example, of horrific scenes), or urges (for example, to jump from a window) and are perceived as unpleasant and involuntary. Compulsions include repetitive behaviors that the person is compelled to carry out ritualistically in response to an obsession or according to a rigid set of rules. Compulsions are carried out in an effort to prevent or reduce anxiety or distress, and yet are clearly excessive or unrealistic. A common example of an OCD symptom is a person who is obsessed with germs and feels compelled to wash their hands excessively. OCD symptoms are time-consuming and cause significant dysfunction in daily life.

Schizophrenia Spectrum and Other Psychotic Disorders

The defining characteristic of schizophrenia and other psychotic disorders is abnormalities in one or more of five domains: delusions, hallucinations, disorganized thinking, grossly disorganized or abnormal motor behavior, and negative symptoms, which include diminished emotional expression and a decrease in the ability to engage in self-initiated activities. Disorders in this category include schizotypal disorder, schizoaffective disorder, and schizophreniform disorder. The most common diagnosis in this category is schizophrenia.

Schizophrenia

Schizophrenia is a brain disorder that impacts the way a person thinks (often described as a "thought disorder"), and is characterized by a range of cognitive, behavioral, and emotional experiences that can include: delusions, hallucinations, disorganized thinking, and grossly disorganized or abnormal motor behavior. These symptoms are chronic and severe, significantly impairing occupational and social functioning.

The lifetime prevalence of schizophrenia is estimated to be about 1percent of the population. Childhood-onset schizophrenia (defined as onset before age 13) is much rarer, affecting approximately 0.01 percent of children. Symptoms of schizophrenia typically manifest between the ages of 16 and 30.

While family history of psychosis is often not predictive of schizophrenia, genetic predisposition correlates to risk for developing the disease. Physiological factors, such as certain pregnancy and birth complications and environmental factors, such as season of birth (late winter/early spring) and growing up in an urban environment may be associated with increased risk for schizophrenia.

People with schizophrenia can experience what are termed positive or negative symptoms. Positive symptoms are psychotic behaviors including:

- Delusions of false and persistent beliefs that are not part of the individual's culture. For example, people with schizophrenia may believe that their thoughts are being broadcast on the radio.

- Hallucinations that include hearing, seeing, smelling, or feeling things that others cannot. Most commonly, people with the disorder hear voices that talk to them or order them to do things.

- Disorganized speech that involves difficulty organizing thoughts, thought-blocking, and making up nonsensical words.

- Grossly disorganized or catatonic behavior.

Negative symptoms may include flat affect, disillusionment with daily life, isolating behavior, lack of motivation, and infrequent speaking, even when forced to interact. As with other forms of serious mental illness, schizophrenia is related to homelessness, involvement with the criminal justice system, and other negative outcomes.

Trauma- and Stressor-Related Disorders

The defining characteristic of trauma- and stressor-related disorders is previous exposure to a traumatic or stressful event. The most common disorder in this category is posttraumatic stress disorder (PTSD).

Posttraumatic Stress Disorder (PTSD)

PTSD is characterized as the development of debilitating symptoms following exposure to a traumatic or dangerous event. These can include re-experiencing symptoms from an event, such as flashbacks or nightmares, avoidance symptoms, changing a personal routine to escape having to be reminded of an event, or being hyper-aroused (easily startled or tense) that makes daily tasks nearly impossible to complete. PTSD was first identified as a result of symptoms experienced by soldiers and those in war; however, other traumatic events, such as rape, child abuse, car accidents, and natural disasters have also been shown to give rise to PTSD.

It is estimated that more than 7.7 million people in the United States could be diagnosed as having a PTSD with women being more likely to have the disorder when compared to men.

Risk for PTSD is separated into three categories, including pretraumatic, peritraumatic, and posttraumatic factors.

Pretraumatic factors include childhood emotional problems by age 6, lower socioeconomic status, lower education, prior exposure to trauma, childhood adversity, lower intelligence, minority racial/ethnic status, and a family psychiatric history. Female gender and younger age at exposure may also contribute to pretraumatic risk.

Peritraumatic factors include the severity of the trauma, perceived life threat, personal injury, interpersonal violence, and dissociation during the trauma that persists afterwards.

Posttraumatic risk factors include negative appraisals, ineffective coping strategies, subsequent exposure to distressing reminders, subsequent adverse life events, and other trauma-related losses.

Diagnosis of PTSD must be preceded by exposure to actual or threatened death, serious injury, or violence. This may entail directly experiencing or witnessing the traumatic event, learning that the traumatic event occurred to a close family member or friend, or repeated exposure to distressing details of the traumatic event. Individuals diagnosed with PTSD experience intrusive symptoms (for example, recurrent upsetting dreams, flashbacks, distressing memories, intense psychological distress), avoidance of stimuli associated with the traumatic event, and negative changes in cognition and mood corresponding with the traumatic event (for example, dissociative amnesia, negative beliefs about oneself, persistent negative affect, feelings of detachment or estrangement). They also experience significant changes in arousal and reactivity associated with the traumatic events, such as hypervigilance, distractibility, exaggerated startle response, and irritable or self-destructive behavior.

Section 1.2

Mental Health Myths and Facts

This section includes text excerpted from "Myths and Facts," MentalHealth.gov, U.S. Department of Health and Human Services (HHS), May 31, 2013. Reviewed September 2017.

Mental Health Problems Affect Everyone

Myth: Mental health problems don't affect me.

Fact: Mental health problems are actually very common. In 2014, about:

- One in five American adults experienced a mental health issue.

- One in 10 young people experienced a period of major depression.

- One in 25 Americans lived with a serious mental illness, such as schizophrenia, bipolar disorder, or major depression.

Suicide is the 10th leading cause of death in the United States. It accounts for the loss of more than 41,000 American lives each year, more than double the number of lives lost to homicide.

Myth: Children don't experience mental health problems.

Fact: Even very young children may show early warning signs of mental health concerns. These mental health problems are often clinically diagnosable, and can be a product of the interaction of biological, psychological, and social factors.

Half of all mental health disorders show first signs before a person turns 14 years old, and three quarters of mental health disorders begin before age 24.

Unfortunately, less than 20 percent of children and adolescents with diagnosable mental health problems receive the treatment they need. Early mental health support can help a child before problems interfere with other developmental needs.

Myth: People with mental health problems are violent and unpredictable.

Fact: The vast majority of people with mental health problems are no more likely to be violent than anyone else. Most people with mental illness are not violent and only 3 percent – 5 percent of violent acts can be attributed to individuals living with a serious mental illness. In fact, people with severe mental illnesses are over 10 times more likely to be victims of violent crime than the general population. You probably know someone with a mental health problem and don't even realize it, because many people with mental health problems are highly active and productive members of our communities.

Myth: People with mental health needs, even those who are managing their mental illness, cannot tolerate the stress of holding down a job.

Fact: People with mental health problems are just as productive as other employees. Employers who hire people with mental health problems report good attendance and punctuality as well as motivation, good work, and job tenure on par with or greater than other employees.

When employees with mental health problems receive effective treatment, it can result in:

- Lower total medical costs

- Increased productivity

- Lower absenteeism

- Decreased disability costs

Myth: Personality weakness or character flaws cause mental health problems. People with mental health problems can snap out of it if they try hard enough.

Fact: Mental health problems have nothing to do with being lazy or weak and many people need help to get better. Many factors contribute to mental health problems, including:

- Biological factors, such as genes, physical illness, injury, or brain chemistry

- Life experiences, such as trauma or a history of abuse

- Family history of mental health problems

People with mental health problems can get better and many recover, completely.

14

Helping Individuals with Mental Health Problems

Myth: There is no hope for people with mental health problems. Once a friend or family member develops mental health problems, he or she will never recover.

Fact: Studies show that people with mental health problems get better and many recover, completely. Recovery refers to the process in which people are able to live, work, learn, and participate fully in their communities. There are more treatments, services, and community support systems than ever before, and they work.

Myth: Therapy and self-help are a waste of time. Why bother when you can just take a pill?

Fact: Treatment for mental health problems varies depending on the individual and could include medication, therapy, or both. Many individuals work with a support system during the healing and recovery process.

Myth: I can't do anything for a person with a mental health problem.

Fact: Friends and loved ones can make a big difference. Only 44 percent of adults with diagnosable mental health problems and less than 20 percent of children and adolescents receive needed treatment. Friends and family can be important influences to help someone get the treatment and services they need by:

- Reaching out and letting them know you are available to help

- Helping them access mental health services

- Learning and sharing the facts about mental health, especially if you hear something that isn't true

- Treating them with respect, just as you would anyone else

- Refusing to define them by their diagnosis or using labels such as "crazy"

Myth: Prevention doesn't work. It is impossible to prevent mental illnesses.

Fact: Prevention of mental, emotional, and behavioral disorders focuses on addressing known risk factors such as exposure to trauma that can affect the chances that children, youth, and young adults will develop mental health problems. Promoting the social-emotional wellbeing of children and youth leads to:

- Higher overall productivity
- Better educational outcomes
- Lower crime rates
- Stronger economies
- Lower healthcare costs
- Improved quality of life
- Increased lifespan
- Improved family life

Chapter 2

Understanding Anxiety Disorders

Occasional anxiety is a normal part of life. You might feel anxious when faced with a problem at work, before taking a test, or making an important decision. But anxiety disorders involve more than temporary worry or fear. For a person with an anxiety disorder, the anxiety does not go away and can get worse over time. The feelings can interfere with daily activities such as job performance, school work, and relationships. There are several different types of anxiety disorders. Examples include generalized anxiety disorder, panic disorder, and social anxiety disorder.

Signs and Symptoms[1]

Generalized Anxiety Disorder

People with generalized anxiety disorder display excessive anxiety or worry for months and face several anxiety-related symptoms.

Generalized anxiety disorder symptoms include:

- Restlessness or feeling wound-up or on edge

This chapter includes text excerpted from documents published by two public domain sources. Text under headings marked 1 are excerpted from "Mental Health Information—Anxiety Disorders," National Institute of Mental Health (NIMH), March 2016; Text under heading marked 2 is excerpted from "Anxiety Disorders," Office on Women's Health (OWH), February 12, 2015.

- Being easily fatigued
- Difficulty concentrating or having their minds go blank
- Irritability
- Muscle tension
- Difficulty controlling the worry
- Sleep problems (difficulty falling or staying asleep or restless, unsatisfying sleep)

Panic Disorder

People with panic disorder have recurrent unexpected panic attacks, which are sudden periods of intense fear that may include palpitations, pounding heart, or accelerated heart rate; sweating; trembling or shaking; sensations of shortness of breath, smothering, or choking; and feeling of impending doom.

Panic disorder symptoms include:

- Sudden and repeated attacks of intense fear
- Feelings of being out of control during a panic attack
- Intense worries about when the next attack will happen
- Fear or avoidance of places where panic attacks have occurred in the past

Social Anxiety Disorder

People with social anxiety disorder (sometimes called "social phobia") have a marked fear of social or performance situations in which they expect to feel embarrassed, judged, rejected, or fearful of offending others.

Social anxiety disorder symptoms include:

- Feeling highly anxious about being with other people and having a hard time talking to them
- Feeling very self-conscious in front of other people and worried about feeling humiliated, embarrassed, or rejected, or fearful of offending others
- Being very afraid that other people will judge them
- Worrying for days or weeks before an event where other people will be

- Staying away from places where there are other people
- Having a hard time making friends and keeping friends
- Blushing, sweating, or trembling around other people
- Feeling nauseous or sick to your stomach when other people are around

Evaluation for an anxiety disorder often begins with a visit to a primary care provider. Some physical health conditions, such as an overactive thyroid or low blood sugar, as well as taking certain medications, can imitate or worsen an anxiety disorder. A thorough mental health evaluation is also helpful, because anxiety disorders often coexist with other related conditions, such as depression or obsessive-compulsive disorder.

Risk Factors[1]

Researchers are finding that genetic and environmental factors, frequently in interaction with one another, are risk factors for anxiety disorders. Specific factors include:

- Shyness, or behavioral inhibition, in childhood
- Being female
- Having few economic resources
- Being divorced or widowed
- Exposure to stressful life events in childhood and adulthood
- Anxiety disorders in close biological relatives
- Parental history of mental disorders
- Elevated afternoon cortisol levels in the saliva (specifically for social anxiety disorder)

Diagnosis[2]

Anxiety disorders are diagnosed when fear and dread of nonthreatening situations, events, places, or objects become excessive and are uncontrollable. Anxiety disorders are also diagnosed if the anxiety has lasted for at least six months and it interferes with social, work, family, or other aspects of daily life.

Treatments and Therapies[1]

Anxiety disorders are generally treated with psychotherapy, medication, or both.

Psychotherapy

Psychotherapy or "talk therapy" can help people with anxiety disorders. To be effective, psychotherapy must be directed at the person's specific anxieties and tailored to his or her needs. A typical "side effect" of psychotherapy is temporary discomfort involved with thinking about confronting feared situations.

Cognitive Behavioral Therapy (CBT)

CBT is a type of psychotherapy that can help people with anxiety disorders. It teaches a person different ways of thinking, behaving, and reacting to anxiety-producing and fearful situations. CBT can also help people learn and practice social skills, which is vital for treating social anxiety disorder.

Two specific stand-alone components of CBT used to treat social anxiety disorder are cognitive therapy and exposure therapy. Cognitive therapy focuses on identifying, challenging, and then neutralizing unhelpful thoughts underlying anxiety disorders.

Exposure therapy focuses on confronting the fears underlying an anxiety disorder in order to help people engage in activities they have been avoiding. Exposure therapy is used along with relaxation exercises and/or imagery. One study, called a meta-analysis because it pulls together all of the previous studies and calculates the statistical magnitude of the combined effects, found that cognitive therapy was superior to exposure therapy for treating social anxiety disorder.

CBT may be conducted individually or with a group of people who have similar problems. Group therapy is particularly effective for social anxiety disorder. Often "homework" is assigned for participants to complete between sessions.

Self-Help or Support Groups

Some people with anxiety disorders might benefit from joining a self-help or support group and sharing their problems and achievements with others. Internet chat rooms might also be useful, but any advice received over the Internet should be used with caution, as Internet acquaintances have usually never seen each other and false identities are common. Talking with a trusted friend or member of the clergy can also provide support, but it is not necessarily a sufficient alternative to care from an expert clinician.

Stress-Management Techniques

Stress management techniques and meditation can help people with anxiety disorders calm themselves and may enhance the effects of therapy. While there is evidence that aerobic exercise has a calming effect, the quality of the studies is not strong enough to support its use as treatment. Since caffeine, certain illicit drugs, and even some over-the-counter cold medications can aggravate the symptoms of anxiety disorders, avoiding them should be considered. Check with your physician or pharmacist before taking any additional medications.

The family can be important in the recovery of a person with an anxiety disorder. Ideally, the family should be supportive but not help perpetuate their loved one's symptoms.

Medication

Medication does not cure anxiety disorders but often relieves symptoms. Medication can only be prescribed by a medical doctor (such as a psychiatrist or a primary care provider), but a few states allow psychologists to prescribe psychiatric medications.

Medications are sometimes used as the initial treatment of an anxiety disorder, or are used only if there is insufficient response to a course of psychotherapy. In research studies, it is common for patients treated with a combination of psychotherapy and medication to have better outcomes than those treated with only one or the other.

The most common classes of medications used to combat anxiety disorders are antidepressants, antianxiety drugs, and beta blockers. Be aware that some medications are effective only if they are taken regularly and that symptoms may recur if the medication is stopped.

Antidepressants

Antidepressants are used to treat depression, but they also are helpful for treating anxiety disorders. They take several weeks to start working and may cause side effects such as headache, nausea, or difficulty sleeping. The side effects are usually not a problem for most people, especially if the dose starts off low and is increased slowly over time.

Antianxiety Medications

Antianxiety medications help reduce the symptoms of anxiety, panic attacks, or extreme fear and worry. The most common antianxiety medications are called benzodiazepines. Benzodiazepines are first-line treatments for generalized anxiety disorder. With panic disorder or social phobia (social anxiety disorder), benzodiazepines are usually second-line treatments, behind antidepressants.

Beta Blockers

Beta blockers, such as propranolol and atenolol, are also helpful in the treatment of the physical symptoms of anxiety, especially social anxiety. Physicians prescribe them to control rapid heartbeat, shaking, trembling, and blushing in anxious situations.

Choosing the right medication, medication dose, and treatment plan should be based on a person's needs and medical situation, and done under an expert's care. Only an expert clinician can help you decide whether the medication's ability to help is worth the risk of a side effect. Your doctor may try several medicines before finding the right one.

You and your doctor should discuss:

- How well medications are working or might work to improve your symptoms

- Benefits and side effects of each medication

- Risk for serious side effects based on your medical history

- The likelihood of the medications requiring lifestyle changes

- Costs of each medication

- Other alternative therapies, medications, vitamins, and supplements you are taking and how these may affect your treatment

- How the medication should be stopped. Some drugs can't be stopped abruptly but must be tapered off slowly under a doctor's supervision

Chapter 3

Prevalence of Anxiety Disorders in United States

Any Anxiety Disorder

Anxiety is a normal reaction to stress and can actually be beneficial in some situations. For some people, however, anxiety can become excessive, and while the person suffering may realize it is excessive they may also have difficulty controlling it and it may negatively affect their day-to-day living. There are a wide variety of anxiety disorders, including posttraumatic stress disorder, obsessive-compulsive disorder, and specific phobias to name a few. Collectively they are among the most common mental disorders experienced by Americans.

This chapter includes text excerpted from "Health and Education—Prevalence—Any Anxiety Disorder among Adults," National Institute of Mental Health (NIMH), October 15, 2014. Reviewed September 2017.

Among Adults

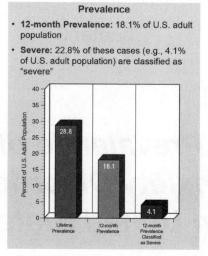

Figure 3.1. *Prevalence of Any Anxiety Disorder among Adults*

Prevalence

- 12-month prevalence: 18.1 percent of U.S. adult population
- Severe: 22.8 percent of these cases (e.g., 4.1% of U.S. adult population) are classified as "severe"

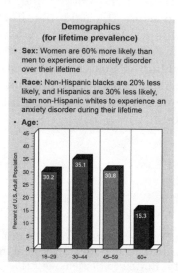

Figure 3.2. *Lifetime Prevalence of Any Anxiety Disorder among Adults*

Demographics (For Lifetime Prevalence)

- Sex: Women are 60 percent more likely than men to experience an anxiety disorder over their lifetime.

- Race: Non-Hispanic blacks are 20 percent less likely, and Hispanics are 30 percent less likely, than non-Hispanic whites to experience an anxiety disorder during their lifetime.

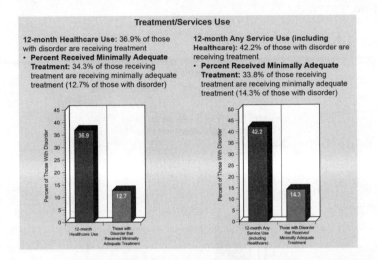

Treatment/Services Use

12-month Healthcare Use: 36.9% of those with disorder are receiving treatment
• **Percent Received Minimally Adequate Treatment:** 34.3% of those receiving treatment are receiving minimally adequate treatment (12.7% of those with disorder)

12-month Any Service Use (including Healthcare): 42.2% of those with disorder are receiving treatment
• **Percent Received Minimally Adequate Treatment:** 33.8% of those receiving treatment are receiving minimally adequate treatment (14.3% of those with disorder)

Figure 3.3. *Treatment/Services for Any Anxiety Disorder among Adults*

Lifetime Prevalence of 13 to 18 Year Olds

- Lifetime prevalence: 25.1 percent of 13 to 18 year olds

- Lifetime prevalence of "severe" disorder: 5.9 percent of 13 to 18 year old have "severe" anxiety disorder

- Average age-of-onset: 11 years old

Among Children

Demographics (For Lifetime Prevalence)

- Sex: Statistically different

- Age: Not statistically different

- Race: Statistically significant differences were found between non-Hispanic whites and other races

Generalized Anxiety Disorder

Generalized anxiety disorder (GAD) is characterized by excessive worry about a variety of everyday problems for at least 6 months. For example, people with GAD may excessively worry about and anticipate problems with their finances, health, employment, and relationships. They typically have difficulty calming their concerns, even though they realize that their anxiety is more intense than the situation warrants.

Among Adults

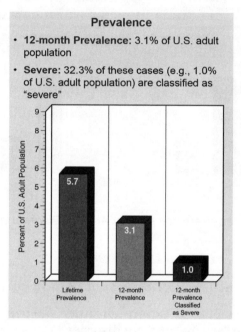

Figure 3.4. *Prevalence of Generalized Anxiety Disorder among Adults*

Prevalence

- 12 month prevalence: 3.1 percent of U.S. adult population

- Severe: 32.3 percent of these cases (e.g., 1.0 % of U.S. adult population) are classified as "severe"

- Average age-of-onset: 31 years old

26

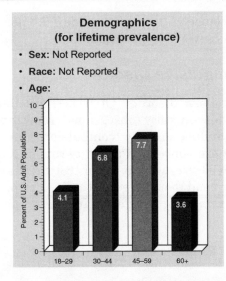

Figure 3.5. *Lifetime Prevalence of Generalized Anxiety Disorder among Adults*

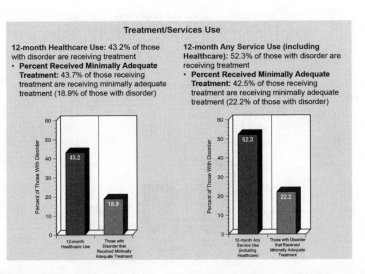

Figure 3.6. *Treatment/Services for Generalized Anxiety Disorder among Adults*

Among Children

Lifetime Prevalence of 13 to 18 Year Olds

- Lifetime prevalence: 1.0 percent of 13 to 18 year olds

- Lifetime prevalence of "severe" disorder: 0.4 percent of 13 to 18 year olds have "severe" hypomania.

Obsessive-Compulsive Disorder

Obsessive-compulsive disorder (OCD) is characterized by intrusive thoughts that produce anxiety (obsessions), repetitive behaviors that are engaged in to reduce anxiety (compulsions), or a combination of both. While many are concerned about germs or leaving their stove on, people with OCD are unable to control their anxiety-producing thoughts and their need to engage in ritualized behaviors. As a result, OCD can have a tremendous negative impact on people's day-to-day functioning.

Among Adults

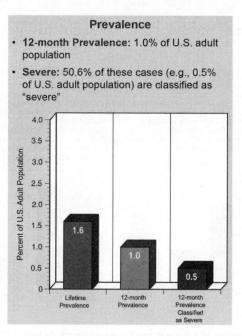

Figure 3.7. *Prevalence of Obsessive-Compulsive Disorder among Adults*

Prevalence

- 12 month prevalence: 1.0 percent of U.S. adult population

- Severe: 50.6 percent of these cases (e.g., 0.5 % of U.S. adult population) are classified as "severe"

28

- Average age-of-onset: 19 years old

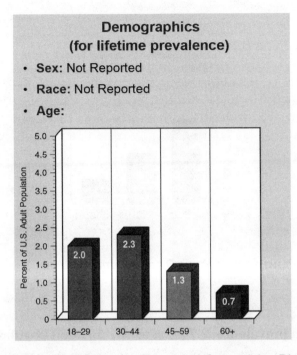

Demographics
(for lifetime prevalence)
- **Sex:** Not Reported
- **Race:** Not Reported
- **Age:**

Figure 3.8. *Lifetime Prevalence of Obsessive-Compulsive Disorder among Adults*

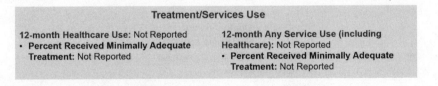

Figure 3.9. *Treatment/Services for Obsessive-Compulsive Disorder among Adults*

Panic Disorder

Panic disorder is an anxiety disorder characterized by unexpected and repeated episodes of intense fear accompanied by physical symptoms that may include chest pain, heart palpitations, shortness of breath, dizziness, or abdominal distress.

Among Adults

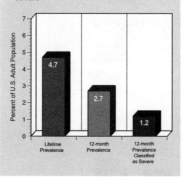

Figure 3.10. *Prevalence of Panic Disorder among Adults*

Prevalence

- 12 month prevalence: 2.7 percent of U.S. adult population

- Severe: 44.8 percent of these cases (e.g., 1.2 % of U.S. adult population) are classified as "severe"

- Average age-of-onset: 24 years old

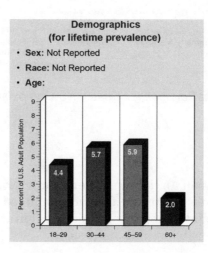

Figure 3.11. *Lifetime Prevalence of Panic Disorder among Adults*

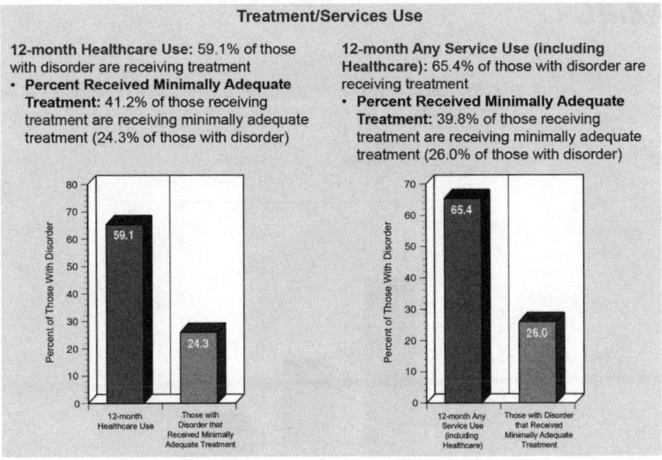
Treatment/Services Use
12-month Healthcare Use: 59.1% of those with disorder are receiving treatment
• Percent Received Minimally Adequate Treatment: 41.2% of those receiving treatment are receiving minimally adequate treatment (24.3% of those with disorder)
12-month Any Service Use (including Healthcare): 65.4% of those with disorder are receiving treatment
• Percent Received Minimally Adequate Treatment: 39.8% of those receiving treatment are receiving minimally adequate treatment (26.0% of those with disorder)
Percent of Those With Disorder
59.1
24.3
12-month Healthcare Use
Those with Disorder that Received Minimally Adequate Treatment
Percent of Those With Disorder
65.4
26.0
12-month Any Service Use (including Healthcare)
Those with Disorder that Received Minimally Adequate Treatment

Figure 3.12. *Treatment/Services for Panic Disorder among Adults*

Among Children

Lifetime Prevalence of 13 to 18 Year Olds

- Lifetime prevalence: 2.3 percent of 13 to 18 year olds
- Lifetime prevalence of "severe" disorder: 2.3 percent of 13 to 18 year olds have "severe" hypomania.

Posttraumatic Stress Disorder (PTSD)

Posttraumatic stress disorder (PTSD) is an anxiety disorder that can develop after exposure to a terrifying event or ordeal in which there was the potential for or actual occurrence of grave physical harm. Traumatic events that may trigger PTSD include violent personal assaults, natural or human-caused disasters, accidents, and military combat. People with PTSD have persistent frightening thoughts and memories of their ordeal, may experience sleep problems, feel detached or numb, or be easily startled.

Among Adults

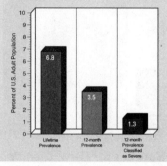

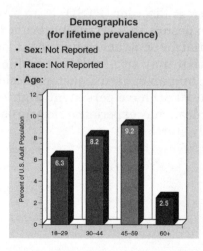

Figure 3.13. *Lifetime Prevalence of Posttraumatic Stress Disorder among Adults*

Prevalence

- 12 month prevalence: 3.5 percent of U.S. adult population

- Severe: 36.6 percent of these cases (e.g., 1.3 % of U.S. adult population) are classified as "severe"

- Average age-of-onset: 23 years old

Figure 3.14. *Lifetime Prevalence of Posttraumatic Stress Disorder (PTSD) among Adults*

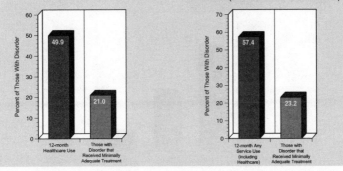

Figure 3.15. *Treatment/Services for Posttraumatic Stress Disorder among Adults*

Among Children

Lifetime Prevalence of 13 to 18 Year Olds

- Lifetime prevalence: 4.0 percent of 13 to 18 year olds

- Lifetime prevalence of "severe" disorder: 1.4 percent of 13 to 18 year olds have "severe" hypomania.

Social Phobia

Social phobia is characterized by a persistent, intense, and chronic fear of being watched and judged by others and feeling embarrassed or humiliated by their actions. This fear may be so severe that it interferes with work, school, and other activities and may negatively affect the person's ability to form relationships.

Among Adults

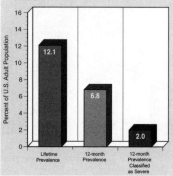

Figure 3.16. *Prevalence of Social Phobia among Adults*

Prevalence

- 12 month Prevalence: 6.8 percent of U.S. adult population

- Severe: 29.9 percent of these cases (e.g., 2.0 % of U.S. adult population) are classified as "severe"

- Average age-of-onset: 13 years old

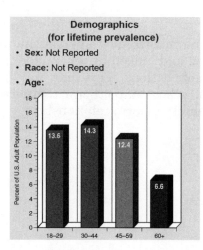

Figure 3.17. *Lifetime Prevalence of Social Phobia among Adults*

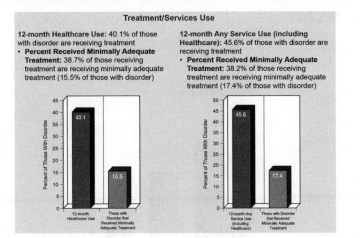

Figure 3.18. *Treatment/Services for Social Phobia among Adults*

Among Children

Lifetime Prevalence of 13 to 18 Year Olds

- Lifetime prevalence: 5.5 percent of 13 to 18 year olds

- Lifetime prevalence of "severe" disorder: 1.3 percent of 13 to 18 year olds have "severe" disorder.

Specific Phobia

Specific phobia involves marked and persistent fear and avoidance of a specific object or situation. This type of phobia includes, but is not limited to, the fear of heights, spiders, and flying.

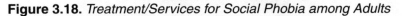

Among Adults

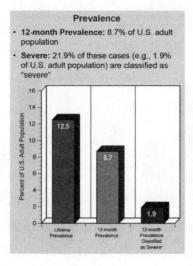

Figure 3.19. *Prevalence of Specific Phobia among Adults*

Prevalence

- 12 month prevalence: 8.7 percent of U.S. adult population

- Severe: 21.9 percent of these cases (e.g., 1.9 % of U.S. adult population) are classified as "severe"

- Average age-of-onset: 7 years old

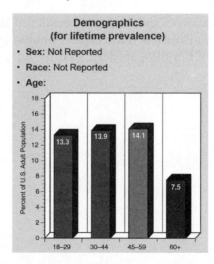

Figure 3.20. *Lifetime Prevalence of Specific Phobia among Adults*

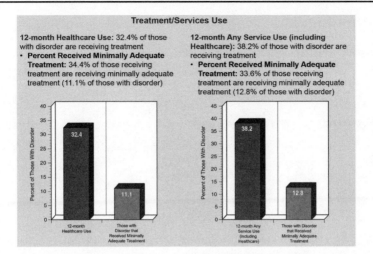

Figure 3.21. *Treatment/Services for Specific Phobia among Adults*

Among Children

Lifetime Prevalence of 13 to 18 Year Olds

- Lifetime prevalence: 15.1 percent of 13 to 18 year olds

- Lifetime prevalence of "severe" disorder: 0.6 percent of 13 to 18 year olds have a "severe" disorder.

Chapter 4

Anxiety Disorders in Specific Populations

Chapter Contents

Section 4.1

Anxiety and Depression among Children

This section includes text excerpted from "Children's Mental Health—Types of Disorders—Anxiety and Depression," Centers for Disease Control and Prevention (CDC), March 23, 2017.

Many children have fears and worries, and will feel sad and hopeless from time to time. Strong fears will appear at different times in development. For example, toddlers are often very distressed about being away from their parents, even if they are safe and cared for. Although fears and worries are typical in children, persistent or extreme forms of fear and sadness feelings could be due to anxiety or depression. Because the symptoms primarily involve thoughts and feelings, they are called internalizing disorders.

Anxiety

When children do not outgrow the fears and worries that are typical in young children, or when there are so many fears and worries that they interfere with school, home, or play activities, the child may be diagnosed with an anxiety disorder. Examples of different types of anxiety disorders include:

- Being very afraid when away from parents (separation anxiety)
- Having extreme fear about a specific thing or situation, such as dogs, insects, or going to the doctor (phobias)
- Being very afraid of school and other places where there are people (social anxiety)
- Being very worried about the future and about bad things happening (general anxiety)
- Having repeated episodes of sudden, unexpected, intense fear that come with symptoms like heart pounding, having trouble breathing, or feeling dizzy, shaky, or sweaty (panic disorder)

Anxiety may present as fear or worry, but can also make children irritable and angry. Anxiety symptoms can also include trouble sleeping, as well as physical symptoms like fatigue, headaches, or stomachaches. Some anxious children keep their worries to themselves and, thus, the symptoms can be missed.

Depression

Occasionally being sad or feeling hopeless is a part of every child's life. However, some children feel sad or uninterested in things that they used to enjoy, or feel helpless or hopeless in situations where they could do something to address the situations. When children feel persistent sadness and hopelessness, they may be diagnosed with depression.

Examples of behaviors often seen when children are depressed include:

- Feeling sad, hopeless, or irritable a lot of the time
- Not wanting to do or enjoy doing fun things
- Changes in eating patterns—eating a lot more or a lot less than usual
- Changes in sleep patterns—sleeping a lot more or a lot less than normal
- Changes in energy—being tired and sluggish or tense and restless a lot of the time
- Having a hard time paying attention
- Feeling worthless, useless, or guilty
- Self-injury and self-destructive behavior

Extreme depression can lead a child to think about suicide or plan for suicide. For youth ages 10–24 years, suicide is the leading form of death.

Some children may not talk about helpless and hopeless thoughts, and they may not appear sad. Depression might also cause a child to make trouble or act unmotivated, so others might not notice that the child is depressed or may incorrectly label the child as a trouble-maker or lazy.

Treatment for Anxiety and Depression

The first step to treatment is to talk with a healthcare provider to get an evaluation. The American Academy of Child and Adolescent

Psychiatry (AACAP) recommends that healthcare providers routinely screen children for behavioral and mental health concerns. Some of the signs and symptoms of anxiety or depression are shared with other conditions, such as trauma. Specific symptoms like having a hard time focusing could be a sign of attention deficit hyperactivity disorder (ADHD). It is important to get a careful evaluation to get the best diagnosis and treatment. Consultation with a health provider can help determine if medication should be part of the treatment. A mental health professional can develop a therapy plan that works best for the child and family. Behavior therapy includes child therapy, family therapy, or a combination of both. The school can also be included in the treatment plan. For very young children, involving parents in treatment is key. Cognitive behavioral therapy (CBT) is one form of therapy that is used to treat anxiety or depression, particularly in older children. It helps the child change negative thoughts into more positive, effective ways of thinking, leading to more effective behavior. Behavior therapy for anxiety may involve helping children cope with and manage anxiety symptoms while gradually exposing them to their fears so as to help them learn that bad things do not occur.

Treatments can also include a variety of ways to help the child feel less stressed and be healthier like nutritious food, physical activity, sufficient sleep, predictable routines, and social support.

Get Help Finding Treatment

Here are tools to find a healthcare provider familiar with treatment options:

- Psychologist Locator, a service of the American Psychological Association (APA) Practice Organization.
- Child and Adolescent Psychiatrist Finder, a research tool by the American Academy of Child and Adolescent Psychiatry (AACAP).
- Find a Cognitive Behavioral Therapist, a search tool by the Association for Behavioral and Cognitive Therapies (ABCT).
- If you need help finding treatment facilities, use the "Treatment Locator" widget.

Managing Symptoms: Staying Healthy

Being healthy is important for all children and can be especially important for children with depression or anxiety. In addition to getting the right treatment, leading a healthy lifestyle can play a role in managing symptoms of depression or anxiety. Here are some healthy behaviors that may help:

- Eating a healthful diet centered on fruits, vegetables, whole grains, legumes (for example, beans, peas, and lentils), lean protein sources, and nuts and seeds

- Participating in physical activity for at least 60 minutes each day

- Getting the recommended amount of sleep each night based on age

- Practicing mindfulness or relaxation techniques

Prevention of Anxiety and Depression

It is not known exactly why some children develop anxiety or depression. Many factors may play a role, including biology and temperament. But it is also known that some children are more likely to develop anxiety or depression when they experience trauma or stress, when they are maltreated, when they are bullied or rejected by other children, or when their own parents have anxiety or depression.

Although these factors appear to increase the risk for anxiety or depression, there are ways to decrease the chance that children experience them. Learn about public health approaches to prevent these risks:

- Bullying prevention

- Child maltreatment prevention

- Youth violence prevention

- Depression after birth

- Caring for children in a disaster

Section 4.2

Anxiety among Teens

This section includes text excerpted from "Your Feelings:
Feeling Anxious or Worried," girlshealth.gov, Office on
Women's Health (OWH), January 7, 2015.

Feeling Anxious or Worried

Everyone feels anxious or worried at some point. Anxiety can be
a very normal reaction to a tough situation. Sometimes, anxiety can
help you rise to a challenge. For example, feeling worried about a test
can make you study for it.

An anxiety disorder is different from normal anxiety. A person
with an anxiety disorder has very strong feelings of worry or dread
for months. These feelings come often, and they get in the way of the
person's everyday life. If you think you have an anxiety disorder, talk
to a trusted adult. You can feel better.

What Are Some Types of Anxiety Disorders?

There are a number of anxiety disorders that young people can
have. Some of them are listed below.

- **Social phobia** is a strong fear of being judged by others and of
  being embarrassed. This fear can be so strong that it gets in the
  way of everyday things like going to school or eating in front of
  others. Of course, most of us may worry a bit about certain social
  situations, but people with social phobia might worry about an
  event for weeks. They also may have physical symptoms like
  blushing, sweating, or shaking in a social situation.

  Most people who have social phobia know that they don't need to
  be so afraid, but they can't stop worrying. Sometimes, they avoid
  places where they might have to do something they fear will be
  uncomfortable. It can be hard for a person with social phobia to
  make and keep friends.

- **Generalized anxiety disorder (GAD)** is when a person
  worries a lot about many things, even though there is little or

44

nothing to worry about. The person may worry about a wide range of things, including school, relationships, money, and health. Sometimes, just the thought of getting through the day makes the person anxious. A person with GAD may have trouble concentrating, headaches, irritability, sleep problems, muscle tension, and other uncomfortable feelings.

- **Panic disorder** means a person has panic attacks, which are sudden, strong feelings of fear that come for no clear reason. An attack can bring a rush of physical feelings like heart-pounding, difficulty breathing, and dizziness. A person having a panic attack may feel like she is going to die.

Because panic attacks can be so scary, someone who has them may worry a lot about when the next one might come.

- **Agoraphobia** is a fear of places that make you feel unsafe. This might be places that seem hard to get out of or where you fear you might not be able to get help if you need it. Examples include a bus, a bridge, a crowd, or someplace far from home.

- **Specific phobias** are very strong fears of particular things or situations. Examples include being very afraid of dogs, flying in a plane, taking an elevator, or driving through a tunnel. A person can't control the fear even if she knows there is no need to be afraid.

- **Obsessive-compulsive disorder (OCD)** causes frequent and upsetting thoughts, which are called obsessions. A person with these thoughts feels a strong urge to do certain behaviors to try to stop the thoughts. These behaviors, which are called compulsions, may be things like repeated counting, cleaning, or hand-washing.

- **Posttraumatic stress disorder (PTSD)** comes from having a terrifying experience, like surviving a hurricane or witnessing an attack. Symptoms of PTSD include having nightmares or feeling like you are reliving the experience.

- **Separation anxiety** involves a very strong fear any time you are being separated from someone important to you, like a parent.

Dealing with Anxiety

Are you thinking about doing something you find scary? One helpful tool is to ask yourself, "What is the worst thing that can happen?"

You may realize that the worst thing that can happen actually is a lot less scary than you thought. And you might also consider the best that can happen—like everything will go fabulously well and you'll have a great time.

Here are some more ways to handle anxiety:

- **Go someplace peaceful.** You might take a walk in nature or lie down someplace quiet in your house.

- **Connect with others.** It can feel great to have support. Friends can get your mind off your worries and onto something fun.

- **Do something soothing.** Try yoga or deep breathing.

- **Find healthy ways to deal with pressure.**

- **Think positive.** Think about the great things in your life—and in yourself! Imagine really good times heading your way.

- **Avoid things that can make your worry worse.** Caffeine and certain drugs can make you feel more on edge, for example. If you're looking for energy, healthy foods and good sleep are much better bets.

If your anxiety is getting in the way of your life or it goes on for too long, you may need treatment. Treatment for anxiety disorders may include medicines or therapy. Treatment can work very well, and you can feel better. Anxiety disorders that aren't treated can get worse, though. You can find out about treatment by talking with your parents or another trusted adult.

If your anxiety is so bad that you are thinking about suicide, get help right away. Contact the National Suicide Prevention Lifeline hotline by chat, or call 800-273-TALK (800-273-8255).

Section 4.3

Anxiety among Pregnant Women

This section includes text excerpted from "Moms' Mental Health Matters: Depression and Anxiety around Pregnancy," *Eunice Kennedy Shriver* National Institute of Child Health and Human Development (NICHD), February 25, 2016.

Pregnancy and a new baby can bring a range of emotions. In fact, many women feel overwhelmed, sad, or anxious at different times during their pregnancy and even after the baby is born. For many women, these feelings go away on their own. But for some women, these emotions are more serious and may stay for some time.

Depression and anxiety that happen during pregnancy or anytime during the first year after the birth of your baby are medical conditions. These feelings are not something you caused by doing or not doing something. And, they can be treated if you seek help.

What Are Depression and Anxiety?

Depression—feeling sad, empty, and/or "down"—and anxiety—feeling nervous, worried, and/or scared—are serious medical conditions that involve the brain and may occur during pregnancy or after birth. These feelings go beyond what people may experience when they have a bad day or are nervous about an upcoming event. They are also more than "just feeling moody" or having the "baby blues."

Depression and anxiety may get in the way of doing everyday activities, like taking care of yourself and your baby. They are long lasting and won't go away on their own. But they are treatable, which is why it's important to get help.

Are You Talking about Postpartum Depression?

Postpartum depression is one name you might hear for depression and anxiety that can happen during and after pregnancy. But it might not be the best way to describe what women feel.

The word "postpartum" means "after birth," so "postpartum depression" is talking only about depression after the baby is born. For many women, this term is correct: they start feeling depression sometime within the first year after they have the baby.

But research shows that some women start to feel depression while they're still pregnant. You might hear the term "perinatal depression" to describe this situation. The word "perinatal" describes the time during pregnancy or just after birth. Researchers believe that depression is one of the most common problems women experience during and after pregnancy.

We now know that women may also experience anxiety around the time of pregnancy, beyond just being nervous about having a baby. Anxiety during and after pregnancy is as common as depression and may even happen at the same time as depression. So, you also may hear "perinatal depression and anxiety" or "perinatal mood and anxiety disorders" used to describe all of what women might feel. No matter what you call them, depression and anxiety that happen during pregnancy or after birth are real medical conditions, and they affect many women.

What Are Some Signs of Depression and Anxiety?

Women, with depression or anxiety around pregnancy, tell us that they feel:

- Extremely sad or angry without warning
- Foggy or have trouble completing tasks
- "Robotic," like they are just going through the motions
- Very anxious around the baby and their other children
- Guilty and like they are failing at motherhood
- Unusually irritable or angry

They also often have:

- Little interest in things they used to enjoy
- Scary, upsetting thoughts that don't go away

How Common Are Depression and Anxiety during Pregnancy or after Birth?

As mentioned above, researchers believe that depression is one of the most common problems women experience during and after pregnancy. According to a national survey, about 1 in 8 women experiences postpartum depression after having a baby. Anxiety during and after pregnancy is as common as depression and may happen at the same time as depression. You may feel like you're the only person in the world who feels depressed and anxious during pregnancy or after your baby is born, but you are not alone.

What Are the Risk Factors for Depression and Anxiety during Pregnancy or after Birth?

Depression and anxiety during pregnancy or after birth can happen to anyone. However, several factors make some women more likely than others to experience one or both of these conditions. These risk factors include:

- A history of depression or anxiety, either during pregnancy or at other times
- Family history of depression or anxiety
- A difficult pregnancy or birth experience
- Giving birth to twins or other multiples
- Experiencing problems in your relationship with your partner
- Experiencing financial problems
- Receiving little or no support from family or friends to help you care for your baby
- Unplanned pregnancy

Depression and anxiety during pregnancy or after birth don't happen because of something you do or don't do—they are medical conditions. Although the causes of these conditions are not fully understood, researchers think depression and anxiety during this time may result from a mix of physical, emotional, and environmental factors.

Can Depression and Anxiety during Pregnancy or after Birth Affect My Baby?

Yes—these medical conditions can affect your baby, but not directly. Early mother-child bonding is important for your baby's development and becoming close to your baby is a big part of that bonding. When you have depression or anxiety during pregnancy or after birth, it can be hard to become close to your baby. You may not be able to respond

49

to what your baby needs. And, if there are older children in the house, they may be missing your support as well.

Early treatment is important for you, your baby, and the rest of your family. The sooner you start, the more quickly you will start to feel better.

Are There Treatments for Depression or Anxiety during Pregnancy or after Birth?

Yes, there are treatments, and they can help you feel better. Treatment can reduce your symptoms or make them go away completely.

Many treatment options are available for depression or anxiety during pregnancy or after birth. Some women may participate in counseling ("talk therapy"); others may need medication. There is no single treatment that works for everyone.

Your provider may ask you a set of questions, called a screening, to learn more about what you are feeling. Together, you can find the treatment that is right for you. Some treatments for depression and anxiety that occur during or after pregnancy are listed below.

Counseling ("Talk Therapy")

Some women find it helpful to talk about their concerns or feelings with a mental health provider. Your provider can help you find ways to manage your feelings and to make changes to help ease the depression or anxiety.

Medication

Several medications can treat depression and anxiety effectively and are safe for pregnant women and for breastfeeding moms and their babies. Talk with a healthcare provider about medications that may be right for you. You can also visit the U.S. Food and Drug Administration (FDA) (www.fda.gov) to learn about drugs and their possible effects on a breastfed baby.

Is There Anything I Can Do in Addition to Treatment?

There are some things you can do, in addition to treatment, that may help you feel better.

- Connect with other moms.

- Make time for yourself.

- Do something you enjoy.
- Be realistic.
- Ask for help.
- Rest when the baby rests.
- Be with others.

Can I Prevent Depression or Anxiety during Pregnancy or after Birth?

Currently, there is no known way to prevent depression or anxiety that occurs during pregnancy or after the birth of your baby. But knowing what signs and symptoms to watch for during and after pregnancy can help you prepare and get help quickly. Here's what you can do:

- Find out whether you have factors that put you at greater risk for depression and anxiety during pregnancy and after birth.
- Talk with a healthcare provider about depression and anxiety around pregnancy and learn what to watch for.
- Learn as much as you can about pregnancy, childbirth, and parenthood so you know what to expect.
- Set realistic expectations for yourself and your family.
- Do things in addition to seeking treatment that may help you feel better
- Plan ahead. While you're pregnant, think about who can give you support and help when your baby comes. Talk with that person about helping you so that you can both prepare.

Remember, depression and anxiety that happen during pregnancy or after the birth of your baby are not things you cause—they are medical conditions that require medical care.

Section 4.4

Anxiety among Older Adults

This section includes text excerpted from "Anxiety
Disorders: About Anxiety Disorders," NIHSeniorHealth,
National Institute on Aging (NIA), January 2016.

Occasional anxiety is a normal part of life. You might feel anxious when faced with a problem at work, before taking a test, or making an important decision. However, anxiety disorders involve more than temporary worry or fear. For a person with an anxiety disorder, the anxiety does not go away and can get worse over time. These feelings can interfere with daily activities such as job performance, school work, and relationships.

Studies estimate that anxiety disorders affect up to 15 percent of older adults in a given year. More women than men experience anxiety disorders. They tend to be less common among older adults than younger adults. But developing an anxiety disorder late in life is not a normal part of aging.

Anxiety disorders commonly occur along with other mental or physical illnesses, including alcohol or substance abuse, which may mask anxiety symptoms or make them worse. In older adults, anxiety disorders often occur at the same time as depression, heart disease, diabetes, and other medical problems. In some cases, these other problems need to be treated before a person can respond well to treatment for anxiety.

There are three types of anxiety disorders:

1. Generalized anxiety disorder (GAD)

2. Social phobia

3. Panic disorder

Generalized Anxiety Disorder (GAD)

All of us worry about things like health, money, or family problems. But people with GAD are extremely worried about these and many other things, even when there is little or no reason to worry about them. They are very anxious about just getting through the day. They think things will always go badly. At times, worrying keeps people with GAD from doing everyday tasks.

Social Phobia

In social phobia, a person fears being judged by others or of being embarrassed. This fear can get in the way of doing everyday things such as going to work, running errands, or meeting with friends. People who have social phobia often know that they shouldn't be so afraid, but they can't control their fear.

Panic Disorder

In panic disorder, a person has sudden, unexplained attacks of terror, and often feels his or her heart pounding. During a panic attack, a person feels a sense of unreality, a fear of impending doom, or a fear of losing control. Panic attacks can occur at any time.

Anxiety Disorders Are Treatable

In general, anxiety disorders are treated with medication, specific types of psychotherapy, or both. Treatment choices depend on the type of disorder, the person's preference, and the expertise of the doctor. If you think you have an anxiety disorder, talk to your doctor.

Section 4.5

Anxiety among Gay and Bisexual Men

This section includes text excerpted from "Gay and Bisexual Men's Health—Mental Health," Centers for Disease Control and Prevention (CDC), February 29, 2016.

The majority of gay and bisexual men have and maintain good mental health, even though research has shown that they are at greater risk for mental health problems. Like everyone else, the majority of gay and bisexual men are able to cope successfully if connected to the right resources.

However, ongoing homophobia, stigma (negative and usually unfair beliefs), and discrimination (unfairly treating a person or group of people) can have negative effects on your health. Research also shows that, compared to other men, gay and bisexual men have higher chances of having:

- Major depression,

- Bipolar disorder, and

- Generalized anxiety disorder.

Gay and bisexual men may also face other health threats that usually happen along with mental health problems. These include more use of illegal drugs and a greater risk for suicide. Gay and bisexual men are more likely than other men to have tried to commit suicide as well as to have succeeded at suicide. Human immunodeficiency virus (HIV) is another issue that has had a huge impact on the mental health of gay and bisexual men. It affects men who are living with HIV; those who are at high risk, but HIV negative; and loved ones of those living with, or who have died from HIV.

Revealing Sexual Orientation

Keeping your sexual orientation hidden from others (being "in the closet") and fear of having your sexual orientation disclosed (being "outed") can add to the stress of being gay or bisexual. In general, research has shown that gay and bisexual men who are open about their sexual orientation with others have better health outcomes than gay and bisexual men who do not. However, being "out" in some settings and to people who react negatively can add to the stress experienced by gay and bisexual men, and can lead to poorer mental health and discrimination.

Keys to Maintaining Good Mental Health

Having a supportive group of friends and family members is often key to successfully dealing with the stress of day-to-day life and maintaining good mental health. If you are unable to get social support from your friends and families, you can try finding support by becoming involved in community, social, athletic, religious, and other groups. Mental health counseling and support groups that are sensitive to the needs of gay and bisexual men can be especially useful if you are coming to terms with your sexual orientation or are experiencing depression, anxiety, or other mental health problems.

While many gay, bisexual, and other men who have sex with men may not seek care from a mental health provider because of a fear of discrimination or homophobia, it is important to keep this as an option and to find a provider that is trustworthy and compatible.

Chapter 5

How Anxiety Affects Quality of Life

Many of us worry from time to time. We fret over finances, feel anxious about job interviews, or get nervous about social gatherings. These feelings can be normal or even helpful. They may give us a boost of energy or help us focus. But for people with anxiety disorders, they can be overwhelming.

Anxiety disorders affect nearly 1 in 5 American adults each year. People with these disorders have feelings of fear and uncertainty that interfere with everyday activities, and last for 6 months or more. Anxiety disorders can also raise your risk for other medical problems such as heart disease, diabetes, substance abuse, and depression.

The good news is that most anxiety disorders get better with therapy. The course of treatment depends on the type of anxiety disorder. Medications, psychotherapy ("talk therapy"), or a combination of both can usually relieve troubling symptoms.

"Anxiety disorders are one of the most treatable mental health problems we see," says Dr. Daniel Pine, an National Institutes of Health

This chapter includes text excerpted from "Understanding Anxiety Disorders—When Panic, Fear, and Worries Overwhelm," *NIH News in Health,* National Institutes of Health (NIH), March 2016.

(NIH) neuroscientist and psychiatrist. "Still, for reasons we don't fully understand, most people who have these problems don't get the treatments that could really help them."

One of the most common types of anxiety disorder is social anxiety disorder, or social phobia. It affects both women and men equally—a total of about 15 million U.S. adults. Without treatment, social phobia can last for years or even a lifetime. People with social phobia may worry for days or weeks before a social event. They're often embarrassed, self-conscious, and afraid of being judged. They find it hard to talk to others. They may blush, sweat, tremble, or feel sick to their stomach when around other people.

Other common types of anxiety disorders include generalized anxiety disorder, which affects nearly 7 million American adults, and panic disorder, which affects about 6 million. Both are twice as common in women as in men.

People with generalized anxiety disorder worry endlessly over everyday issues—like health, money, or family problems—even if they realize there's little cause for concern. They startle easily, can't relax, and can't concentrate. They find it hard to fall asleep or stay asleep. They may get headaches, muscle aches, or unexplained pains. Symptoms often get worse during times of stress.

People with panic disorder have sudden, repeated bouts of fear—called panic attacks—that last several minutes or more. During a panic attack, they may feel that they can't breathe or that they're having a heart attack. They may fear loss of control or feel a sense of unreality. Not everyone who has panic attacks will develop panic disorder. But if the attacks recur without warning, creating fear of having another attack at any time, then it's likely panic disorder.

Anxiety disorders tend to run in families. But researchers aren't certain why some family members develop these conditions while others don't. No specific genes have been found to actually cause an anxiety disorder. "Many different factors—including genes, stress, and the environment—have small effects that add up in complex ways to affect a person's risk for these disorders," Pine says.

"Many kids with anxiety disorders will outgrow their conditions. But most anxiety problems we see in adults started during their childhood," Pine adds.

"Anxiety disorders are among the most common psychiatric disorders in children, with an estimated 1 in 3 suffering anxiety at some point during childhood or adolescence," says Dr. Susan Whitfield-Gabrieli, a brain imaging expert at the Massachusetts Institute of Technology (MIT). "About half of diagnosable mental health disorders start by age 14, so there's a lot of interest in uncovering the factors that might influence the brain by those early teen years."

Part Two

Types of Anxiety Disorders

Chapter 6

Agoraphobia

The word agoraphobia literally means "fear of wide, open spaces." However, people with a diagnosis of agoraphobia might also have extreme fear or anxiety of other types of situations, such as such as being out of their home alone or being in a crowd. Individuals with agoraphobia often try to avoid these feared situations because of their high levels of anxiety. If avoidance is not possible, they need to be accompanied by another person, and/or they endure the situations with extreme anxiety. These situations are often avoided for fear of having a panic attack. Thus many people with a diagnosis of agoraphobia also have a diagnosis of panic disorder.

Panic disorder and agoraphobia are two separate psychiatric disorders that often occur together. Panic disorder is characterized by recurrent and sometimes unexpected panic attacks. A panic attack, or "fight or flight" response, is a sudden rush of intense anxiety with symptoms such as rapid heart rate, difficulty breathing, numbness or tingling, and/or a fear of dying. Panic attacks usually reach their peak within minutes, but people sometimes continue to feel anxious or exhausted after one occurs. In some cases, people with panic disorder experience nocturnal panic attacks, which wake them up from

---

This chapter includes text excerpted from "What Are Panic Disorder and Agoraphobia?" Mental Illness Research, Education, and Clinical Centers (MIRECC), U.S. Department of Veterans Affairs (VA), 2016.

sleep. It is common for individuals with panic disorder to worry about having another panic attack and to make behavioral changes as a result, such as avoiding people, places, or things they associate with the attacks.

Prevalence

Nearly 5 percent of people in the United States will have panic disorder at some point in their lifetimes, and it is about twice as common in women. It is estimated that approximately one quarter to one third of the population will experience panic-like symptoms at some point in their lifetime, but these subclinical symptoms never progress to the full severity of panic disorder. Nonetheless, subclinical panic symptoms are often associated with high degrees of distress. The prevalence of agoraphobia is similar to that of panic disorder, with about 5 percent of people experiencing it at some point in their lifetime.

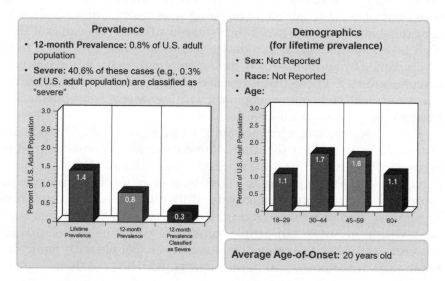

Figure 6.1. *Prevalence and Demographics of Agoraphobia among Adults*

(Source: "Agoraphobia among Adults," National Institute of Mental Health (NIMH).)

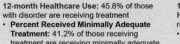

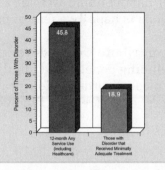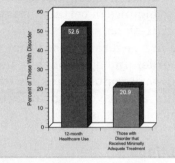

Figure 6.2. *Treatment/Service Use for Agoraphobia among Adults*

(Source: "Agoraphobia among Adults," National Institute of Mental Health (NIMH).)

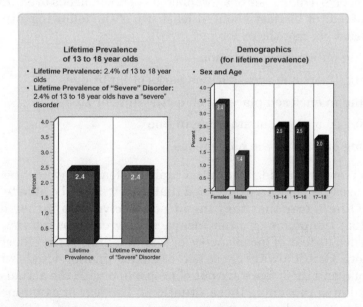

Figure 6.3. *Prevalence and Demographics of Agoraphobia among Children*

(Source: "Agoraphobia among Children," National Institute of Mental Health (NIMH).)

Causes

The causes for agoraphobia are very similar to those of panic disorder, and it is likely that genetic, biological, personality, and environmental stressors all play a role in the development of the disorder. For those who develop agoraphobia after having panic attacks, the stated cause of avoidance of certain situations is usually a fear of panicking in those situations.

There are several factors that contribute to the development of panic disorder and agoraphobia, including genetic and family history of panic disorder or other anxiety or mood disorders, biological factors, personality and psychological factors, and stressful life events and environmental stressors.

Diagnosis

Panic disorder and agoraphobia cannot be diagnosed with a blood test, CAT scan, or any other laboratory test. The only way to diagnose these disorders is with a thorough clinical interview. A medical evaluation is also important to rule out underlying medical causes of the symptoms.

To receive a diagnosis of agoraphobia, a person needs to exhibit high levels of fear or anxiety about at least two of the following situations, for at least six months or longer:

* Using public transportation
* Being in open spaces, such as parks or on bridges
* Being in enclosed places such as theaters or stores
* Being in a crowd or standing in line
* Being outside of the home alone

A person with a diagnosis of agoraphobia fears or avoids these situations because they are concerned that they will not be able to escape them. Others fear that they might not receive help if they develop panic-like symptoms or other incapacitating or embarrassing symptoms (such as fear of incontinence or fear of falling in the elderly). The situations almost always cause fear or anxiety in individuals with agoraphobia, and their fears are out of proportion with the actual danger involved in approaching these situations. The fear or avoidance must cause significant distress or impairment in major areas of functioning in order to receive a diagnosis of agoraphobia. If a person is avoiding these situations because of concerns related to a medical condition, the anxiety and avoidance must be clearly excessive.

Finally, to receive a diagnosis of agoraphobia, the clinician must determine that the symptoms are not better explained by another mental health diagnosis. For example, if the person only avoids social situations, social anxiety disorder might be diagnosed. If they avoid places that remind them of a traumatic event, posttraumatic stress disorder might be diagnosed. Other disorders associated with avoidance, such as major depression, specific phobias, and separation anxiety disorder, might be diagnosed instead of agoraphobia if symptoms are better accounted for by those disorders.

Course of Illness in Agoraphobia

Between one-third to one-half of people will have panic attacks prior to the onset of agoraphobia; the average age of onset for those individuals is late teens. For those who do not have panic attacks prior to the onset of agoraphobia, the average age of onset is later—in the mid to late 20's. While most develop the disorder at a younger age, a third of individuals will have an onset after age 40. Agoraphobia tends to be a chronic illness if left untreated. Most individuals with agoraphobia also have co-occurring psychiatric disorders, such as anxiety, mood, and/or substance use disorders.

How Family Members Can Help

Family members of individuals with panic disorder and/or agoraphobia can support their relative's recovery in many ways. It is important for the person who is experiencing anxiety to first visit a medical doctor for a thorough evaluation. If possible, family members could also attend to help answer questions and to provide support. If medication is prescribed, family members can provide support in regularly taking those medications. Family members can also support attendance to psychotherapy appointments by giving reminders and providing transportation to the clinic.

If the individual with panic disorder and/or agoraphobia is in therapy, it might be helpful for family members to talk with the therapist to learn specifics about the illness and how they can provide support. CBT includes homework assignments, and family members can encourage their relative to engage in the homework and offer to help, if relevant. For example, family members can help reinforce the concept that panic attacks are not dangerous and work with their relative to consider alternative, nonscary thoughts about the attacks. If the person is engaging in a relaxation or mindfulness practice as part of treatment, family members can help by giving the time and space for their relative to engage in such a practice at home. Studies have shown that partner-assisted exposure therapy helps reduce symptoms of panic and agoraphobia. Family members can encourage exposure practice with their relative. If there are situations that the person is completely avoiding, family members can offer to initially accompany them into those situations, with the goal being that the person would eventually go into those situations by themselves. Lastly, family members can provide emotional support. Some aspects of panic disorder and agoraphobia can be quite frustrating to relatives. For example, a person with these disorders might avoid making plans, cancel at the last minute for fear of having a panic attack, frequently ask for reassurance about whether or not their symptoms are dangerous, or have difficulty doing things that are easy for most people (e.g., going to the store, driving on the freeway, or going out to restaurants). Family members who understand that these types of behaviors are a part of the disorder may feel less frustration and more warmth and empathy towards their relative.

Cognitive Behavior Therapy (CBT)

One of the most effective treatments for panic disorder and agoraphobia is cognitive behavioral therapy (CBT), which can be used alone or in conjunction with medications. CBT can often be utilized effectively on its own for milder cases, whereas a combination is often preferred for more severe cases. CBT is a structured treatment that can be provided in an individual or group format, usually on a weekly basis. There are also some self help books and manuals that are based on the principles of CBT. The goal of CBT is to significantly reduce or eliminate panic attacks, as well as significantly decrease the fear and behavior changes associated with them. Much of the work of CBT is done between sessions in the form of "homework," so that the person can monitor their panic symptoms and apply the techniques learned in therapy sessions.

CBT for panic disorder is based on the assumptions that:

1. Individuals with panic disorder misinterpret their panic attacks as dangerous or scary,

2. They are overly attuned to their bodily sensations, making them more vulnerable to experiencing attacks, and

3. They often make changes in their behaviors, such as avoidance of situations that they associate with the attacks. One of

the goals of treatment is to help the person have a more realistic view of their panic attacks, in order to help make them less scary. This is done through providing education about panic disorder, teaching people to be aware of their scary thoughts about the attacks, and instructing them on how to change these thoughts to make them more realistic and less frightening.

A technique called interoceptive exposure is used to help people overcome their fear of the bodily sensations associated with panic attacks. Interoceptive exposure involves engaging in specific exercises to bring on the symptoms of anxiety and panic in a controlled way. Although often uncomfortable at first, these exposure exercises are very effective for alleviating the distress of experiencing symptoms of panic and eventually the symptoms themselves. Finally, CBT utilizes in vivo exposures, in which a person systematically starts to face the people, places, and activities that they might be avoiding as a result of the panic attacks. For example, if someone is avoiding exercising or drinking caffeine for fear of having an attack, the therapist will work with them to strategically plan on introducing and continuing these avoided activities.

With CBT for agoraphobia, the emphasis would likely be on the in vivo exposure element of treatment. By engaging in in vivo exposure therapy, individuals with agoraphobia will systematically and frequently approach feared situations and learn that they are not scary or dangerous.

Relaxation Training

Some therapists use relaxation training as a method of reducing anxiety and panic attacks. It can be used in conjunction with CBT and/or medication, but most professionals agree that relaxation training alone is probably not sufficient to fully alleviate panic symptoms for most people. One type of relaxation strategy often used for panic disorder is diaphragmatic breathing, or belly breathing. This type of breathing, which leads to deeper breaths and more oxygen in the lungs, might be particularly helpful for those who experience shortness of breath, chest pain, or dizziness during their panic attacks. Diaphragmatic breathing is also a relaxation strategy for treating more generalized anxiety, which might then reduce one's susceptibility to having a panic attack. Likewise, progressive muscle relaxation, a type of relaxation which involves tensing and relaxing different muscles in the body, can also lead to reducing generalized anxiety.

Mindfulness and Acceptance Practices

Mindfulness is another technique often used in conjunction with CBT and/or medication. Contrary to what some people think, mindfulness and relaxation are not the same thing, although many people find practicing mindfulness to be relaxing. There are many ways to practice mindfulness. One common way is to sit quietly and focus attention on one's breath, without actually trying to change the breath. People who regularly practice mindfulness can learn to be less reactive to their emotions and changes in their bodies. They can learn to be more accepting of negative emotional states, such as anxiety. For those with panic disorder and agoraphobia, mindfulness can teach people to observe their anxiety, rather than feeding into it with negative thoughts and avoidance behaviors. Thus, acceptance of one's anxiety can cause the anxiety to lessen and feel less scary.

Medication: What You Should Know

- There are different types of medications that are very effective for panic disorder and agoraphobia. These include antidepressant medications, benzodiazepines, and anticonvulsants.

- These medications work by modulating gamma-aminobutyric acid (GABA), serotonin, norepinephrine, or dopamine; neurotransmitters believed to regulate anxiety and mood.

- Sometimes the medication you first try may not lead to the improvements you desire with regard to your anxiety. What works well for one person may not do as well for another. Be open to trying another medication or combination of medications in order to find a good fit. Let your doctor know if your symptoms have not improved and do not give up searching for the right medication!

- All medications may cause side effects, but many people have no side effects or minor side effects. The side effects people typically experience are tolerable and subside in a few days. Check with your doctor if any of the common side effects listed persist or become bothersome. In rare cases, these medications can cause severe side effects. Contact your doctor immediately if you experience one or more severe symptoms.

Antidepressant Medications

- Antidepressant medications, while initially developed for depression, have been found to be successful in treating anxiety disorders and are commonly used to treat panic disorder. While many available antidepressants are listed here, the evidence for their effectiveness in treating panic disorder varies considerably. You should discuss medication choices with your doctor.

- Antidepressant medications work to increase the following neurotransmitters: serotonin, norepinephrine, and/or dopamine.

- Antidepressants must be taken as prescribed for three to four weeks before you can expect to see positive changes in your symptoms. So don't stop taking your medication because you think it's not working. Give it time!

- Once you have responded to treatment, it is important to continue treatment. It is typical for treatment to continue for 6-9 months. Discontinuing treatment earlier may lead to a relapse of symptoms. If you have a more severe case of panic disorder, the doctor might recommend longer term treatment.

- To prevent the panic disorder from coming back or worsening, do not abruptly stop taking your medications, even if you are feeling better. Stopping your medication can cause a relapse. Medication should only be stopped under your doctor's supervision. If you want to stop taking your medication, talk to your doctor about how to correctly stop it.

- When taking antidepressant medications for panic disorder, if you forget to take a dose, a safe rule of thumb is: if you missed your regular time by three hours or less, you should take that dose when you remember it. If it is more than three hours after the dose should have been taken, just skip the forgotten dose and resume your medication at the next regularly scheduled time. Never double up on doses of your antidepressant to "catch up" on those you have forgotten.

Benzodiazepines

- Benzodiazepines are a different type of medication that are used for anxiety. Benzodiazepines work by enhancing the effects of the neurotransmitter GABA, which has a calming effect.

71

- Benzodiazepines can be taken on an as needed basis or might be prescribed to be taken on a regular schedule.

- Users of these medications can feel the effects quite quickly (sometimes in less than a half hour), and the effects can last for several hours up to a day, depending on what medication is being taken.

- While benzodiazepines can be effective in the short term, for most people, they are not the best long-term treatment strategy. Many doctors prescribe a benzodiazepine as a person is getting started on an antidepressant. Use of an antidepressant is usually a better long-term medication management strategy than benzodiazepines. Hence, the doctor might taper the individual off the benzodiazepine once they are experiencing the benefits of the antidepressant.

- The use of benzodiazepines on an as needed basis should be avoided. One of the goals of psychotherapy for panic disorder, especially CBT, is for the panic sufferer to learn that while panic attacks are uncomfortable and unpleasant, they are not dangerous and can be tolerated. Becoming less fearful of the panic attack is instrumental in recovering from panic disorder. When a person takes a benzodiazepine on an as needed basis, such as when they have a panic attack or feel increased anxiety, they are depriving themselves the chance to learn that panic attacks are not dangerous. In fact, they are giving themselves the opposite message: I can't tolerate this, so I must take a medication immediately.

- Benzodiazepines may be habit-forming. Those who take benzodiazepines on a regular basis are at risk for dependency and withdrawal. Individuals might need to increase the dosage of their medication in order to get the desired effect. They may also experience symptoms of withdrawal when coming off the medication. Because of these addictive properties, benzodiazepines might not be prescribed to people with a history of substance abuse problems.

- Benzodiazepines can cause drowsiness, impair coordination and concentration, and reduce short-term memory. They should not be used simultaneously with alcohol or opiate medications.

Anticonvulsant Medications

- Anticonvulsant medications are usually used to treat seizures, but they also help control mood and are helpful for individuals with panic disorder. They are generally reserved for patients who do not respond to a trial of antidepressants.

- Anticonvulsants are believed to work by increasing the neurotransmitter, GABA, which has a calming effect on the brain. It is also believed that they decrease glutamate, which is an excitatory neurotransmitter.

Chapter 7

General Anxiety Disorder

What Is Generalized Anxiety Disorder (GAD)?

Occasional anxiety is a normal part of life. You might worry about things like health, money, or family problems. But people with generalized anxiety disorder (GAD) feel extremely worried or feel nervous about these and other things—even when there is little or no reason to worry about them. People with GAD find it difficult to control their anxiety and stay focused on daily tasks.

The good news is that GAD is treatable. Call your doctor to talk about your symptoms so that you can feel better.

What Are the Signs and Symptoms of GAD?

GAD develops slowly. It often starts during the teen years or young adulthood. People with GAD may:

- Worry very much about everyday things
- Have trouble controlling their worries or feelings of nervousness
- Know that they worry much more than they should
- Feel restless and have trouble relaxing
- Have a hard time concentrating

This chapter includes text excerpted from "Generalized Anxiety Disorder: When Worry Gets out of Control," National Institute of Mental Health (NIMH), 2016.

- Be easily startled
- Have trouble falling asleep or staying asleep
- Feel easily tired or tired all the time
- Have headaches, muscle aches, stomach aches, or unexplained pains
- Have a hard time swallowing
- Tremble or twitch
- Be irritable or feel "on edge"
- Sweat a lot, feel light-headed or out of breath
- Have to go to the bathroom a lot

Children and teens with GAD often worry excessively about:

- Their performance, such as in school or in sports
- Catastrophes, such as earthquakes or war

Adults with GAD are often highly nervous about everyday circumstances, such as:

- Job security or performance
- Health
- Finances
- The health and wellbeing of their children
- Being late
- Completing household chores and other responsibilities

Both children and adults with GAD may experience physical symptoms that make it hard to function and that interfere with daily life.

Symptoms may get better or worse at different times, and they are often worse during times of stress, such as with a physical illness, during exams at school, or during a family or relationship conflict.

What Causes GAD?

GAD sometimes runs in families, but no one knows for sure why some family members have it while others don't. Researchers have found that several parts of the brain, as well as biological processes, play a key role in fear and anxiety. By learning more about how the brain and body function in people with anxiety disorders, researchers may be able to create better treatments. Researchers are also looking for ways in which stress and environmental factors play a role.

How Is GAD Treated?

First, talk to your doctor about your symptoms. Your doctor should do an exam and ask you about your health history to make sure that an unrelated physical problem is not causing your symptoms. Your doctor may refer to you a mental health specialist, such as a psychiatrist or psychologist.

GAD is generally treated with psychotherapy, medication, or both. Talk with your doctor about the best treatment for you.

Psychotherapy. A type of psychotherapy called cognitive behavioral therapy (CBT) is especially useful for treating GAD. CBT teaches a person, different ways of thinking, behaving, and reacting to situations that help him or her feel less anxious and worried.

Medication. Doctors may also prescribe medication to help treat GAD. Your doctor will work with you to find the best medication and dose for you. Different types of medication can be effective in GAD:

- Selective serotonin reuptake inhibitors (SSRIs)
- Serotonin norepinephrine reuptake inhibitors (SNRIs)
- Other serotonergic medication
- Benzodiazepines

Doctors commonly use SSRIs and SNRIs to treat depression, but they are also helpful for the symptoms of GAD. They may take several weeks to start working. These medications may also cause side effects, such as headaches, nausea, or difficulty sleeping. These side effects are usually not severe for most people, especially if the dose starts off low and is increased slowly over time. Talk to your doctor about any side effects that you have.

Buspirone is another serotonergic medication that can be helpful in GAD. Buspirone needs to be taken continuously for several weeks for it to be fully effective.

Benzodiazepines, which are sedative medications, can also be used to manage severe forms of GAD. These medications are powerfully effective in rapidly decreasing anxiety, but they can cause tolerance and dependence if you use them continuously. Therefore, your doctor will only prescribe them for brief periods of time if you need them.

Don't give up on treatment too quickly. Both psychotherapy and medication can take some time to work. A healthy lifestyle can also help combat anxiety. Make sure to get enough sleep and exercise, eat a healthy diet, and turn to family and friends who you trust for support.

Chapter 8

Illness Anxiety Disorder

What Is Illness Anxiety Disorder?

Illness anxiety disorder is a condition in which a person is preoccupied with having or acquiring a serious disease. The person misinterprets normal body sensations, or minor symptoms, as indications of major illness, even though a thorough medical examination fails to reveal any serious disease. People with a high risk of acquiring a medical condition, in particular, become consumed with worry and often assume various normal bodily sensations are symptoms of the disease. This leads to anxiety that is more severe than the physical symptoms themselves and causes distress that can affect a person's daily life. The disorder occurs in early adulthood and may be seen in both men and women.

The condition that was previously known as hypochondriasis has been reclassified in the *Diagnostic and Statistical Manual of Mental Disorders, 5th Edition* (DSM-5) of the American Psychiatric Association (APA) under the following two disorders:

1   **Illness anxiety disorder**, which manifests with mild or no physical symptoms.

2. **Somatic symptom disorder,** which manifests with multiple, sometimes major, physical symptoms.

Note that illness anxiety disorder and somatic symptom disorder are different conditions in that physical symptoms are usually not seen

---

"Illness Anxiety Disorder," © 2018 Omnigraphics. Reviewed September 2017.

in illness anxiety disorder, while they are present, and significantly so, in somatic symptom disorder.

What Are the Symptoms of Illness Anxiety Disorder?

People with illness anxiety disorder worry about getting a serious disease and so are preoccupied with related thoughts, causing distress that can impair work, family, and social life. Physical symptoms may or may not be present, although they are usually relatively mild. Patients are generally more concerned about the implications of the symptoms rather than the symptoms themselves.

They get easily alarmed about their health, and negative medical test results fail to provide any reassurance. Patients may frequently consult many healthcare professionals for reassurance, or they might avoid medical care altogether for fear of being diagnosed with a serious illness. Some patients examine themselves obsessively for new symptoms by looking in the mirror or checking their skin for lesions. They think that any new symptom or sensation is a sign of serious illness.

Illness anxiety disorder is chronic, sometimes fluctuating in some people while remaining steady in others. Some patients are able to understand their fears are unreasonable and unfounded, and many of these individuals tend to recover.

What Causes Illness Anxiety Disorder?

The exact causes of illness anxiety disorder are not known, but the following factors likely play a role:

- **Lack of education.** A poor understanding of disease and what body sensations actually mean could contribute to misinterpretation of symptoms.

- **Learned behavior.** A parent or other family member with excessive anxiety about health issues could promote similar behavior in relatives.

- **Past experiences.** Serious illnesses in childhood could make individuals susceptible to frightening thoughts about physical sensations.

What Are the Risk Factors of Illness Anxiety Disorder?

The following are some of the risk factors of illness anxiety disorder:

- A period of life spent with high stress.

- The threat of illness that existed but did not become serious.
- A history of child abuse.
- A history of illness in childhood or a parent with serious illness.
- The personality trait of being a worrier.
- The tendency to check the Internet obsessively, searching for illnesses.

How Is Illness Anxiety Disorder Diagnosed?

As part of diagnosis, a healthcare professional will conduct a complete physical examination and routine medical tests to find out if the patient has any condition that requires treatment. In the absence of any such condition, the patient will likely be referred to a mental healthcare professional for further diagnosis.

A psychiatrist, psychologist, or other mental-health specialist will conduct a psychological evaluation and elicit information on symptoms, family history, fears and concerns, stress factors, relationship problems and other issues in the patient's life. The diagnosis will then be made based on criteria defined in the DSM-5. Some factors considered for diagnosis include preoccupation with symptoms lasting for at least six months, no somatic symptoms or minimal somatic symptoms, fear of acquiring a serious illness, and the absence of any other mental health condition.

How Is Illness Anxiety Disorder Treated?

The goal of treatment is to help the patient lead a normal life. Psychotherapy, especially cognitive behavioral therapy (CBT), is used to deal with emotional aspects of the disorder. The patient is taught to recognize symptoms, deal with them, and lead an active life even if symptoms persist. Sometimes antidepressants or other medications are prescribed to help relieve symptoms.

What Is the Prognosis for Illness Anxiety Disorder?

Illness anxiety disorder could become a chronic condition unless the psychological factors causing the disorder are treated, so continuing to work with trained professionals is key to a successful outcome. Stress management and relaxation techniques may help reduce anxiety, and staying physically active can improve mood and reduce stress.

In addition, the use of alcohol and recreational drugs can aggravate symptoms and increase anxiety, so these should be avoided.

References

1. "Illness Anxiety Disorder," Mayo Foundation for Medical Education and Research (MFMER), July 2, 2015.

2. Dimsdale, Joel E., MD. "Illness Anxiety Disorder," Merck & Co., August 2016.

3. Berger, Fred K., MD. "Illness Anxiety Disorder," A.D.A.M., Inc., July 29, 2016.

Chapter 9

Obsessive-Compulsive Disorder

Chapter Contents

Section 9.1

Obsessive-Compulsive Disorder (OCD) among Children

This section includes text excerpted from "Children's Mental Health—Obsessive-Compulsive Disorder," Centers for Disease Control and Prevention (CDC), March 23, 2017.

Many children occasionally have thoughts that bother them, and they might feel like they have to do something about those thoughts, even if their actions don't actually make sense. For example, they might worry about having bad luck if they don't wear a favorite piece of clothing. For some children, the thoughts and the urges to perform certain actions persist, even if they try to ignore them or make them go away. Children may have an obsessive-compulsive disorder (OCD) when unwanted thoughts, and the behaviors they feel they must do because of the thoughts, happen frequently, take up a lot of time (more than an hour a day), interfere with their activities, or make them very upset. The thoughts are called obsessions. The behaviors are called compulsions.

Symptoms

Having OCD means having obsessions, compulsions, or both. Examples of obsessive or compulsive behaviors include:

- Having unwanted thoughts, impulses, or images that occur over and over and which cause anxiety or distress.

- Having to think about or say something over and over (for example, counting, or repeating words over and over silently or out loud)

- Having to do something over and over (for example, handwashing, placing things in a specific order, or checking the same things over and over, like whether a door is locked)

- Having to do something over and over according to certain rules that must be followed exactly in order to make an obsession go away.

Children do these behaviors because they have the feeling that the behaviors will prevent bad things from happening or will make them feel better. However, the behavior is not typically connected to actual danger of something bad happening, or the behavior is extreme, such as washing hands multiple times per hour.

A common myth is that OCD means being really neat and orderly. Sometimes, OCD behaviors may involve cleaning, but many times someone with OCD is too focused on one thing that must be done over and over, rather than on being organized. Obsessions and compulsions can also change over time.

Treatment for OCD

The first step to treatment is to talk with a healthcare provider to arrange an evaluation. A comprehensive evaluation by a mental health professional will determine if the anxiety or distress involves memories of a traumatic event that actually happened, or if the fears are based on other thoughts or beliefs. The mental health professional should also determine whether someone with OCD has a current or past tic disorder. Anxiety or depression and disruptive behaviors may also occur with OCD.

Treatments can include behavior therapy and medication. Behavior therapy, specifically cognitive behavioral therapy, helps the child change negative thoughts into more positive, effective ways of thinking, leading to more effective behavior. Behavior therapy for OCD can involve gradually exposing children to their fears in a safe setting; this helps them learn that bad things do not really occur when they don't do the behavior, which eventually decreases their anxiety. Behavior therapy alone can be effective, but some children are treated with a combination of behavior therapy and medication. Families and schools can help children manage stress by being part of the therapy process and learning how to respond supportively without accidentally making obsessions or compulsions more likely to happen again.

Get Help Finding Treatment

Here are tools to find a healthcare provider familiar with treatment options:

- Psychologist Locator, a service of the American Psychological Association (APA) Practice Organization.

- Child and Adolescent Psychiatrist Finder, a research tool by the American Academy of Child and Adolescent Psychiatry (AACAP).

- Find a Cognitive Behavioral Therapist, a search tool by the Association for Behavioral and Cognitive Therapies (ABCT).

- If you need help finding treatment facilities, use the "Treatment Locator" widget.

Prevention of OCD

It is not known exactly why some children develop OCD. There is likely to be a biological and neurological component, and some children with OCD also have Tourette syndrome or other tic disorders. There are some studies that suggest that health problems during pregnancy and birth may make OCD more likely, which is one of many important reasons to support the health of women during pregnancy.

Section 9.2

Obsessive-Compulsive Disorder among Adults

This section includes text excerpted from "Obsessive-Compulsive Disorder: When Unwanted Thoughts or Irresistible Actions Take Over," National Institute of Mental Health (NIMH), November 2016.

Do you constantly have disturbing uncontrollable thoughts? Do you feel the urge to repeat the same behaviors or rituals over and over? Are these thoughts and behaviors making it hard for you to do things you enjoy?

If so, you may have obsessive-compulsive disorder (OCD). The good news is that, with treatment, you can overcome the fears and behaviors that may be putting your life on hold.

What Is Obsessive-Compulsive Disorder (OCD)?

OCD is a common, chronic (long-lasting) disorder in which a person has uncontrollable, reoccurring thoughts (obsessions) and behaviors (compulsions) that he or she feels the urge to repeat over and over in response to the obsession.

While everyone sometimes feels the need to double check things, people with OCD have uncontrollable thoughts that cause them anxiety, urging them to check things repeatedly or perform routines and rituals for at least 1 hour per day. Performing the routines or rituals may bring brief but temporary relief from the anxiety. However, left untreated, these thoughts and rituals cause the person great distress and get in the way of work, school, and personal relationships.

What Are the Signs and Symptoms of OCD?

People with OCD may have obsessions, compulsions, or both. Some people with OCD also have a tic disorder. Motor tics are sudden, brief, repetitive movements, such as eye blinking, facial grimacing, shoulder shrugging, or head or shoulder jerking. Common vocal tics include repetitive throat-clearing, sniffing, or grunting sounds.

Obsessions may include:

- Fear of germs or contamination

- Fear of losing or misplacing something

- Worries about harm coming towards oneself or others

- Unwanted and taboo thoughts involving sex, religion, or others

- Having things symmetrical or in perfect order

Compulsions may include:

- Excessively cleaning or washing a body part

- Keeping or hoarding unnecessary objects

- Ordering or arranging items in a particular, precise way

- Repeatedly checking on things, such as making sure that the door is locked or the oven is off

- Repeatedly counting items

- Constantly seeking reassurance

What Causes OCD?

OCD may have a genetic component. It sometimes runs in families, but no one knows for sure why some family members have it while others don't. OCD usually begins in adolescence or young adulthood, and tends to appear at a younger age in boys than in girls. Researchers have found that several parts of the brain, as well as biological processes, play a key role in obsessive thoughts and compulsive behavior, as well as the fear and anxiety related to them. Researchers also know that people who have suffered physical or sexual trauma are at an increased risk for OCD.

How Is OCD Treated?

The first step is to talk with your doctor or healthcare provider about your symptoms. The clinician should do an exam and ask you about your health history to make sure that a physical problem is not causing your symptoms. Your doctor may refer you to a mental health specialist, such as a psychiatrist, psychologist, social worker, or counselor for further evaluation or treatment.

OCD is generally treated with cognitive behavior therapy, medication, or both. Speak with your mental health professional about the best treatment for you.

Cognitive Behavioral Therapy (CBT)

In general, CBT teaches you different ways of thinking, behaving, and reacting to the obsessions and compulsions.

Exposure and Response Prevention (EX/RP) is a specific form of CBT which has been shown to help many patients recover from OCD. EX/RP involves gradually exposing you to your fears or obsessions and teaching you healthy ways to deal with the anxiety they cause.

Other therapies, such as habit reversal training, can also help you overcome compulsions.

Medication

Doctors also may prescribe different types of medications to help treat OCD including selective serotonin reuptake inhibitors (SSRIs) and a type of serotonin reuptake inhibitor (SRI) called clomipramine.

SSRIs and SRIs are commonly used to treat depression, but they are also helpful for the symptoms of OCD. SSRIs and SRIs may take 10–12 weeks to start working, longer than is required for the treatment of depression. These medications may also cause side effects, such as headaches, nausea, or difficulty sleeping.

People taking clomipramine, which is in a different class of medication from the SSRIs, sometimes experience dry mouth, constipation, rapid heartbeat, and dizziness on standing. These side effects are usually not severe for most people and improve as treatment continues, especially if the dose starts off low and is increased slowly over time. Talk to your doctor about any side effects that you have. Don't stop taking your medication without talking to your doctor first. Your doctor will work with you to find the best medication and dose for you.

Don't give up on treatment too quickly. Both psychotherapy and medication can take some time to work. While there is no cure for OCD, current treatments enable most people with this disorder to control their symptoms and lead full, productive lives. A healthy lifestyle that involves relaxation and managing stress can also help combat OCD. Make sure to also get enough sleep and exercise, eat a healthy diet, and turn to family and friends whom you trust for support.

Section 9.3

Hoarding Disorder: A Form of OCD

This section contains text excerpted from the following sources: Text under the heading "What Is Compulsive Hoarding?" is excerpted from "Treatment of Compulsive Hoarding," ClinicalTrials. gov, National Institutes of Health (NIH), June 19, 2013. Reviewed September 2017; Text under the heading "What Does Research Reveal about People Suffering from Compulsive Hoarding Disorder?" is excerpted from "Distinct Brain Activity in Hoarders," National Institutes of Health (NIH), August 20, 2012. Reviewed September 2017.

What Is Compulsive Hoarding?

Compulsive hoarding is a form of obsessive-compulsive disorder (OCD) that is characterized by excessive acquisition of possessions, difficulty discarding possessions, and excessive clutter. This condition is resistant to both pharmacological and psychotherapeutic interventions that are effective in treating other symptoms of OCD.

What Does Research Reveal about People Suffering from Compulsive Hoarding Disorder?

Certain brain regions under-activate in people with hoarding disorder when dealing with others' possessions but over-activate when deciding whether to keep or discard their own things. The findings give insight into the biology of hoarding and may guide future treatment strategies.

People with hoarding disorder have trouble making decisions about when to throw things away. Possessions can pile up and result in debilitating clutter.

Previous studies of brain function in hoarders implicated regions associated with decision-making, attachment, reward processing, impulse control, and emotional regulation. But the patient populations and research methods varied between the studies, making it difficult to draw clear conclusions.

In a study, a research team, led by Dr. David Tolin of Hartford Hospital and Yale University, used functional magnetic resonance imaging (fMRI) to investigate the neural basis for hoarding disorder. They compared the brains of patients with hoarding disorder to patients with OCD and healthy controls as they decided whether to keep or discard possessions. The study was funded by National Institutes of Health's (NIH) National Institute of Mental Health (NIMH).

The researchers analyzed brain images of 43 hoarders, 31 people with OCD and 33 healthy controls. Participants were given 6 seconds to make a decision about whether to keep or discard junk mail that either belonged to them or to someone else. Participants later watched as the items they chose to discard were placed in a paper shredder. They were then asked to rate their emotions and describe how they felt during the decision-making tasks. The results appeared in the August 2012 issue of the *Archives of General Psychiatry.*

The hoarders chose to keep more mail that belonged to them than those in the OCD or healthy control groups. Hoarders also took longer to make decisions and reported greater anxiety, indecisiveness and sadness than the other groups.

The imaging analysis revealed that hoarders differ from both healthy controls and patients with OCD in 2 specific brain regions: the anterior cingulate cortex and insula. Scientists believe that these areas are part of a brain network involved in processing emotion. Both regions were more active in hoarders when they were making decisions about mail that belonged to them, but less active when making decisions about mail that didn't belong to them.

90

These results suggest that hoarders' decisions about possessions are hampered by abnormal activity in brain regions used to identify the emotional significance of things. "They lose the ability to make relative judgments, so the decision becomes absolutely overwhelming and aversive to them," Tolin says.

The scientists believe that these brain abnormalities are specific to hoarding and separate the disorder from OCD. In addition to further exploring the unique traits of hoarders, the researchers are now using this information to help assess potential treatments.

Chapter 10

Panic Disorder

Do you sometimes have sudden attacks of anxiety and overwhelming fear that last for several minutes? Maybe your heart pounds, you sweat, and you feel like you can't breathe or think. Do these attacks occur at unpredictable times with no obvious trigger, causing you to worry about the possibility of having another one at any time?

If so, you may have a type of anxiety disorder called panic disorder. Left untreated, panic disorder can lower your quality of life because it may lead to other fears and mental health disorders, problems at work or school, and social isolation.

What Is Panic Disorder?

People with panic disorder have sudden and repeated attacks of fear that last for several minutes or longer. These are called **panic attacks.** Panic attacks are characterized by a fear of disaster or of losing control even when there is no real danger. A person may also have a strong physical reaction during a panic attack. It may feel like having a heart attack. Panic attacks can occur at any time, and many people with panic disorder worry about and dread the possibility of having another attack.

A person with panic disorder may become discouraged and feel ashamed because he or she cannot carry out normal routines like going to school or work, going to the grocery store, or driving.

This chapter includes text excerpted from "Panic Disorder: When Fear Overwhelms," National Institute of Mental Health (NIMH), September 2016.

Panic disorder often begins in the late teens or early adulthood. More women than men have panic disorder. But not everyone who experiences panic attacks will develop panic disorder.

What Causes Panic Disorder?

Panic disorder sometimes runs in families, but no one knows for sure why some family members have it while others don't. Researchers have found that several parts of the brain, as well as biological processes, play a key role in fear and anxiety. Some researchers think that people with panic disorder misinterpret harmless bodily sensations as threats. Researchers are also looking for ways in which stress and environmental factors may play a role.

What Are the Signs and Symptoms of Panic Disorder?

People with panic disorder may have:

- Sudden and repeated panic attacks of overwhelming anxiety and fear.
- A feeling of being out of control, or a fear of death or impending doom during a panic attack.
- Physical symptoms during a panic attack, such as a pounding or racing heart, sweating, chills, trembling, breathing problems, weakness or dizziness, tingly or numb hands, chest pain, stomach pain, and nausea.
- An intense worry about when the next panic attack will happen.
- A fear or avoidance of places where panic attacks have occurred in the past.

How Is Panic Disorder Treated?

First, talk to your doctor about your symptoms. Your doctor should do an exam and ask you about your health history to make sure that an unrelated physical problem is not causing your symptoms. Your doctor may refer to you a mental health specialist, such as a psychiatrist or psychologist.

Panic disorder is generally treated with psychotherapy, medication, or both. Talk with your doctor about the best treatment for you.

Psychotherapy. A type of psychotherapy called cognitive behavioral therapy (CBT) is especially useful as a first-line treatment for panic disorder. CBT teaches you different ways of thinking, behaving, and reacting to the feelings that come on with a panic attack. The attacks can begin to disappear once you learn to react differently to the physical sensations of anxiety and fear that occur during panic attacks.

Medication. Doctors also may prescribe different types of medications to help treat panic disorder:

- Selective serotonin reuptake inhibitors (SSRIs)
- Serotonin-norepinephrine reuptake inhibitors (SNRIs)
- Beta blockers
- Benzodiazepines

SSRIs and SNRIs are commonly used to treat depression, but they are also helpful for the symptoms of panic disorder. They may take several weeks to start working. These medications may also cause side effects, such as headaches, nausea, or difficulty sleeping. These side effects are usually not severe for most people, especially if the dose starts off low and is increased slowly over time. Talk to your doctor about any side effects that you have.

Another type of medication called beta blockers can help control some of the physical symptoms of panic disorder, such as rapid heart rate. Although doctors do not commonly prescribe beta blockers for panic disorder, they may be helpful in certain situations that precede a panic attack.

Benzodiazepines, which are sedative medications, are powerfully effective in rapidly decreasing panic attack symptoms, but they can cause tolerance and dependence if you use them continuously. Therefore, your doctor will only prescribe them for brief periods of time if you need them. Your doctor will work with you to find the best medication and dose for you.

Don't give up on treatment too quickly. Both psychotherapy and medication can take some time to work. A healthy lifestyle can also help combat panic disorder. Make sure to get enough sleep and exercise, eat a healthy diet, and turn to family and friends who you trust for support.

Chapter 11

Posttraumatic Stress Disorder

Chapter Contents

Section 11.1

Posttraumatic Stress Disorder

This section includes text excerpted from "Posttraumatic Stress Disorder," National Institute of Mental Health (NIMH), July 4, 2017.

What Is Posttraumatic Stress Disorder (PTSD)?

Posttraumatic stress disorder (PTSD) is a disorder that some people develop after experiencing a shocking, scary, or dangerous event. It is natural to feel afraid during and after a traumatic situation. This fear triggers many split-second changes in the body to respond to danger and help a person avoid danger in the future. This "fight-or-flight" response is a typical reaction meant to protect a person from harm. Nearly everyone will experience a range of reactions after trauma, yet most people will recover from those symptoms naturally. Those who continue to experience problems may be diagnosed with PTSD. People who have PTSD may feel stressed or frightened even when they are no longer in danger.

Who Develops PTSD?

Anyone can develop PTSD at any age. This includes war veterans as well as survivors of physical and sexual assault, abuse, car accidents, disasters, terror attacks, or other serious events. Not everyone with PTSD has been through a dangerous event. Some experiences, like the sudden or unexpected death of a loved one, can also cause PTSD.

According to the National Center for PTSD, about seven or eight of every 100 people will experience PTSD at some point in their lives. Women are more likely to develop PTSD than men. Some traumas may put an individual at a higher risk and biological factors like genes may make some people more likely to develop PTSD than others.

What Are the Symptoms of PTSD?

Symptoms usually begin within 3 months of the traumatic incident, but sometimes they begin later. For symptoms to be considered PTSD, they must last more than a month and be severe enough to interfere with functioning in relationships or work. The course of the illness varies from person to person. Some people recover within 6 months, while others have symptoms that last much longer. In some people, the condition becomes chronic (ongoing). A doctor who has experience helping people with mental illnesses, such as a psychiatrist or psychologist, can diagnose PTSD.

To be diagnosed with PTSD, an adult must have all of the following for at least 1 month:

- At least one re-experiencing symptom
- At least one avoidance symptom
- At least two arousal and reactivity symptoms
- At least two cognition and mood symptoms

Re-experiencing symptoms:

- Flashbacks—reliving the trauma over and over, including physical symptoms like a racing heart or sweating
- Bad dreams
- Frightening thoughts

Re-experiencing symptoms may cause problems in a person's everyday routine. They can start from the person's own thoughts and feelings. Words, objects, or situations that are reminders of the event can also trigger re-experiencing symptoms.

Avoidance symptoms:

- Staying away from places, events, or objects that are reminders of the experience
- Avoiding thoughts or feelings related to the traumatic event

Things or situations that remind a person of the traumatic event can trigger avoidance symptoms. These symptoms may cause a person to change his or her personal routine. For example, after a bad car accident, a person who usually drives may avoid driving or riding in a car.

Arousal and reactivity symptoms:

- Being easily startled
- Feeling tense or "on edge"
- Having difficulty sleeping, and/or having angry outbursts

Arousal symptoms are usually constant, instead of being triggered by something that brings back memories of the traumatic event. They can make the person feel stressed and angry. These symptoms may make it hard to do daily tasks, such as sleeping, eating, or concentrating.

Cognition and mood symptoms:

• Trouble remembering key features of the traumatic event

• Negative thoughts about oneself or the world

• Distorted feelings like guilt or blame

• Loss of interest in enjoyable activities

Cognition and mood symptoms can begin or worsen after the traumatic event. These symptoms can make the person feel alienated or detached from friends or family members.

After a dangerous event, it's natural to have some of the symptoms mentioned on previous pages. Sometimes people have very serious symptoms that go away after a few weeks. This is called acute stress disorder, or ASD. When the symptoms last more than a month, seriously affect a person's ability to function and are not due to substance use, medical illness, or anything except the event itself, the person might be experiencing PTSD. Some people with PTSD don't show any symptoms for weeks or months. PTSD is often accompanied by depression, substance abuse, or one or more anxiety disorders.

Do Children React Differently than Adults?

Children and teens can have extreme reactions to trauma, but their symptoms may not be the same as adults. In very young children (less than 6 years of age), these symptoms can include:

• Wetting the bed after having learned to use the toilet

• Forgetting how or being unable to talk

• Acting out the scary event during playtime

• Being unusually clingy with a parent or other adult

Older children and teens usually show symptoms more like those seen in adults. They may also develop disruptive, disrespectful, or destructive behaviors. Older children and teens may feel guilty for not preventing injury or deaths. They may also have thoughts of revenge.

Why Do Some People Develop PTSD and Other People Do Not?

It is important to remember that not everyone who lives through a dangerous event develops PTSD. In fact, most will recover quickly without intervention.

Many factors play a part in whether a person will develop PTSD. Some of these are risk factors that make a person more likely to develop PTSD. Other factors, called resilience factors, can help reduce the risk of developing the disorder. Some of these risk and resilience factors are present before the trauma and others become important during and after a traumatic event.

Risk factors for PTSD include:

- Living through dangerous events and traumas
- Getting hurt
- Seeing people hurt or killed
- Childhood trauma
- Feeling horror, helplessness, or extreme fear
- Having little or no social support after the event
- Dealing with extra stress after the event, such as loss of a loved one, pain and injury, or loss of a job or home
- Having a history of mental illness or substance abuse

Resilience factors that may reduce the risk of PTSD include:

- Seeking out support from other people, such as friends and family
- Finding a support group after a traumatic event
- Learning to feel good about one's own actions in the face of danger
- Having a coping strategy, or a way of getting through the bad event and learning from it
- Being able to act and respond effectively despite feeling fear

How Is PTSD Treated?

It is important for anyone with PTSD to be treated by a mental health professional who is experienced with PTSD. The main treatments are psychotherapy ("talk" therapy), medications, or both. Everyone is different, and PTSD affects people differently, so a treatment that works for one person may not work for another. People with PTSD need to work with a mental health professional to find the best treatment for their symptoms.

If someone with PTSD is living through an ongoing trauma, such as being in an abusive relationship, both of the problems need to be addressed. Other ongoing problems can include panic disorder, depression, substance abuse, and feeling suicidal. Research shows that support from family and friends can be an important part of recovery.

Psychotherapy

Psychotherapy is "talk" therapy. There are many types of psychotherapy but all of them involve talking with a mental health professional to treat a mental illness. Psychotherapy can occur one-on-one or in a group and usually lasts 6 to 12 weeks, but can take more time.

Many types of psychotherapy can help people with PTSD. Some types target PTSD symptoms while others focus on social, family, or job-related problems. The doctor or therapist may combine different therapies depending on each person's needs.

Effective psychotherapies tend to emphasize a few key components, including education about symptoms, teaching skills to help identify the triggers of symptoms, and skills to manage the symptoms. One type of psychotherapy is called cognitive behavioral therapy, or CBT. CBT can include:

- **Exposure therapy.** This therapy helps people face and control their fear. It gradually exposes them to the trauma they experienced in a safe way. It uses mental imagery, writing, or visits to the place where the event happened. The therapist uses these tools to help people with PTSD cope with their feelings.

- **Cognitive restructuring.** This therapy helps people make sense of the bad memories. Sometimes people remember the event differently than how it happened. They may feel guilt or shame about what is not their fault. The therapist helps people with PTSD look at what happened in a realistic way.

Other talk therapies teach people helpful ways to react to frightening events that trigger their PTSD symptoms. Based on this general goal, different types of therapy may:

- Teach about trauma and its effects

- Use relaxation and anger control skills
- Provide tips for better sleep, diet, and exercise habits
- Help people identify and deal with guilt, shame, and other feelings about the event
- Focus on changing how people react to their PTSD symptoms.

Medications

The most studied medications for treating PTSD include antidepressants, which may help control PTSD symptoms such as sadness, worry, anger, and feeling numb inside. Antidepressants and other medications may be prescribed along with psychotherapy. Other medications may be helpful for specific PTSD symptoms. For example, although it is not currently FDA-approved, research has shown that Prazosin may be helpful with sleep problems, particularly nightmares, commonly experienced by people with PTSD. Doctors and patients can work together to find the best medication or medication combination, as well as the right dose.

How Can I Help a Friend or Relative Who Has PTSD?

If you know someone who may be experiencing PTSD, the first and most important thing you can do is to help him or her get the right diagnosis and treatment. You may need to help the person make an appointment and then visit the doctor together. Encourage the person to stay in treatment, or to seek different treatment if symptoms don't get better after six to eight weeks.

To help a friend or relative, you can:

- Offer emotional support, understanding, patience, and encouragement.
- Learn about PTSD so you can understand what your friend is experiencing.
- Listen carefully. Pay attention to your relative's feelings and the situations that may trigger PTSD symptoms.
- Share positive distractions such as walks, outings, and other activities.
- Remind your friend or relative that, with time and treatment, he or she can get better.

Never ignore comments about death or wanting to die. Contact your friend's or relative's therapist or doctor for help or call the National Suicide Prevention Lifeline (800-273-8255) or 911 in an emergency.

There are other types of treatment that can help as well. People with PTSD should talk about all treatment options with their mental health professional. Treatment should provide people with the skills to manage their symptoms and help them participate in activities that they enjoyed before developing PTSD.

How Can I Help Myself?

It may be very hard to take that first step to help yourself. It is important to realize that although it may take some time, with treatment, you can get better.

To help yourself:

- Talk with your doctor about treatment options.

- Engage in mild physical activity or exercise to help reduce stress.

- Set realistic goals for yourself.

- Break up large tasks into small ones, set some priorities, and do what you can as you can.

- Try to spend time with other people and confide in a trusted friend or relative.

- Tell others about things that may trigger symptoms.

- Expect your symptoms to improve gradually, not immediately.

- Identify and seek out comforting situations, places, and people.

Where Can I Go for Help?

If you are unsure of where to go for help, ask your family doctor, or contact someone from one of the groups listed below:

- Mental health specialists, such as psychiatrists, psychologists, social workers, or mental health counselors

- Health maintenance organizations

- Community mental health centers

- Hospital psychiatry departments and outpatient clinics

- Mental health programs at universities or medical schools
- State hospital outpatient clinics
- Family services, social agencies, or clergy
- Peer support groups
- Private clinics and facilities
- Employee assistance programs
- Local medical and/or psychiatric societies
- Visit NIMH's Help for Mental Illnesses page (www.nimh.nih. gov/findhelp)

What If I or Someone I Know Is in Crisis?

If you are thinking about harming yourself, or know someone who is, get help immediately:

- In a crisis, an emergency room doctor can provide temporary help and can tell you where and how to get further support.
- Call 911 or go to a hospital emergency room or ask a friend or family member to help you do these things.
- Call the toll-free, 24-hour National Suicide Prevention Lifeline at 800-273-TALK (800-273-8255); TTY: 800-799-4TTY (800-799-4889) to talk to a trained counselor.
- Call your doctor.
- Do not leave the suicidal person alone.

Section 11.2

PTSD in Children and Teens

This section contains text excerpted from the following sources:
Text in this section begins with excerpts from "PTSD: National
Center for PTSD—PTSD in Children and Teens," National Center
for Posttraumatic Stress Disorder (NCPTSD), U.S. Department of
Veterans Affairs (VA), August 13, 2015; Text under the heading
"Helping Kids Cope with Disaster" is excerpted from "Coping with
Disaster," Federal Emergency Management
Agency (FEMA), February 28, 2017.

This section provides an overview of how trauma affects school-aged
children and teens. You will also find information on treatments for
posttraumatic stress disorder (PTSD) in children.

What Events Cause PTSD in Children?

Children and teens could have PTSD if they have lived through an
event that could have caused them or someone else to be killed or badly
hurt. Such events include sexual or physical abuse or other violent
crimes. Disasters such as floods, school shootings, car crashes, or fires
might also cause PTSD. Other events that can cause PTSD are war, a
friend's suicide, or seeing violence in the area they live.

Child protection services in the United States get around three
million reports each year. This involves 5.5 million children. Of the
reported cases, there is proof of abuse in about 30 percent. From these
cases, we get an idea how often different types of abuse occur:

- 65 percent neglect
- 18 percent physical abuse
- 10 percent sexual abuse
- 7 percent psychological (mental) abuse

Also, three to ten million children witness family violence each
year. Around 40 percent to 60 percent of those cases involve child
physical abuse. It is thought that two-thirds of child abuse cases are
not reported.

How Many Children Get PTSD?

Studies show that about 15 percent to 43 percent of girls and 14 percent to 43 percent of boys go through at least one trauma. Of those children and teens who have had a trauma, 3 percent to 15 percent of girls and 1 percent to 6 percent of boys develop PTSD. Rates of PTSD are higher for certain types of trauma survivors.

What Are the Risk Factors for PTSD?

Three factors have been shown to raise the chances that children will get PTSD. These factors are:

- How severe the trauma is

- How the parents react to the trauma

- How close or far away the child is from the trauma

Children and teens that go through the most severe traumas tend to have the highest levels of PTSD symptoms. The PTSD symptoms may be less severe if the child has more family support and if the parents are less upset by the trauma. Lastly, children and teens who are farther away from the event report less distress.

Other factors can also affect PTSD. Events that involve people hurting other people, such as rape and assault, are more likely to result in PTSD than other types of traumas. Also, the more traumas a child goes through, the higher the risk of getting PTSD. Girls are more likely than boys to get PTSD.

It is not clear whether a child's ethnic group may affect PTSD. Some research shows that minorities have higher levels of PTSD symptoms. Other research suggests this may be because minorities may go through more traumas.

Another question is whether a child's age at the time of the trauma has an effect on PTSD. Researchers think it may not be that the effects of trauma differ according to the child's age. Rather, it may be that PTSD looks different in children of different ages.

What Does PTSD Look Like in Children?

School-Aged Children (Ages 5–12)

These children may not have flashbacks or problems remembering parts of the trauma, the way adults with PTSD often do. Children, though, might put the events of the trauma in the wrong order. They might also think there were signs that the trauma was going to happen. As a result, they think that they will see these signs again before another trauma happens. They think that if they pay attention, they can avoid future traumas.

Children of this age might also show signs of PTSD in their play. They might keep repeating a part of the trauma. These games do not make their worry and distress go away. For example, a child might always want to play shooting games after he sees a school shooting. Children may also fit parts of the trauma into their daily lives. For example, a child might carry a gun to school after seeing a school shooting.

Teens (Ages 12–18)

Teens are in between children and adults. Some PTSD symptoms in teens begin to look like those of adults. One difference is that teens are more likely than younger children or adults to show impulsive and aggressive behaviors.

What Are the Other Effects of Trauma on Children?

Besides PTSD, children and teens that have gone through trauma often have other types of problems. Much of what we know about the effects of trauma on children comes from the research on child sexual abuse. This research shows that sexually abused children often have problems with:

- Fear, worry, sadness, anger, feeling alone, and apart from others, feeling as if people are looking down on them, low self-worth, and not being able to trust others.

- Behaviors such as aggression, out-of-place sexual behavior, self-harm, and abuse of drugs or alcohol.

How Is PTSD Treated in Children and Teens?

For many children, PTSD symptoms go away on their own after a few months. Yet some children show symptoms for years if they do not get treatment. There are many treatment options, described below:

Cognitive Behavioral Therapy (CBT)

CBT is the most effective approach for treating children. One type of CBT is called Trauma-Focused CBT (TF-CBT). In TF-CBT, the child may talk about his or her memory of the trauma. TF-CBT also includes techniques to help lower worry and stress. The child may learn how to assert himself or herself. The therapy may involve learning to change thoughts or beliefs about the trauma that are not correct or true. For example, after a trauma, a child may start thinking, "the world is totally unsafe."

Some may question whether children should be asked to think about and remember events that scared them. However, this type of treatment approach is useful when children are distressed by memories of the trauma. The child can be taught at his or her own pace to relax while they are thinking about the trauma. That way, they learn that they do not have to be afraid of their memories. Research shows that TF-CBT is safe and effective for children with PTSD.

CBT often uses training for parents and caregivers as well. It is important for caregivers to understand the effects of PTSD. Parents need to learn coping skills that will help them help their children.

Psychological First Aid / Crisis Management

Psychological First Aid (PFA) has been used with school-aged children and teens that have been through violence where they live. PFA can be used in schools and traditional settings. It involves providing comfort and support, and letting children know their reactions are normal. PFA teaches calming and problem solving skills. PFA also helps caregivers deal with changes in the child's feelings and behavior. Children with more severe symptoms may be referred for added treatment.

Eye Movement Desensitization and Reprocessing (EMDR)

EMDR combines cognitive therapy with directed eye movements. EMDR is effective in treating both children and adults with PTSD, yet studies indicate that the eye movements are not needed to make it work.

Play Therapy

Play therapy can be used to treat young children with PTSD who are not able to deal with the trauma more directly. The therapist uses games, drawings, and other methods to help children process their traumatic memories.

Other Treatments

Special treatments may be needed for children who show out-of-place sexual behaviors, extreme behavior problems, or problems with drugs or alcohol.

Helping Kids Cope with Disaster

- Disasters can leave children feeling frightened, confused, and insecure. Whether a child has personally experienced trauma, has merely seen the event on television or has heard it discussed by adults, it is important for parents and teachers to be informed and ready to help if reactions to stress begin to occur.

- Children may respond to disaster by demonstrating fears, sadness or behavioral problems. Younger children may return to earlier behavior patterns, such as bedwetting, sleep problems and separation anxiety. Older children may also display anger, aggression, school problems or withdrawal. Some children who have only indirect contact with the disaster but witness it on television may develop distress.

Recognize Risk Factors

For many children, reactions to disasters are brief and represent normal reactions to "abnormal events." A smaller number of children can be at risk for more enduring psychological distress as a function of three major risk factors:

- Direct exposure to the disaster, such as being evacuated, observing injuries or death of others, or experiencing injury along with fearing one's life is in danger.

- Loss/grief: This relates to the death or serious injury of family or friends.

- On-going stress from the secondary effects of disaster, such as temporarily living elsewhere, loss of friends and social networks, loss of personal property, parental unemployment, and costs incurred during recovery to return the family to predisaster life and living conditions.

Vulnerabilities in Children

In most cases, depending on the risk factors above, distressing responses are temporary. In the absence of severe threat to life, injury, loss of loved ones, or secondary problems such as loss of home, moves, etc., symptoms usually diminish over time. For those that were directly exposed to the disaster, reminders of the disaster such as high winds, smoke, cloudy skies, sirens, or other reminders of the disaster may cause upsetting feelings to return. Having a prior history of some type of traumatic event or severe stress may contribute to these feelings.

Children's coping with disaster or emergencies is often tied to the way parents cope. They can detect adults' fears and sadness. Parents and adults can make disasters less traumatic for children by taking steps to manage their own feelings and plans for coping. Parents are almost always the best source of support for children in disasters. One way to establish a sense of control and to build confidence in children before a disaster is to engage and involve them in preparing a family disaster plan. After a disaster, children can contribute to a family recovery plan.

Meeting the Child's Emotional Needs

Children's reactions are influenced by the behavior, thoughts, and feelings of adults. Adults should encourage children and adolescents to share their thoughts and feelings about the incident. Clarify misunderstandings about risk and danger by listening to children's concerns and answering questions. Maintain a sense of calm by validating children's concerns and perceptions and with discussion of concrete plans for safety.

Listen to what the child is saying. If a young child is asking questions about the event, answer them simply without the elaboration needed for an older child or adult. Some children are comforted by knowing more or less information than others; decide what level of information your particular child needs. If a child has difficulty expressing feelings, allow the child to draw a picture or tell a story of what happened.

Try to understand what is causing anxieties and fears. Be aware that following a disaster, children are most afraid that:

- The event will happen again.
- Someone close to them will be killed or injured.
- They will be left alone or separated from the family.

Reassuring Children after a Disaster

Suggestions to help reassure children include the following:

- Personal contact is reassuring. Hug and touch your children.

111

- Calmly provide factual information about the recent disaster and current plans for insuring their safety along with recovery plans.

- Encourage your children to talk about their feelings.

- Spend extra time with your children such as at bedtime.

- Re-establish your daily routine for work, school, play, meals, and rest.

- Involve your children by giving them specific chores to help them feel they are helping to restore family and community life.

- Praise and recognize responsible behavior.

- Understand that your children will have a range of reactions to disasters.

- Encourage your children to help update your a family disaster plan.

If you have tried to create a reassuring environment by following the steps above, but your child continues to exhibit stress, if the reactions worsen over time, or if they cause interference with daily behavior at school, at home, or with other relationships, it may be appropriate to talk to a professional. You can get professional help from the child's primary care physician, a mental health provider specializing in children's needs, or a member of the clergy.

Monitor and Limit Exposure to the Media

News coverage related to a disaster may elicit fear and confusion and arouse anxiety in children. This is particularly true for large-scale disasters or a terrorist event where significant property damage and loss of life has occurred. Particularly for younger children, repeated images of an event may cause them to believe the event is recurring over and over.

If parents allow children to watch television or use the Internet where images or news about the disaster are shown, parents should be with them to encourage communication and provide explanations. This may also include parent's monitoring and appropriately limiting their own exposure to anxiety-provoking information.

Use Support Networks

Parents help their children when they take steps to understand and manage their own feelings and ways of coping. They can do this by building and using social support systems of family, friends, community organizations and agencies, faith-based institutions, or other resources that work for that family. Parents can build their own unique social support systems so that in an emergency situation or when a disaster strikes, they can be supported and helped to manage their reactions. As a result, parents will be more available to their children and better able to support them. Parents are almost always the best source of support for children in difficult times. But to support their children, parents need to attend to their own needs and have a plan for their own support.

Preparing for disaster helps everyone in the family accept the fact that disasters do happen, and provides an opportunity to identify and collect the resources needed to meet basic needs after disaster. Preparation helps; when people feel prepared, they cope better and so do children.

Section 11.3

Issues Related to Women

This section includes text excerpted from "PTSD:
National Center for PTSD—Women, Trauma, and PTSD,"
National Center for Posttraumatic Stress Disorder (NCPTSD),
U.S. Department of Veterans Affairs (VA), August 13, 2015.

Trauma is common in women; five out of ten women experience a traumatic event. Women tend to experience different traumas than men. While both men and women report the same symptoms of PTSD (hyperarousal, reexperiencing, avoidance, and numbing), some symptoms are more common for women or men.

Most early information on trauma and PTSD came from studies of male Veterans, mostly Vietnam Veterans. Researchers began to study the effects of sexual assault and found that women's reactions were similar to male combat Veterans. Women's experiences of trauma can also cause PTSD. This finding led to more research on women's exposure to trauma and PTSD.

113

Risk of Experiencing Trauma

Findings from a large national mental health study show that a little more than half of all women will experience at least one traumatic event in their life. Women are slightly less likely to experience trauma than men. The most common trauma for women is sexual assault or child sexual abuse. About one in three women will experience a sexual assault in their lifetime. Rates of sexual assault are higher for women than men. Women are also more likely to be neglected or abused in childhood, to experience domestic violence, or to have a loved one suddenly die.

What Happens after Trauma

After a trauma, some women may feel depressed, start drinking or using drugs, or develop PTSD. Women are more than twice as likely to develop PTSD than men (10% for women and 4% for men). There are a few reasons women might get PTSD more than men:

- Women are more likely to experience sexual assault.
- Sexual assault is more likely to cause PTSD than many other events.
- Women may be more likely to blame themselves for trauma experiences than men.

Why Are Some Women at Higher Risk for PTSD?

Not all women who experience a traumatic event develop PTSD. Women are more likely to develop PTSD if they:

- Have a past mental health problem (for example depression or anxiety)
- Experienced a very severe or life-threatening trauma
- Were sexually assaulted
- Were injured during the event
- Had a severe reaction at the time of the event
- Experienced other stressful events afterwards
- Do not have good social support

What PTSD Is Like for Women

Some PTSD symptoms are more common in women than men. Women are more likely to be jumpy, to have more trouble feeling emotions, and to avoid things that remind them of the trauma than men. Men are more likely to feel angry and to have trouble controlling their anger than women. Women with PTSD are more likely to feel depressed and anxious, while men with PTSD are more likely to have problems with alcohol or drugs. Both women and men who experience PTSD may develop physical health problems.

Treatment for PTSD

There are good treatments for PTSD. However, not everyone who experiences a trauma seeks treatment. Women may be more likely than men to seek help after a traumatic event. At least one study found that women respond to treatment as well as or better than men. This may be because women are generally more comfortable sharing feelings and talking about personal things with others than men.

Section 11.4

How Is Posttraumatic Stress Disorder Measured?

This section includes text excerpted from "PTSD: National Center for PTSD—How Is PTSD Measured?" National Center for Posttraumatic Stress Disorder (NCPTSD), U.S. Department of Veterans Affairs (VA), August 10, 2015.

To develop PTSD, a person must have gone through a trauma. Almost all people who go through trauma have some symptoms for a short time after the trauma. Yet most people do not get PTSD. A certain pattern of symptoms is involved in PTSD. There are four major types of symptoms: re-experiencing, avoidance, arousal, and negative changes in beliefs and feelings.

Deciding if someone has PTSD can involve several steps. The diagnosis of PTSD is most often made by a mental health provider. To diagnose PTSD, a mental health provider "measures," "assesses," or "evaluates" PTSD symptoms you may have had since the trauma.

What Is a PTSD Screen?

A person who went through trauma might be given a screen to see if he or she could have PTSD. A screen is a very short list of questions just to see if a person needs to be assessed further. The results of the screen do not show whether a person has PTSD. A screen can only show whether this person should be assessed further.

What Can I Expect from an Assessment for PTSD?

The length of a PTSD assessment can vary widely depending on the purpose as well as the training of the evaluator. While some evaluations may take as little as 15 minutes, a more thorough evaluation takes about one hour. Some PTSD assessments can take eight or more one-hour sessions. This is more likely when the information is needed for legal reasons or disability claims.

You can expect to be asked questions about events that may have been traumatic for you. You will be asked about symptoms you may have had since these events. Assessments that are more complete are likely to involve structured sets of questions. You may be asked to complete surveys that ask about your thoughts and feelings. Your spouse or partner may be asked to provide extra information. Although it is uncommon, you may also be asked to go through a test that looks at how your body reacts to mild reminders of your trauma.

No matter what your case involves, you should always be able to ask questions in advance. The evaluator should be able to tell you what the assessment will include, how long it will take, and how the results of the assessment will be used.

What Are Some of the Common Measures Used?

There are two main types of measures used in PTSD evaluations:

Structured Interviews

A structured interview is a standard set of questions that an interviewer asks. Some examples of structured interviews are:

- Clinician-Administered PTSD Scale (CAPS). Created by the National Center for PTSD staff, the CAPS is one of the most widely used PTSD interviews. The questions ask how often you have PTSD symptoms and how intense they are. The CAPS also asks about other symptoms that commonly occur with PTSD.

- Structured Clinical Interview for DSM (SCID). The SCID is another widely used interview. The SCID can be used to assess a range of mental health disorders including PTSD.

Other interviews include:

- Anxiety Disorders Interview Schedule-Revised (ADIS)

- PTSD-Interview

- Structured Interview for PTSD (SI-PTSD)

- PTSD Symptom Scale Interview (PSS-I)

Each has special features that might make it a good choice for a particular evaluation.

Self-Report Questionnaires

A self-report questionnaire is a set of questions, usually printed out, that you are given to answer. This kind of measure often takes less time and may be less costly than an interview. An example of a self-report measure is:

- PTSD Checklist (PCL). The PCL is another widely used measure developed by National Center for PTSD staff.

Other self-report measures are:

- Impact of Events Scale-Revised (IES-R)

- Keane PTSD Scale of the MMPI-2

- Mississippi Scale for Combat Related PTSD and the Mississippi Scale for Civilians

- Posttraumatic Diagnostic Scale (PDS)

- Penn Inventory for Posttraumatic Stress

- Los Angeles Symptom Checklist (LASC)

Section 11.5

Coping with Traumatic Stress Reactions

This section includes text excerpted from "PTSD: National
Center for PTSD—Coping with Traumatic Stress Reactions,"
National Center for Posttraumatic Stress Disorder (NCPTSD),
U.S. Department of Veterans Affairs (VA), August 14, 2015.

When trauma survivors take direct action to cope with their stress reactions, they put themselves in a position of power. Active coping with the trauma makes you begin to feel less helpless.

- Active coping means accepting the impact of trauma on your life and taking direct action to improve things.

- Active coping occurs even when there is no crisis. Active coping is a way of responding to everyday life. It is a habit that must be made stronger.

Know That Recovery Is a Process

Following exposure to a trauma most people experience stress reactions. Understand that recovering from the trauma is a process and takes time. Knowing this will help you feel more in control.

- Having an ongoing response to the trauma is normal.

- Recovery is an ongoing, daily process. It happens little by little. It is not a matter of being cured all of a sudden.

- Healing doesn't mean forgetting traumatic events. It doesn't mean you will have no pain or bad feelings when thinking about them.

- Healing may mean fewer symptoms and symptoms that bother you less.

- Healing means more confidence that you will be able to cope with your memories and symptoms. You will be better able to manage your feelings.

Positive Coping Actions

Certain actions can help to reduce your distressing symptoms and make things better. Plus, these actions can result in changes that last into the future. Here are some positive coping methods:

Learn about Trauma and PTSD

It is useful for trauma survivors to learn more about common reactions to trauma and about PTSD. Find out what is normal. Find out what the signs are that you may need assistance from others. When you learn that the symptoms of PTSD are common, you realize that you are not alone, weak, or crazy. It helps to know your problems are shared by hundreds of thousands of others. When you seek treatment and begin to understand your response to trauma, you will be better able to cope with the symptoms of PTSD.

Talk to Others for Support

When survivors talk about their problems with others, something helpful often results. It is important not to isolate yourself. Instead make efforts to be with others. Of course, you must choose your support people with care. You must also ask them clearly for what you need. With support from others, you may feel less alone and more understood. You may also get concrete help with a problem you have.

Practice Relaxation Methods

Try some different ways to relax, including:

- Muscle relaxation exercises
- Breathing exercises
- Meditation
- Swimming, stretching, yoga
- Prayer
- Listening to quiet music
- Spending time in nature

While relaxation techniques can be helpful, in a few people they can sometimes increase distress at first. This can happen when you focus attention on disturbing physical sensations and you reduce contact with the outside world. Most often, continuing with relaxation in small amounts that you can handle will help reduce negative reactions. You may want to try mixing relaxation in with music, walking, or other activities.

Distract Yourself with Positive Activities

Pleasant recreational or work activities help distract a person from his or her memories and reactions. For example, art has been a way for many trauma survivors to express their feelings in a positive, creative way. Pleasant activities can improve your mood, limit the harm caused by PTSD, and help you rebuild your life.

Talking to Your Doctor or a Counselor about Trauma and PTSD

Part of taking care of yourself means using the helping resources around you. If efforts at coping don't seem to work, you may become fearful or depressed. If your PTSD symptoms don't begin to go away or get worse over time, it is important to reach out and call a counselor who can help turn things around. Your family doctor can also refer you to a specialist who can treat PTSD. Talk to your doctor about your trauma and your PTSD symptoms. That way, he or she can take care of your health better.

Many with PTSD have found treatment with medicines to be helpful for some symptoms. By taking medicines, some survivors of trauma are able to improve their sleep, anxiety, irritability, and anger. It can also reduce urges to drink or use drugs.

Coping with the Symptoms of PTSD

Here are some direct ways to cope with these specific PTSD symptoms:

Unwanted Distressing Memories, Images, or Thoughts

- Remind yourself that they are just that, memories.
- Remind yourself that it's natural to have some memories of the trauma(s).
- Talk about them to someone you trust.
- Remember that, although reminders of trauma can feel over-whelming, they often lessen with time.

Sudden Feelings of Anxiety or Panic

Traumatic stress reactions often include feeling your heart pounding and feeling lightheaded or spacey. This is usually caused by rapid breathing. If this happens, remember that:

These reactions are not dangerous. If you had them while exercising, they most likely would not worry you.

- These feelings often come with scary thoughts that are not true. For example, you may think, "I'm going to die," "I'm having a heart attack," or "I will lose control." It is the scary thoughts that make these reactions so upsetting.

- Slowing down your breathing may help.

- The sensations will pass soon and then you can go on with what you were doing.

Each time you respond in these positive ways to your anxiety or panic, you will be working toward making it happen less often. Practice will make it easier to cope.

Feeling Like the Trauma Is Happening Again (Flashbacks)

- Keep your eyes open. Look around you and notice where you are.

- Talk to yourself. Remind yourself where you are, what year you're in, and that you are safe. The trauma happened in the past, and you are in the present.

- Get up and move around. Have a drink of water and wash your hands.

- Call someone you trust and tell them what is happening.

- Remind yourself that this is a common response after trauma.

- Tell your counselor or doctor about the flashback(s).

Dreams and Nightmares Related to the Trauma

- If you wake up from a nightmare in a panic, remind yourself that you are reacting to a dream. Having the dream is why you are in a panic, not because there is real danger now.

- You may want to get up out of bed, regroup, and orient yourself to the here and now.

- Engage in a pleasant, calming activity. For example, listen to some soothing music.

- Talk to someone if possible.

- Talk to your doctor about your nightmares. Certain medicines can be helpful.

Difficulty Falling or Staying Asleep

- Keep to a regular bedtime schedule.

- Avoid heavy exercise for the few hours just before going to bed.

- Avoid using your sleeping area for anything other than sleeping or sex.

- Avoid alcohol, tobacco, and caffeine. These harm your ability to sleep.

- Do not lie in bed thinking or worrying. Get up and enjoy something soothing or pleasant. Read a calming book, drink a glass of warm milk or herbal tea, or do a quiet hobby.

Irritability, Anger, and Rage

- Take a time out to cool off or think things over. Walk away from the situation.

- Get in the habit of exercise daily. Exercise reduces body tension and relieves stress.

- Remember that staying angry doesn't work. It actually increases your stress and can cause health problems.

- Talk to your counselor or doctor about your anger. Take classes in how to manage anger.

- If you blow up at family members or friends, find time as soon as you can to talk to them about it. Let them know how you feel and what you are doing to cope with your reactions.

Difficulty Concentrating or Staying Focused

- Slow down. Give yourself time to focus on what it is you need to learn or do.

- Write things down. Making "to do" lists may be helpful.

- Break tasks down into small do-able chunks.

- Plan a realistic number of events or tasks for each day.

- You may be depressed. Many people who are depressed have trouble concentrating. Again, this is something you can discuss with your counselor, doctor, or someone close to you.

Trouble Feeling or Expressing Positive Emotions

- Remember that this is a common reaction to trauma. You are not doing this on purpose. You should not feel guilty for something you do not want to happen and cannot control.

- Make sure to keep taking part in activities that you enjoy or used to enjoy. Even if you don't think you will enjoy something, once you get into it, you may well start having feelings of pleasure.

- Take steps to let your loved ones know that you care. You can express your caring in little ways: write a card, leave a small gift, or phone someone and say hello.

Chapter 12

Selective Mutism

What Is Selective Mutism?

Selective mutism (SM) is a social anxiety disorder that is most often seen in children. Individuals with SM are unable to speak in certain social settings and with certain people. A child with SM may speak normally with parents and a few others but have difficulty speaking, or speaking above a whisper, in specific settings, such as school, public places, or family gatherings. The condition is quite rare, with fewer than 1 percent of cases documented in school, clinical, and child-guidance casework.

Children with SM typically fail to talk in school, which can interfere with academic and social performance. They sometimes communicate nonverbally by nodding, pointing, or writing, but some children remain motionless and expressionless until others correctly guess what they need. SM can cause considerable distress in certain instances, such as when the child does not communicate in times of pain or when needing to use the bathroom.

Children with SM possess the desire to speak but hold back because of anxiety, embarrassment, and shyness. It is important to understand that the child does not willfully refuse to speak but rather is unable to do so in particular situations. As a result, they often fail to participate in age-appropriate activities in and outside of school. SM is not to be confused with such behavior as shyness during the first few weeks of school or reticence to speak when a child is adapting to a new language.

"Selective Mutism," © 2018 Omnigraphics. Reviewed September 2017.

What Are the Signs and Symptoms of Selective Mutism?

The diagnostic criteria laid down in the *Diagnostic and Statistical Manual of Mental Disorders,* 5th Edition (DSM-5) include:

- Consistent failure to talk in social situations in which the child is expected to speak—in school, for example—despite speaking in other situations.

- The inability to talk interferes with educational and occupational achievements or social interaction.

- The problem lasts for at least one month in duration but is not limited to the first month in school.

- The failure to speak in social situations cannot be attributed to lack of knowledge or comfort with using language.

- The condition cannot be explained by communication disorders or mental-health issues, such as autism or schizophrenia.

Children with SM may also display symptoms related to social anxiety and social phobia, such as:

- being overly attached to parents
- hiding, running away, freezing, and crying
- being traumatized when asked to respond verbally in public
- becoming anxious when a picture or video is taken
- avoiding eating in public
- being anxious about using public restrooms

Children with SM avoid conversations in many situations, and if they are able to express themselves, frequently do so by gesturing, nodding, and pointing. They often fear being ignored, ridiculed, or harshly evaluated if they try to speak.

What Are the Causes and Risk Factors of Selective Mutism?

The causes of SM are not yet definitively known, but multiple factors may play a role. For example, some research studies point to genetic influence as a possible cause for a predisposition to the condition. In many cases, it has been found that parents or other family members currently or previously have had symptoms related to extreme shyness, panic attacks, and social anxiety.

Some of the risk factors associated with SM include extreme shyness, a family history of the condition, or an anxiety disorder, such as panic disorder, or obsessive-compulsive behavior. In addition, research has shown that SM is four times more common in immigrant children than in the general population.

How Is Selective Mutism Diagnosed?

Diagnosis of SM is based on the crucial observation that the child can comprehend language and speak normally but consistently fails to do so in specific settings. For instance, the child typically displays appropriate verbal skills at home with parents and certain other individuals with whom they are comfortable. In order to arrive at a diagnosis, a doctor or mental-health professional will rely on reports from parents and other adults who are in contact with the child to determine patterns across a variety of situations. Sometimes the diagnostician may ask for videos of the child in places where he or she is able to speak normally.

Specifically, the diagnosis is based on the child having the ability to speak in some settings and not in others, and in particular it must not relate to such temporary situations as the first month of school. For the diagnosis to be confirmed, the inability to speak must interfere with schooling and other social activities that most children are otherwise able to negotiate easily.

How Is Selective Mutism Treated?

Early intervention is crucial for the successful treatment of SM. The most effective treatment has been shown to be behavioral therapy using controlled exposure. The therapist works with the child and parents and systematically approaches the settings in which the child cannot speak. The therapist gradually builds the child's confidence, one situation at a time, during which he or she is never pressured to speak. Instead, the child is encouraged with positive reinforcement. The therapist provides the parents with specialized techniques to apply in real-life settings. The predictability and control that therapy gives the child helps reduce anxiety and improves self-image as a result of the mastery of speaking skills in various settings.

Medication may be prescribed, but this is not required in all cases of SM. However, if conditions are severe, a physician may prescribe antianxiety medications. In addition, a history of similar disorders in the family and lack of response to behavioral therapy and other forms of psychotherapy may prompt the need for pharmacological intervention. In many cases, when medication has been prescribed, children are better able to deal with exposure tasks in behavior therapy, which can help lead to successful treatment. The classes of medications prescribed for SM include selective serotonin reuptake inhibitors (SSRIs) and other antidepressants. Some children respond well to SSRIs in the case of anxiety, but they need to be monitored carefully for side effects.

What Are Other Concerns Related to SM?

At one time, a common theory held that SM was often closely related to child abuse, but according to the Selective Mutism Foundation, research has since discarded this line of thinking. The suggestion of child abuse is devastating to families, and it has deterred many parents from seeking appropriate help for their child's SM. Child abuse can cause similar symptoms in children, but it may not be specific to immediate family members and could be due to other adults or even children. It is best to contact appropriate agencies in suspected cases of child abuse.

SM is sometimes mistaken for autism, since many children with this disorder also experience speech and language problems. The crucial difference is that children with SM have the ability to speak and function normally in some settings.

SM is not necessarily limited to children. Most children who experience SM at a young age do so for a short period, but others may find that it continues over many years. If misdiagnosed or improperly treated, SM could persist into adulthood. Studies have shown that some adults report struggling with the symptoms of SM and having to deal with residual symptoms, such as shyness, social anxiety, depression, and panic attacks for many years.

Parents can help children with SM by providing them with opportunities to socialize and speak in low-stress settings. They can implement behavioral techniques in all social situations in which the child finds it difficult to speak. To do this properly, parents should enlist the assistance of school authorities, teachers, school psychologists, guidance counsellors, and social workers to implement a consistent treatment plan.

References

1. "Selective Mutism (SM) Basics," Child Mind Institute, n.d.

2. "Understanding Selective Mutism Brochure. A Silent Cry for Help!" Selective Mutism Foundation, n.d.

3. "Selective Mutism," The American Speech-Language-Hearing Association (ASHA), n.d.

Chapter 13

Separation Anxiety Disorder

What Is Separation Anxiety Disorder (SAD)?

Individuals with separation anxiety disorder (SAD) worry excessively when they anticipate or experience separation from parents or loved ones. Children with SAD experience extreme distress when they are away from parents or caregivers and fear they could get lost from their family or think something bad is happening to their family while they are apart. Separation anxiety is normal in early childhood, but it becomes a disorder when anxiety interferes with age-appropriate activities and behavior. SAD is most often diagnosed in children during preschool and the early school years, but in rare cases, it can become a problem in early adolescence. It is estimated that about 4 percent of all children have this disorder, which can be treated with behavioral and pharmacological therapy if identified early.

What Are the Characteristics of SAD?

Symptoms exhibited with SAD tend to vary with each individual, but some common characteristics include:

- Overattachment to parents or loved ones and a perception of danger to family during separation.

"Separation Anxiety Disorder," © 2018 Omnigraphics. Reviewed September 2017.

- Worry and stress before or during separation from parents or loved ones.

- Complaints of headache, nausea, dizziness, or other physical symptoms when separation is anticipated.

- Having a hard time saying goodbye to parents, throwing tantrums when faced with separation, feeling afraid of staying alone in one part of a house, or fear of sleeping in a darkened room.

- Being afraid of staying home in the absence of parents or loved ones.

- Worrisome thoughts of harm to parents or loved ones (e.g., accident, illness, or death).

- Persistent thoughts of the dangers of being separated from loved ones, such as being kidnapped or getting lost.

- An overwhelming need to know where parents are when apart, often phoning or texting.

- Difficulty falling asleep away from home.

- Nightmares with themes of separation from parents or loved ones.

- Avoiding playtime, birthday parties, and other activities away from loved ones.

- Obsessively shadowing a parent at home or elsewhere.

- Refusal to leave home or go to school.

What Causes SAD?

Biological and environmental factors could all contribute to SAD. Other causes can include chemical imbalances, possibly of such substances as norepinephrine and serotonin in the brain. There could be a biological tendency to feel anxious, but the disorder could also be the result of behavior learned from family members who display elevated anxiety levels around the child. It's also possible that SAD could result from a traumatic childhood experience.

Who Is Affected by SAD?

A certain degree of separation anxiety is normal in children, and dealing with it is a natural part of growing up. SAD is identified when anxiety about being apart from home and family is far beyond that of typical child development. It occurs equally in both sexes, and symptoms usually surface in children following a break from school, such as after Christmas vacation or a period of extended illness. Children of parents with this disorder have a higher than average likelihood of developing the same condition.

How Is SAD Diagnosed?

A child psychiatrist or other mental-health professional diagnoses SAD on the basis of a psychological evaluation. Diagnosis involves identifying and quantifying the distress experienced by the individual during separation from parents or loved ones. Among other factors, the child must experience the symptoms for at least four weeks to meet the technical criteria for SAD. A clinician will be able to determine if the symptoms are otherwise only a temporary response to a stressful life situation.

What Is the Treatment for SAD?

The diagnostician will evaluate the condition of the child and decide on treatment based on the severity of symptoms, age of the child, health and medical history, tolerance for medication and therapy, and personal preference for mode of treatment. The first line of treatment in SAD is psychotherapy. Cognitive behavioral therapy (CBT), in particular, has been very successful in mild to moderate cases.

The focus of treatment is to provide the child with the skills to manage anxiety and master the situations that contribute to the symptoms of SAD. Exposure therapy, a modified version of CBT is recommended in certain cases. Here, the child is exposed to separation in small, controlled doses, which helps reduce anxiety gradually over time. In severe cases that do not respond to psychotherapy, medication may be required. In such cases, selective serotonin reuptake inhibitors (SSRIs), antidepressants, and antianxiety medications are often prescribed to make the child feel calmer.

How Is SAD Prevented?

Preventive measures are presently unknown. Instead of prevention, the focus is on early detection and intervention, which can successfully reduce the severity of the disorder and enhance normal growth and development patterns, while improving the quality of life for affected children.

References

1. "Separation Anxiety Disorder," Jane and Terry Semel Institute for Neuroscience and Human Behavior, n.d.

2. "Separation Anxiety Disorder," Stanford Children's Health, n.d.

3. "Separation Anxiety Disorder," Child Mind Institute, n.d.

Chapter 14

Social Anxiety Disorder

Chapter Contents

Section 14.1

What Is Social Anxiety Disorder?

This section includes text excerpted from "Social Anxiety Disorder: More Than Just Shyness," National Institute of Mental Health (NIMH), November 2016.

Are you extremely afraid of being judged by others?

Are you very self-conscious in everyday social situations?

Do you avoid meeting new people?

If you have been feeling this way for at least six months and these feelings make it hard for you to do everyday tasks—such as talking to people at work or school—you may have a social anxiety disorder.

Social anxiety disorder (also called social phobia) is a mental health condition. It is an intense, persistent fear of being watched and judged by others. This fear can affect work, school, and your other day-to-day activities. It can even make it hard to make and keep friends. But social anxiety disorder doesn't have to stop you from reaching your potential. Treatment can help you overcome your symptoms.

Social anxiety disorder is a common type of anxiety disorder. A person with social anxiety disorder feels symptoms of anxiety or fear in certain or all social situations, such as meeting new people, dating, being on a job interview, answering a question in class, or having to talk to a cashier in a store. Doing everyday things in front of people—such as eating or drinking in front of others or using a public restroom—also causes anxiety or fear. The person is afraid that he or she will be humiliated, judged, and rejected.

The fear that people with social anxiety disorder have in social situations is so strong that they feel it is beyond their ability to control. As a result, it gets in the way of going to work, attending school, or doing everyday things. People with social anxiety disorder may worry about these and other things for weeks before they happen. Sometimes, they end up staying away from places or events where they think they might have to do something that will embarrass them.

Some people with the disorder do not have anxiety in social situations but have performance anxiety instead. They feel physical symptoms of anxiety in situations such as giving a speech, playing a sports game, or dancing or playing a musical instrument on stage.

Social anxiety disorder usually starts during youth in people who are extremely shy. Social anxiety disorder is not uncommon; research suggests that about 7 percent of Americans are affected. Without treatment, social anxiety disorder can last for many years or a lifetime and prevent a person from reaching his or her full potential.

What Are the Signs and Symptoms of Social Anxiety Disorder?

When having to perform in front of or be around others, people with social anxiety disorder tend to:

- Blush, sweat, tremble, feel a rapid heart rate, or feel their "mind going blank"
- Feel nauseous or sick to their stomach
- Show a rigid body posture, make little eye contact, or speak with an overly soft voice
- Find it scary and difficult to be with other people, especially those they don't already know, and have a hard time talking to them even though they wish they could
- Be very self-conscious in front of other people and feel embarrassed and awkward
- Be very afraid that other people will judge them
- Stay away from places where there are other people

What Causes Social Anxiety Disorder?

Social anxiety disorder sometimes runs in families, but no one knows for sure why some family members have it while others don't. Researchers have found that several parts of the brain are involved in fear and anxiety. Some researchers think that misreading of others' behavior may play a role in causing or worsening social anxiety. For example, you may think that people are staring or frowning at you when they truly are not. Underdeveloped social skills are another possible contributor to social anxiety. For example, if you have underdeveloped social skills, you may feel discouraged after talking with people and may worry about doing it in the future. By learning more about fear and anxiety in the brain, scientists may be able to create better treatments. Researchers are also looking for ways in which stress and environmental factors may play a role.

How Is Social Anxiety Disorder Treated?

First, talk to your doctor or healthcare professional about your symptoms. Your doctor should do an exam and ask you about your health history to make sure that an unrelated physical problem is not causing your symptoms. Your doctor may refer you to a mental health specialist, such as a psychiatrist, psychologist, clinical social worker, or counselor. The first step to effective treatment is to have a diagnosis made, usually by a mental health specialist.

Social anxiety disorder is generally treated with psychotherapy (sometimes called "talk" therapy), medication, or both. Speak with your doctor or healthcare provider about the best treatment for you. If your healthcare provider cannot provide a referral, visit the National Institute of Mental Health (NIMH) Help for Mental Illnesses webpage at www.nimh.nih.gov/findhelp for resources you may find helpful.

Psychotherapy

A type of psychotherapy called cognitive behavioral therapy (CBT) is especially useful for treating social anxiety disorder. CBT teaches you different ways of thinking, behaving, and reacting to situations that help you feel less anxious and fearful. It can also help you learn and practice social skills. CBT delivered in a group format can be especially helpful.

Support Groups

Many people with social anxiety also find support groups helpful. In a group of people who all have social anxiety disorder, you can receive unbiased, honest feedback about how others in the group see you. This way, you can learn that your thoughts about judgment and rejection are not true or are distorted. You can also learn how others with social anxiety disorder approach and overcome the fear of social situations.

Medication

There are three types of medications used to help treat social anxiety disorder:

- Antianxiety medications

- Antidepressants

- Beta blockers

Antianxiety medications are powerful and begin working right away to reduce anxious feelings; however, these medications are usually not taken for long periods of time. People can build up a tolerance if they are taken over a long period of time and may need higher and higher doses to get the same effect. Some people may even become dependent on them. To avoid these problems, doctors usually prescribe antianxiety medications for short periods, a practice that is especially helpful for older adults.

Antidepressants are mainly used to treat depression, but are also helpful for the symptoms of social anxiety disorder. In contrast to antianxiety medications, they may take several weeks to start working. Antidepressants may also cause side effects, such as headaches, nausea, or difficulty sleeping. These side effects are usually not severe for most people, especially if the dose starts off low and is increased slowly over time. Talk to your doctor about any side effects that you have.

Beta blockers are medicines that can help block some of the physical symptoms of anxiety on the body, such as an increased heart rate, sweating, or tremors. Beta blockers are commonly the medications of choice for the "performance anxiety" type of social anxiety.

Your doctor will work with you to find the best medication, dose, and duration of treatment. Many people with social anxiety disorder obtain the best results with a combination of medication and CBT or other psychotherapies.

Don't give up on treatment too quickly. Both psychotherapy and medication can take some time to work. A healthy lifestyle can also help combat anxiety. Make sure to get enough sleep and exercise, eat a healthy diet, and turn to family and friends who you trust for support.

Finding Help

Mental Health Treatment Program Locator

The Substance Abuse and Mental Health Services Administration (SAMHSA) provides this online resource for locating mental health treatment facilities and programs. The Mental Health Treatment Locator section of the Behavioral Health Treatment Services Locator lists facilities providing mental health services to persons with mental illness.

Find a facility in your state at www.findtreatment.samhsa.gov/.

For additional resources, visit www.nimh.nih.gov/findhelp.

Section 14.2

Brain Imaging Predicts Psychotherapy Success in Patients with Social Anxiety Disorder

This section includes text excerpted from "Brain
Imaging Predicts Psychotherapy Success in Patients with Social
Anxiety Disorder," National Institute of Mental Health (NIMH),
February 1, 2013. Reviewed September 2017.

Treatment for social anxiety disorder or social phobia has entered the personalized medicine arena—brain imaging can provide neuro-markers to predict whether traditional options such as cognitive behavioral therapy will work for a particular patient, reported a National Institute of Mental Health (NIMH)-funded study that was published in a *JAMA Psychiatry*.

The Study

Social anxiety disorder (SAD)—the fear of being judged by others and humiliated—is the third most prevalent psychiatric disorder in Americans, after depression and alcohol dependence, according to the National Comorbidity Survey, a U.S. poll on mental health. This fear can be so strong that it interferes with daily life activities like going to work or school. If left untreated, some sufferers use alcohol, food, or drugs to reduce the fear at social events, which often leads to other disorders such as alcoholism, eating disorders, and depression. The NIMH claims that 6.8 percent of U.S. adults and 5.5 percent of 13- to 15-year-olds, the age of onset for this chronic disorder, are annually afflicted.

Although psychotherapy and drugs, such as antidepressants and benzodiazepines, exist as treatments for SAD, current behavioral measures poorly predict which would work better for individual patients. "Half of social anxiety disorder patients have satisfactory response to treatment. There is little evidence about which patient would benefit from a particular form of treatment," said John D. Gabrieli, Ph.D., lead author of the study. "There is no rational basis for prescribing one treatment over the other. Which treatment a patient gets depends on whom they see."

Enter personalized medicine, the use of genetic or other biological markers to tailor treatments to those who would actually benefit from them, thus sparing the expense and side effects for those who would not. Brain imaging could identify neuromarkers or targeted areas of the brain that could one day optimize treatment for individual patients. Neuromarkers are being used in other areas of mental illness, for instance, to predict the onset of psychosis in schizophrenia and the likelihood of relapse in drug addiction.

In this study, Gabrieli, at the Massachusetts Institute of Technology (MIT) in Cambridge, and his colleagues, used functional magnetic resonance imaging (fMRI) in 39 SAD patients before a 12-week course of cognitive behavioral therapy (CBT). The patients viewed angry versus neutral faces and scenes while undergoing fMRI examination. Compared to neutral faces, angry faces convey disapproval and are likely to prompt excessive fear responses and negative connotations in SAD patients; CBT teaches these patients ways to downregulate their responses. The patients' brain images were then compared to their scores on a conventional clinical measure, the Liebowitz Social Anxiety Scale (LSAS), a questionnaire which they took before and after therapy completion.

Results of the Study

SAD patients responded more to the images of faces and not scenes, which is characteristic for the social basis of this disorder. Patients whose brains reacted strongly to the facial images before treatment benefitted more from the therapy than those who reacted to these the least. Specifically, changes in two occipitotemporal brain regions—areas involved in early processing of visual cues such as faces—correlated with positive cognitive behavioral therapy outcome. These neuromarkers predicted treatment outcome better than the currently used LSAS.

Significance

This study is the first of its kind to use neuroimaging to predict treatment response in SAD patients. Neuromarkers may become a practical clinical tool to guide the selection of optimal treatments for individual patients. Integration of neuromarkers with genetic, behavioral, and other biomarkers is likely to further refine the prediction.

What's Next

A larger study comparing people with SAD with normal participants is needed to verify the results. fMRI studies using other facial expressions (disgust or fear) might be better predictors. Studies that look at other treatment options, such as drugs, are also needed to confirm which treatment is optimal.

Chapter 15

Somatic Symptom Disorder

What Is Somatic Symptom Disorder?

Somatic symptom disorder (formerly known as hypochondria) is a condition in which an individual worries to an intense degree about having a physical illness that cannot be verified medically. The person becomes obsessed with the idea that physical symptoms, such as pain, shortness of breath, or weakness, are due to serious disease, causing major distress to the point of disrupting daily life. The symptoms are not usually faked. They may or may not be related to a serious illness, but they do exist, and the individual truly believes he or she is sick. Somatic symptom disorder can occur at any age but is usually seen in early adulthood, affecting men and women equally. The disorder causes significant emotional and physical suffering, but its symptoms can be eased and the quality of life improved with proper treatment.

What Are the Symptoms of Somatic Symptom Disorder?

Symptoms can vary considerably but typically may include:

- pain
- fatigue

"Somatic Symptom Disorder," © 2018 Omnigraphics. Reviewed September 2017.

- weakness
- shortness of breath
- difficulty swallowing
- nausea
- dizziness
- paralysis
- vision problems
- amnesia

The thoughts, feelings, and behaviors related to somatic symptom disorder can include one or more of the following:

- Significant worry that a potential illness exists.
- Thoughts that physical symptoms are a sign of severe illness.
- Frequently checking the body for symptoms.
- Feeling that physical activity could worsen the condition.
- Frequent healthcare visits that do not improve the condition.
- Belief that doctors are failing to make an accurate diagnosis.
- Consulting many doctors or "shopping around" for a doctor who agrees that the person has a serious illness.
- Severe emotional and/or physical impairment unrelated to a medical condition.
- Anxiety, nervousness, or depression that negatively affect everyday life.

What Are the Risk Factors for Somatic Symptom Disorder?

The following are some risk factors that are often associated with somatic symptom disorder.

- An existing medical condition or ongoing recovery from one.
- Family history of disease or otherwise susceptible to a disease.
- Genetic and biological factors that cause increased sensitivity to pain.

- Anxiety or depression.

- Recent stressful life events, such as violence, or trauma.

- History of childhood sexual abuse or other trauma.

- Low socio-economic status or education.

- Learned behavior, such as receiving attention or other benefits from having an illness.

- Problems in processing emotions, which causes pain to become the focus rather than the emotional problems.

How Is Somatic Symptom Disorder Diagnosed?

It is difficult to diagnose somatic symptom disorder, in part because patients are convinced about the cause of their symptoms. Depending on the patient's symptoms, a healthcare professional will order tests and conduct a complete physical examination to rule out illness. In the absence of any detectable medical condition, the patient will likely be referred to a psychiatrist or other mental-health professional. The psychologist or psychiatrist will assess the person's attitude and behavior and will likely administer a personality assessment. The diagnosis of somatic symptom disorder is made on the basis of detailed criteria present in the *Diagnostic and Statistical Manual of Mental Disorders* (DSM-5), published by the American Psychiatric Association (APA).

How Is Somatic Symptom Disorder Treated?

Somatic symptom disorder is treated with psychotherapy, usually cognitive behavioral therapy, as well as with psychiatric medications.

Psychotherapy

The goal of psychotherapy is to help the patient live a productive life, even if the condition persists. It attempts to alter the thinking and behavior that lead to the symptoms. Treatment could be difficult because the patient firmly believes that symptoms are due to a physical illness and not the result of emotional or mental disturbances. Cognitive behavioral therapy (CBT) helps patients reduce their preoccupation with symptoms and helps them cope with the ongoing condition. With stress-reduction techniques, patients are often able to improve their daily functioning at home, work, and in family life.

Medications

Psychiatric medications can help improve the condition of patients by reducing the symptoms associated with depression, anxiety, and pain. It may take several weeks for the medications to have the desired effect, and certain medicines may not be suitable in specific cases. The doctor may switch medications or alter combinations of drugs to improve their effectiveness.

How Can Somatic Symptom Disorder Be Prevented?

Although not much information is available on the prevention of somatic symptom disorder, the following recommendations may be helpful:

- Seek professional help if you have anxiety or depression.

- Understand how stress affects the body, and learn to de-stress yourself by using stress-reduction techniques.

- If you think you might have somatic symptom disorder, seek medical help as early as possible to avoid worsening of symptoms and to ensure early recovery.

- Stick to the treatment plan.

References

1. "Somatic Symptom Disorder," American Psychiatric Association (APA), 2017.

2. "Somatic Symptom Disorder," Mayo Foundation for Medical Education and Research (MFMER), May 21, 2015.

3. Goldberg, Joseph, MD. "Somatic Symptom Disorder," WebMD, February 9, 2017.

Chapter 16

Specific Phobia

What Is Specific Phobia?

A specific phobia is an intense, irrational fear of something that poses little or no actual danger. Some of the more common specific phobias are centered around closed-in places, heights, escalators, tunnels, highway driving, water, flying, dogs, and injuries involving blood. Such phobias aren't just extreme fear; they are irrational fear of a particular thing. You may be able to ski the world's tallest mountains with ease but be unable to go above the 5th floor of an office building. While adults with phobias realize that these fears are irrational, they often find that facing, or even thinking about facing, the feared object or situation brings on a panic attack or severe anxiety.

Prevalence of Specific Phobia

Specific phobias affect an estimated 19.2 million adult Americans and are twice as common in women as men. They usually appear in childhood or adolescence and tend to persist into adulthood. The causes

---

This chapter contains text excerpted from the following sources: Text beginning with the heading "What Is Specific Phobia?" is excerpted from "Anxiety Disorders—Specific Phobias," National Institute of Mental Health (NIMH), July 31, 2013. Reviewed September 2017; Text beginning with the heading "Some Common Specific Phobias" is excerpted from "Mental Health—Specific Phobias," Office on Women's Health (OWH), U.S. Department of Health and Human Services (HHS), March 29, 2010. Reviewed September 2017.

of specific phobias are not well understood, but there is some evidence that the tendency to develop them may run in families.

If the feared situation or feared object is easy to avoid, people with specific phobias may not seek help; but if avoidance interferes with their careers or their personal lives, it can become disabling and treatment is usually pursued.

Specific phobias respond very well to carefully targeted psychotherapy.

Some Common Specific Phobias

Some of the more common specific phobias are:

- Closed-in places

- Heights

- Escalators

- Tunnels

- Highway driving

- Water

- Flying

- Dogs

- Injuries involving blood

Such phobias aren't just extreme fear; they are irrational fear of a particular thing. You may be able to ski the world's tallest mountains with ease but be unable to go above the fifth floor of an office building. While adults with phobias realize that these fears are irrational, they often find that facing, or even thinking about facing, the feared object or situation brings on a panic attack or severe anxiety.

Treatment

If you think you have an anxiety disorder such as specific phobia, the first person you should see is your family doctor. A physician can determine whether the symptoms that alarm you are due to an anxiety disorder, another medical condition, or both.

Specific phobias respond very well to carefully targeted psychotherapy.

Chapter 17

Test Anxiety

What Is Test Anxiety?

Test anxiety occurs when a person is excessively apprehensive about taking a test. The condition causes distress that can negatively affect performance on the exam, sometimes making the individual forget what he or she previously learned. Someone with test anxiety might lose concentration, become tense, and completely lose focus.

It is normal to be apprehensive before a test, and being nervous can actually have some benefits. For example, a small degree of stress can help you get started on a task and keep you going until you complete it. And it can help you focus better and complete the task properly. But when facing a test, some people become overly nervous to the point where performance suffers, and they experience symptoms that make it difficult to concentrate. When teens have test anxiety their mental faculties may become clouded, and studies show that all kinds of students, regardless of age or ability, can be prone to this condition. Preparation might be affected by insufficient study, lack of time, difficult material, physical exhaustion, or lack of sleep the night before the test. The feeling that you have not prepared properly and will not perform well can result in the symptoms of test anxiety.

Test anxiety is a kind of performance anxiety. This is something that people often experience when they need to go on stage or do something in front of others. In such situations, there is pressure to

"Test Anxiety," © 2018 Omnigraphics. Reviewed September 2017.

do well, which creates a high level of anxiety. This is commonly seen when someone has to perform in a play, give a speech, appear for a job interview, or play in front of a crowd.

Performing poorly on a test because of personal issues or crises at home should not be confused with test anxiety. Some of these issues, such as the death of a close relative, would naturally interfere with concentration in a test and would not be considered test anxiety.

What Are the Signs of Text Anxiety?

Test anxiety affects you mentally and physically. If you have the condition, you could completely forget what you learned and have difficulty concentrating. You can become overwhelmed with negative thoughts about how you are going to complete the test and what will happen if you fail. You might also dwell on how others are performing on the test, imaging them having much less trouble than you.

Physically, people with test anxiety may feel a fluttering known as "butterflies" in their stomach, and might also experience sweating and shaking. They might have a tension headache or feel like fainting or throwing up. Other symptoms associated with the condition include nausea, cramps, dry mouth, muscle tension, and increased breathing and heart rates. These symptoms can have an additional negative impact on test preparation and performance.

What Causes Test Anxiety?

Typically, anxiety occurs when you anticipate something stressful. This is the result of an evolutionary mechanism built into human beings known as the "fight-or-flight" response. The body prepares either to defend itself or flee from a potential threat by releasing a hormone known as adrenaline. Adrenaline causes the physical symptoms associated with test anxiety, such as shaking, sweating, muscle tension, heavy breathing, and a pounding heart. Negative thoughts, such as thinking that you will forget the answers or fail the test, adds to the anxiety and creates a vicious cycle that further worsens performance.

Who Can Suffer from Text Anxiety?

Anyone can be overcome with test anxiety, but perfectionists tend to be most prone to the condition. For them anything less than a perfect score is unacceptable, and they can be extremely fearful of making mistakes. They put pressure on themselves to perform better, which in turn creates a perfect environment for test anxiety. For many people, failing to prepare well enough can lead to test anxiety.

How Can You Cope with Test Anxiety?

Most students with test anxiety worry that they are not smart enough or sufficiently prepared to succeed. Such a mindset can be paralyzing when taking tests. Students must overcome these thoughts and view themselves as competent learners to overcome test anxiety.

Below are some strategies that can help teens deal with test anxiety more effectively.

1. Mental Preparation

Students can do several things to prepare themselves better, some of which are listed below.

- Develop good study habits. There's much more to learning than just attending classes. It is impossible to prepare for a test just by sitting in a classroom. It's equally important to develop good study habits and review schedules.

- Be thorough. Rather than just memorizing, concentrate on the major ideas, main events, and most important issues covered in the material. Avoid anxiety with a solid understanding of the subject matter.

- Review the material. Go over what you've learned by covering it throughout the week. This helps in committing the material to memory.

- Don't cram. It is not advisable to study hard just before the exam. You cannot digest an entire chapter or term in just one night. Plan your study routine in advance, and review accordingly to avoid last-minute tension.

- Know the test format clearly in advance. Doing this takes the initial shock you might experience when you see the test for the first time.

- Write out your own possible questions and answers before the test. This will help you master the topics and feel more prepared.

- Don't think negatively. Negative thoughts can disrupt your study schedule. Always think about positive outcomes.

- Don't expect perfection. You don't have to know everything about a topic or the answer to every possible question.

- Arrive early. Be at the test location well ahead of the test starting time, so you have time to relax with your friends. And don't discuss the test material. Last minute reviews can only serve to confuse you.

2. Planning

Having a strategy in place before you take the test can help reduce anxiety. Some helpful strategies include the following:

- When the test paper is handed out, it is normal to feel tense. Once you have the paper in hand, take a few seconds to calm down before you start.

- Plan your time so you can answer all the questions. Allow more time for the most difficult questions. And don't dwell on any one question. Move on to the next item, and can come back to it later.

- If you are surprised by a question, don't lose your cool. Try answering something easy, and then come back after you've calmed down and can give it more time.

- If you felt confident answering a question the first time around, don't second-guess yourself and change the answer. This fosters negativity and could just be a waste of time.

- If you don't know the answer to a question, just accept that. If you feel the questions shouldn't have been on the test, you can discuss it with your teacher later.

3. Physical Preparation

It is important to take care of your health and pay attention to how you behave prior to a test in order to avoid anxiety-related problems. For example:

- Eat well. Adequate nutrition is an important part of studying before tests. Feeling weak and cranky during study time can lead to frustration and anxiety.

- Make time for physical activity. Exercising regularly helps you maintain a positive attitude. Do not disrupt your exercise schedule during test preparation.

- Get plenty of sleep. Lack of sleep affects memory and concentration. Staying up late studying and then getting up early can be counterproductive at exactly the wrong time.

- Socialize with friends and family and take regular breaks. Social interaction minimizes anxiety and helps reenergize you for additional study. Blend with people with a positive attitude. In particular, avoid those who think negatively, especially about tests.

- Don't procrastinate. If you put off your study schedule, you might be setting yourself up for cramming. And it's possible that you could be waiting until the last minute so you have an excuse for not doing well.

4. Relaxation Techniques

A number of relaxation techniques can help relieve anxiety, improve memory and enhance test performance. Some suggestions:

- When you start to feel anxious, try deep breathing exercises. With your eyes closed, inhale slowly and deeply through your nose, and exhale very slowly through your mouth. Repeat until you feel yourself begin to feel less tense.

- Progressive muscle relaxation can help reduce stress. For example, contract your shoulders for ten seconds, then slowly loosen up and let your muscles relax. Repeat with hands, arms, legs, and feet. Concentrate on how the actions feel and try to become more relaxed with each repetition.

- Visualization exercises may help ease anxiety. Close your eyes and imagine yourself in a calm environment, such as a beach, a forest, or a spa. Combine this with a deep-breathing routine to increase the effect.

- If you regularly practice yoga, tai chi, or meditation, use these techniques to take a break from study. They can help you return to your work in a more relaxed frame of mind.

Being Successful

It takes time and practice to learn how to reduce test anxiety. A good attitude towards studying determines how well you perform on a test, so the best way to deal with test anxiety is to study well and be prepared in all respects. Since test anxiety thrives on the unknown, it is important to use good study techniques and learn the material thoroughly. When students feel confident of their knowledge and develop effective test-taking strategies, they can overcome test anxiety.

References

1. Ehmke, Rachel. "Tips for Beating Test Anxiety," Child Mind Institute, Inc., n.d.

2. Lyness, D'Arcy, PhD. "Test Anxiety," The Nemours Foundation, July, 2013.

3. "Reducing Test Anxiety," Educational Testing Service (ETS), n.d.

4. "Reducing Test Anxiety," Pittsburg State University, n.d.

Part Three

Causes, Risk Factors, and Treatment for Anxiety Disorders

Chapter 18

Anxiety: Signs and Symptoms

Excessive, Irrational Fear

Each anxiety disorder has different symptoms, but all the symptoms cluster around excessive, irrational fear and dread. Unlike the relatively mild, brief anxiety caused by a specific event (such as speaking in public or a first date), severe anxiety that lasts at least six months is generally considered to be problem that might benefit from evaluation and treatment.

Anxiety disorders commonly occur along with other mental or physical illnesses, including alcohol or substance abuse, which may mask anxiety symptoms or make them worse. In older adults, anxiety disorders often occur at the same time as depression, heart disease, diabetes, and other medical problems. In some cases, these other problems need to be treated before a person can respond well to treatment for anxiety.

Symptoms of Generalized Anxiety Disorder (GAD)

Generalized anxiety disorder (GAD) develops slowly. It often starts during the teen years or young adulthood. Symptoms may get

This chapter includes text excerpted from "Anxiety Disorders—Symptoms of Anxiety Disorders," NIHSeniorHealth, National Institute on Aging (NIA), January 2016.

157

better or worse at different times, and often are worse during times of stress.

People with GAD can't seem to get rid of their concerns, even though they usually realize that their anxiety is more intense than the situation warrants. They can't relax, startle easily, and have difficulty concentrating. Often, they have trouble falling asleep or staying asleep.

Physical symptoms that often accompany the anxiety include:

- fatigue
- headaches
- muscle tension
- muscle aches
- difficulty swallowing
- trembling
- twitching
- irritability
- sweating
- nausea
- lightheadedness
- having to go to the bathroom frequently
- feeling out of breath
- hot flashes

When their anxiety level is mild, people with GAD can function socially and hold down a job. Although they don't avoid certain situations as a result of their disorder, people with GAD can have difficulty carrying out the simplest daily activities if their anxiety is severe.

Symptoms of Social Phobia

In social phobia, a person fears being judged by others or of being embarrassed. This fear can get in the way of doing everyday things such as going to work, running errands or meeting with friends. People who have social phobia often know that they shouldn't be so afraid, but they can't control their fear.

People with social phobia tend to:

- be very anxious about being with other people and have a hard time talking to them, even though they wish they could

- be very self-conscious in front of other people and feel embarrassed

- be very afraid that other people will judge them

- worry for days or weeks before an event where other people will be

- stay away from places where there are other people

- have a hard time making friends and keeping friends

- blush, sweat, or tremble around other people

- feel nauseous or sick to their stomach when with other people

Symptoms of Panic Disorder

In panic disorder, a person has sudden, unexplained attacks of terror, and often feels his or her heart pounding. During a panic attack, a person feels a sense of unreality, a fear of impending doom, or a fear of losing control. Panic attacks can occur at any time.

People with panic disorder may have:

- sudden and repeated attacks of fear

- a feeling of being out of control during a panic attack

- an intense worry about when the next attack will happen

- a fear or avoidance of places where panic attacks have occurred in the past

- physical symptoms during an attack, such as a pounding or racing heart, sweating, breathing problems, weakness or dizziness, feeling hot or a cold chill, tingly or numb hands, chest pain, or stomach pain

Seeking Treatment

Anxiety disorders are treatable. If you think you have an anxiety disorder, talk to your doctor. If your doctor thinks you may have an anxiety disorder, the next step is usually seeing a mental health professional. It is advisable to seek help from professionals who have particular expertise in diagnosing and treating anxiety. Certain kinds of cognitive and behavioral therapy and certain medications have been found to be especially helpful for anxiety.

Chapter 19

Risk Factors of Anxiety Disorders

Anxiety disorders are mental disorders that can occur at any age. Everyone feels worried and fearful at times. People with anxiety disorders worry a lot and are fearful and nervous. These feelings cause distress and impair daily life. The person may avoid situations such as work, school, and social activities.

There are several types of anxiety disorders. This chapter focuses on generalized anxiety disorder, panic disorder, and social anxiety disorder.

Signs and Symptoms

Generalized Anxiety Disorder (GAD)

A person with generalized anxiety disorder (GAD) has excessive feelings, thoughts, emotions, and actions. He or she has anxiety or worrying most of the time for at least six months. The worry may be related to job performance, money, health, and other activities. Sometimes the worry shifts from one focus to another. An adult with GAD has several of the following symptoms; a child may have just one symptom:

- Restlessness, or feeling wound up or on edge

This chapter includes text excerpted from "Anxiety Disorders," Substance Abuse and Mental Health Services Administration (SAMHSA), April 5, 2017.

- Being easily tired
- Trouble concentrating, or feeling that their "mind goes blank"
- Irritability
- Muscle tension, aching, or soreness
- Sleep problems, such as trouble falling asleep or staying asleep, restlessness at night, or unsatisfying sleep
- A person with GAD also may have a change in appetite and frequent sweating, nausea, or diarrhea

Panic Disorder

A person with panic disorder has unexpected or expected panic attacks. Panic attacks are sudden periods of intense fear, anxiety, or discomfort. The attack reaches a peak within minutes. It may cause an urge to escape or flee. During a panic attack, a person has several of the following symptoms:

- Pounding heart or fast heart rate
- Sweating
- Trembling or shaking
- Shortness of breath
- Feelings of choking
- Chest pain or discomfort
- Nausea or abdominal distress
- Dizziness or feeling lightheaded
- Chills or feeling overheated
- Numbness or tingling
- Feelings of unreality or being unconnected to oneself
- Fear of going crazy or losing control
- Fear of dying

After one or more panic attacks, he or she usually has one or both of:

- Worry that another panic attack might occur, and irrational fear that this will lead to loss of control of thoughts and feelings, a heart attack, or dying

- Trying to avoid panic attacks, such as by avoiding certain situations or places, or by stopping exercise or other activities.

Social Anxiety Disorder

Social anxiety disorder is sometimes called "social phobia." The person fears being embarrassed or negatively judged by others in a social setting. This worry often causes him or her to withdraw or avoid certain situations. This causes problems at work, at school, or in relationships.

A person with social anxiety disorder often has the following symptoms for more than six months:

- Being afraid of or worrying about social situations, such as meeting new people or eating in front of others

- Feeling very self-conscious in front of others and worrying about offending others or being humiliated, embarrassed, or rejected

- Avoiding social situations that cause fear and anxiety, feeling dread or doom leading up to a feared situation, or being very uncomfortable if able to stay in the situation

- Feeling fear or worry about a situation greater than the actual threat and beyond what most people would feel

- Having problems at work, school, or in relationships due to the symptoms

- Changing the daily routine in response to the symptoms

A person with social anxiety disorder sometimes feels nauseous. They may blush, tremble, sweat, or say their mind "goes blank" in feared situations. A small subgroup of people with social anxiety disorder fear having to perform, present, or talk in front of a group.

Risk Factors

There is no single cause of anxiety disorders. Genetics, brain structure and function, and environmental factors all seem to be involved.

General Anxiety Disorder (GAD)

About 3 percent of adults and 1 percent of adolescents have GAD. Females are much more likely than males to have GAD. Most people with GAD develop symptoms between childhood and middle age.

Panic Disorder

About 3 percent of adults and adolescents have panic disorder. Females are more likely than males to have panic disorder. Most people develop panic disorder between ages 20–24. It can occur much earlier, but rarely starts after age 45.

About 25–50 percent of people with panic disorder also have agoraphobia. They start avoiding places such as crowded areas, buses, and elevators. Agoraphobia can occur without panic disorder.

Risk factors for panic disorder include having stressors in the months before the first panic attack. Stressors can include marriage problems, health problems, use of illicit drugs, misuse of medications, or death of a close family member.

Social Anxiety Disorder

About 7 percent of adults have social anxiety disorder in a given year. Children may have social anxiety symptoms. The rate of social anxiety disorder decreases with age. It is more common in women than in men.

All Anxiety Disorders

Genetics and biological factors. Anxiety disorders tend to run in families. A person who has a close relative with an anxiety disorder or depression is more likely to develop an anxiety disorder. It is unclear whether one or more genes are involved. In some people, an overactive thyroid can contribute to anxiety disorders. A person who tends to feel distress and withdraw from unfamiliar situations, people, and places may be more likely to develop an anxiety disorder.

Brain structure and function. Certain brain structures seem to play a role in anxiety disorders. The amygdala, the part of the brain that controls emotion, may be involved.

Environment factors. Environmental factors that may lead to anxiety disorders include:

- Smoking or using tobacco products, and nicotine withdrawal

- Having a parent with anxiety, depression, or bipolar disorder

- Having breathing problems, such as asthma, and fearing suffocation

- Withdrawal from alcohol or a medication such as a benzodiazepine

- Exposure to stressful life events in childhood and/or adulthood

- Physical or mental abuse, death of a loved one, desertion, divorce, or isolation

- Caffeine, prescription medications, and over-the-counter medicines such as diet pills and allergy medications that contain pseudoephedrine

Evidence-Based Treatments

Anxiety disorders do not go away on their own, but they are among the most treatable mental disorders. If untreated, anxiety disorders can become chronic. Anxiety disorders can be treated with a combination of psychotherapy, sometimes called "talk therapy," and medication. The treatment plan should consider each person's needs and choices. A person should consult a healthcare professional when choosing the right treatment and consider their own gender, race, ethnicity, language, and culture.

Psychotherapy

Cognitive behavioral therapy (CBT) can help people with anxiety disorders. It teaches a person new ways of thinking, acting, and reacting to situations that cause anxiety. It can also help people learn social skills, which is vital for treating social anxiety disorder. Cognitive behavioral therapy may be done one-on-one or with a group of people who have similar problems. Two helpful approaches are cognitive therapy and exposure therapy. Cognitive therapy focuses on challenging unhelpful thoughts related to anxiety. Exposure therapy focuses on confronting fears so people no longer feel they must avoid certain activities.

Family therapy helps family members improve communication and resolve conflicts. Family therapy is usually short-term. It is sometimes used if a person's family may be contributing to their anxiety. The family members learn to avoid doing so.

Acceptance and commitment therapy (ACT) is helpful for people with anxiety disorders. Unlike cognitive behavioral therapy (which aims to reduce problematic thoughts and actions), ACT focuses on acceptance. The person gains insight into patterns of thinking, patterns of avoidance, and the presence or absence of action that is in line with chosen life values. The goal is to reduce the struggle to control or do away with these things, and to increase involvement in meaningful activities. ACT is especially helpful for people with GAD, and may be a good fit for older adults.

Medication

Medications are helpful in treating anxiety disorders. Medications do not cure anxiety disorders but often relieve symptoms. Medication and psychotherapy can be used separately or in combination. Medication may be used if psychotherapy alone is not effective, or if a person does not have access to psychotherapy.

The most common medications for anxiety disorders are antidepressants, benzodiazepines, and beta blockers.

Antidepressants can be helpful for treating anxiety disorders. A doctor should closely monitor anyone who recently started taking an antidepressant. In some cases, children, teenagers, and young adults (under age 25) may have more suicidal thoughts or actions when taking antidepressants. This is more likely in the first few weeks after starting a medication, or when the dose is changed. Women who are pregnant, planning to become pregnant, or breastfeeding should talk to their prescriber about possible health risks to herself, the fetus, or her nursing child. It is important to consult with a healthcare prescriber before stopping an antidepressant. Stopping these medications abruptly can cause serious health problems.

Benzodiazepines are often prescribed to people with anxiety disorders to help reduce worrying, panic attacks, or extreme fear. Benzodiazepines should be monitored by the prescriber. They can lead to physical dependency.

Beta blockers are helpful in treating the physical symptoms of anxiety, especially social anxiety. Physicians prescribe them to control rapid heartbeat, shaking, trembling, and blushing.

For basic information about medications, visit Mental Health Medications at the National Institute of Mental Health. For up-to-date information on medications, side effects, and warnings, visit the Food and Drug Administration.

Complementary Therapies and Activities

Complementary therapies and activities can help people with mental disorders improve their well-being and are meant to be used along with evidence-based treatments. For more information on natural products or mind-body practices, access the National Center for Complementary and Integrative Health.

Stress-management techniques, mindfulness, and meditation can help people with anxiety disorders learn to calm their thoughts and may enhance the effects of therapy.

Progressive muscle relaxation management includes forms of meditation and exercises that help reduce muscle tension and anxiety. These guided exercises help break the cycle of muscle tensions tied to anxiety.

Daily exercise, healthy nutrition, and adequate sleep improve a person's motivation and ability to participate in treatment and reduce stress levels.

Chamomile capsules may have some benefits for some people with mild to moderate GAD.

Chapter 20

Anxiety due to Quitting Smoking

What Are Some of the Withdrawal Symptoms Associated with Quitting Smoking?

Quitting smoking may cause short-term problems, especially for those who have smoked heavily for many years. These temporary changes can result in withdrawal symptoms.

Common withdrawal symptoms associated with quitting include the following:

- Anxiety.

- Nicotine cravings (nicotine is the substance in tobacco that causes addiction).

- Anger, frustration, and irritability.

- Depression.

- Weight gain.

Studies have shown that about half of smokers report experiencing at least four withdrawal symptoms (such as anger, anxiety, or

This chapter includes text excerpted from "How to Handle Withdrawal Symptoms and Triggers When You Decide to Quit Smoking," National Cancer Institute (NCI), October 29, 2010. Reviewed September 2017.

depression) when they quit. People have reported other symptoms, including dizziness, increased dreaming, and headaches.

The good news is that there is much you can do to reduce cravings and manage common withdrawal symptoms. Even without medication, withdrawal symptoms and other problems subside over time. It may also help to know that withdrawal symptoms are usually worst during the first week after quitting. From that point on, the intensity usually drops over the first month. However, everyone is different, and some people have withdrawal symptoms for several months after quitting.

What Can I Do about Anger, Frustration, and Irritability?

After you quit smoking, you may feel edgy and short-tempered, and you may want to give up on tasks more quickly than usual. You may be less tolerant of others and get into more arguments.

Studies have found that the most common negative feelings associated with quitting are feelings of anger, frustration, and irritability. These negative feelings peak within 1 week of quitting and may last 2 to 4 weeks.

Here are some tips for managing these negative feelings:

- Remind yourself that these feelings are temporary.

- Engage in a physical activity, such as taking a walk.

- Reduce caffeine by limiting or avoiding coffee, soda, and tea.

- Try meditation or other relaxation techniques, such as getting a massage, soaking in a hot bath, or breathing deeply through your nose and out through your mouth for 10 breaths.

Ask your doctor about nicotine replacement products or other medications.

What Can I Do about Anxiety?

Within 24 hours of quitting smoking, you may feel tense and agitated. You may feel a tightness in your muscles—especially around the neck and shoulders. Studies have found that anxiety is one of the most common negative feelings associated with quitting. If anxiety occurs, it builds over the first 3 days after quitting and may last 2 weeks.

Here are some tips for managing anxiety:

- Remind yourself that anxiety will pass with time.

- Set aside some quiet time every morning and evening—a time when you can be alone in a quiet environment.

- Engage in physical activity, such as taking a walk.

- Reduce caffeine by limiting or avoiding coffee, soda, and tea.

- Try meditation or other relaxation techniques, such as getting a massage, soaking in a hot bath, or breathing deeply through your nose and out through your mouth for 10 breaths.

- Ask your doctor about nicotine replacement products or other medications.

How Can I Resist the Urge to Smoke When I'm Feeling Stressed?

Most smokers report that one reason they smoke is to handle stress. This happens because smoking cigarettes actually relieves some of your stress by releasing powerful chemicals in your brain. Temporary changes in brain chemistry cause you to experience decreased anxiety, enhanced pleasure, and alert relaxation. Once you stop smoking, you may become more aware of stress.

Everyday worries, responsibilities, and hassles can all contribute to stress. As you go longer without smoking, you will get better at handling stress, especially if you learn stress reduction and relaxation techniques.

Here are some tips:

- Know the causes of stress in your life (your job, traffic, your children, money) and identify the stress signals (headaches, nervousness, or trouble sleeping). Once you pinpoint high-risk trigger situations, you can start to develop new ways to handle them.

- Create peaceful times in your everyday schedule. For example, set aside an hour where you can get away from other people and your usual environment.

- Try relaxation techniques, such as progressive relaxation or yoga, and stick with the one that works best for you.

- Rehearse and visualize your relaxation plan. Put your plan into action. Change your plan as needed.

- You may find it helpful to read a book about how to handle stress.

Chapter 21

Bullying and Its Impact on Children

Who's at Risk of Being Bullied

No single factor puts a child at risk of being bullied or bullying others. Bullying can happen anywhere—cities, suburbs, or rural towns. Depending on the environment, some groups—such as lesbian, gay, bisexual, or transgendered (LGBT) youth, youth with disabilities, and socially isolated youth—may be at an increased risk of being bullied.

Children at Risk of Being Bullied

Generally, children who are bullied have one or more of the following risk factors:

- Are perceived as different from their peers, such as being overweight or underweight, wearing glasses or different clothing, being new to a school, or being unable to afford what kids consider "cool"

- Are perceived as weak or unable to defend themselves

This chapter includes text excerpted from "Effects of Bullying," StopBullying. gov, U.S. Department of Health and Human Services (HHS), March 17, 2012. Reviewed September 2017.

- Are depressed, anxious, or have low self esteem

- Are less popular than others and have few friends

- Do not get along well with others, seen as annoying or provoking, or antagonize others for attention.

Warning Signs for Bullying

There are many warning signs that may indicate that someone is affected by bullying—either being bullied or bullying others. Recognizing the warning signs is an important first step in taking action against bullying. Not all children who are bullied or are bullying others ask for help.

It is important to talk with children who show signs of being bullied or bullying others. These warning signs can also point to other issues or problems, such as depression or substance abuse. Talking to the child can help identify the root of the problem.

Signs a Child Is Being Bullied

Look for changes in the child. However, be aware that not all children who are bullied exhibit warning signs.

Some signs that may point to a bullying problem are:

- Unexplainable injuries

- Lost or destroyed clothing, books, electronics, or jewelry

- Frequent headaches or stomach aches, feeling sick or faking illness

- Changes in eating habits, like suddenly skipping meals or binge eating. Kids may come home from school hungry because they did not eat lunch.

- Difficulty sleeping or frequent nightmares

- Declining grades, loss of interest in schoolwork, or not wanting to go to school

- Sudden loss of friends or avoidance of social situations

- Feelings of helplessness or decreased self esteem

- Self-destructive behaviors such as running away from home, harming themselves, or talking about suicide.

Why Don't Kids Ask for Help?

Statistics from the *Indicators of School Crime and Safety* show that an adult was notified in less than half (40%) of bullying incidents. Kids don't tell adults for many reasons:

- Bullying can make a child feel helpless. Kids may want to handle it on their own to feel in control again. They may fear being seen as weak or a tattletale.

- Kids may fear backlash from the kid who bullied them.

- Bullying can be a humiliating experience. Kids may not want adults to know what is being said about them, whether true or false. They may also fear that adults will judge them or punish them for being weak.

- Kids who are bullied may already feel socially isolated. They may feel like no one cares or could understand.

- Kids may fear being rejected by their peers. Friends can help protect kids from bullying, and kids can fear losing this support.

Effects of Bullying

Bullying can affect everyone—those who are bullied, those who bully, and those who witness bullying. Bullying is linked to many negative outcomes including impacts on mental health, substance use, and suicide. It is important to talk to kids to determine whether bullying—or something else—is a concern.

Kids Who Are Bullied

Kids who are bullied can experience negative physical, school, and mental health issues. Kids who are bullied are more likely to experience:

- Depression and anxiety, increased feelings of sadness and loneliness, changes in sleep and eating patterns, and loss of interest in activities they used to enjoy. These issues may persist into adulthood.

- Health complaints

- Decreased academic achievement—GPA and standardized test scores—and school participation. They are more likely to miss, skip, or drop out of school.

175

A very small number of bullied children might retaliate through extremely violent measures. In 12 of 15 school shooting cases in the 1990s, the shooters had a history of being bullied.

Considerations for Specific Groups

Schools and communities that respect diversity can help protect children against bullying behavior. However, when children perceived as different are not in supportive environments, they may be at a higher risk of being bullied. When working with kids from different groups—including lesbian, gay, bisexual, or transgender (LGBT) youth and youth with disabilities or special healthcare needs—there are specific things you can do to prevent and address bullying.

LGBT Youth

Lesbian, gay, bisexual, or transgender (LGBT) youth and those perceived as LGBT are at an increased risk of being bullied. Families of and people who work with LGBT youth have important and unique considerations for strategies to prevent and intervene in bullying.

Youth with Disabilities or Other Special Health Needs

Children with disabilities or other special health needs may be at higher risk of being bullied. There are specific ways you can support these groups.

Chapter 22

Diagnosis for People with Anxiety

Anxiety disorders sometimes run in families, but no one knows for sure why some people have them while others don't. Anxiety disorders are more common among younger adults than older adults, and they typically start in early life. However, anyone can develop an anxiety disorder at any time.

Diagnosis Can Be Difficult

There are a number of reasons why it can be difficult to accurately diagnose an anxiety disorder in older adults.

- Anxiety disorders among older adults frequently occur at the same time as other illnesses such as depression, diabetes, heart disease, or a number of other medical illnesses. Problems with cognition (thinking) and changes in life circumstances can also complicate matters. Sometimes the physical signs of these illnesses can get mixed up with the symptoms of anxiety, making it difficult to determine if a person has a true anxiety disorder. For instance, a person with heart disease sometimes has chest pain, which can also be a symptom of a panic disorder.

This chapter includes text excerpted from "Anxiety Disorders—Risk Factors and Diagnosis," NIHSeniorHealth, National Institute on Aging (NIA), January 2016.

- Doctors can have difficulty distinguishing between anxiety caused by adapting to difficult life changes, and a true anxiety disorder. For example, if you fell and broke a hip, you may be justifiably fearful of going out for a while. But that would not mean you have developed an anxiety disorder.

- Sometimes the worrying symptoms of a medical illness can lead to an anxiety disorder. Or, sometimes the side effects of medication can cause anxiety. Also, a disability or a change in lifestyle caused by a medical illness may lead to an anxiety disorder. Muscle tightness, feeling very tense all the time, and difficulty sleeping can also be symptoms of a physical illness or an anxiety disorder, complicating diagnosis.

Generalized Anxiety Disorder (GAD)—Diagnosis

Generalized anxiety disorder (GAD) can be diagnosed once a person worries excessively about a variety of everyday problems for at least 6 months.

People with GAD may visit a doctor many times before they find out they have this disorder. They ask their doctors to help them with headaches or trouble falling asleep, which can be symptoms of GAD, but they don't always get the help they need right away. It may take doctors some time to be sure that a person has GAD instead of something else.

Social Phobia—Diagnosis

A doctor can tell that a person has social phobia if the person has had symptoms for at least 6 months. Social phobia usually starts during youth. Without treatment, it can last for many years or a lifetime.

Panic Disorder—Diagnosis

People with panic disorder may sometimes go from doctor to doctor for years and visit the emergency room repeatedly before someone correctly diagnoses their condition. This is unfortunate, because panic disorder is one of the most treatable of all the anxiety disorders, responding in most cases to certain kinds of medication or certain kinds of cognitive psychotherapy, which help change thinking patterns that lead to fear and anxiety.

If You Have Symptoms

Anxiety disorders are treatable. If you think you have an anxiety disorder, talk to your family doctor. Your doctor should do an exam to make sure that another physical problem isn't causing the symptoms. The doctor may refer you to a mental health specialist.

You should feel comfortable talking with the mental health specialist you choose. If you do not, seek help elsewhere. Once you find a mental health specialist you are comfortable with, you should work as a team and make a plan to treat your anxiety disorder together.

Talk about Past Treatment

People with anxiety disorders who have already received treatment for an anxiety disorder should tell their doctor about that treatment in detail. If they received medication, they should tell their doctor what medication was used, what the dosage was at the beginning of treatment, whether the dosage was increased or decreased while they were under treatment, what side effects may have occurred, and whether the treatment helped them become less anxious. If they received psychotherapy, they should describe the type of therapy, how often they attended sessions, and whether the therapy was useful.

Chapter 23

Treatment Options for People with Anxiety

Anxiety Disorders Are Treatable. If You Think You Have an Anxiety Disorder, Talk to Your Doctor

Sometimes a physical evaluation is advisable to determine whether a person's anxiety is associated with a physical illness. If anxiety is diagnosed, the pattern of co-occurring symptoms should be identified, as well as any coexisting conditions, such as depression or substance abuse. Sometimes alcoholism, depression, or other coexisting conditions have such a strong effect on the individual that treating the anxiety should wait until the coexisting conditions are brought under control.

If your doctor thinks you may have an anxiety disorder, the next step is usually seeing a mental health professional. It is advisable to seek help from professionals who have particular expertise in diagnosing and treating anxiety. Certain kinds of cognitive and behavioral therapy and certain medications have been found to be especially helpful for anxiety.

This chapter contains text excerpted from the following sources: Text in this chapter begins with excerpts from "Types, Diagnosis, and Treatment," Medline-Plus, National Institutes of Health (NIH), 2015; Text under the heading "Ask Your Health Professional" is excerpted from "Treating Anxiety Disorders," MedlinePlus, National Institutes of Health (NIH), 2010. Reviewed September 2017.

You should feel comfortable talking with the mental health professional you choose. If you do not, you should seek help elsewhere. Once you find a clinician with whom you are comfortable, the two of you should work as a team and make a plan to treat your anxiety disorder together.

In general, anxiety disorders are treated with medication, specific types of psychotherapy, or both. Treatment choices depend on the type of disorder, the person's preference, and the expertise of the clinician. Most insurance plans, including health maintenance organizations (HMOs), will cover treatment for anxiety disorders.

What Medications Are Used to Treat Anxiety Disorders?

Medication does not necessarily cure anxiety disorders, but it often reduces the symptoms. Medication typically must be prescribed by a doctor. A psychiatrist is a doctor who specializes in mental disorders. Many psychiatrists offer psychotherapy themselves or work as a team with psychologists, social workers, or counselors who provide psychotherapy. The principal medications used for anxiety disorders are antidepressants, antianxiety drugs, and beta blockers. Be aware that some medications are effective only if they are taken regularly and that symptoms may recur if the medication is stopped.

Choosing the right medication, medication dose, and treatment plan should be based on a person's individual needs and medical situation, and done under an expert's care. Only an expert clinician can help you decide whether the medicine's ability to help is worth the risk of a side effect. Your doctor may try several medicines before finding the right one.

Antidepressants

Antidepressants were developed to treat depression, but they also help people with anxiety disorders. They are commonly prescribed for panic disorder, obsessive-compulsive disorder (OCD), posttraumatic stress disorder (PTSD), and social anxiety disorder.

Some tricyclic antidepressants work well for anxiety. Monoamine oxidase inhibitors (MAOIs) are also used for anxiety disorders.

Benzodiazepines (Antianxiety Medications)

The antianxiety medications called benzodiazepines can start working more quickly than antidepressants.

Beta Blockers

Beta blockers control some of the physical symptoms of anxiety, such as trembling and sweating.

Ask Your Health Professional

1. How will you find out whether or not I have an anxiety disorder?

2. What are my treatment options?

3. Are there any medications that might help?

4. How long before we know if the medication is helping?

5. Are there any lifestyle changes I can make to help?

6. How long will it take before I notice some improvement?

7. How long will I have to take medication?

8. How often should I see you about this disorder?

9. Do I need to see a counselor to help with this?

Chapter 24

Therapies for Anxiety

Chapter Contents

Section 24.1

Cognitive Behavioral Therapy (CBT)

This section includes text excerpted from "Types, Diagnosis and Treatment," MedlinePlus, National Institutes of Health (NIH), 2015.

Cognitive behavioral therapy (CBT) (sometimes called "talk therapy" or psychotherapy) involves talking with a trained clinician, such as a psychiatrist, psychologist, social worker, or counselor, to understand what caused an anxiety disorder and how to deal with it.

CBT can be useful in treating anxiety disorders. It can help people change the thinking patterns that support their fears and change the way they react to anxiety-provoking situations.

For example, CBT can help people with panic disorder learn that their panic attacks are not really heart attacks and help people with social phobia learn how to overcome the belief that others are always watching and judging them. When people are ready to confront their fears, they are shown how to use exposure techniques to desensitize themselves to situations that trigger their anxieties.

Exposure-based treatment has been used for many years to treat specific phobias. The person gradually encounters the object or situation that is feared, perhaps at first only through pictures or tapes, then later face-to-face. Sometimes the therapist will accompany the person to a feared situation to provide support and guidance. Exposure exercises are undertaken once the patient decides he is ready for it and with his cooperation.

To be effective, therapy must be directed at the person's specific anxieties and must be tailored to his or her needs. A typical "side effect" is temporary discomfort involved with thinking about confronting feared situations.

CBT may be conducted individually or with a group of people who have similar problems. Group therapy is particularly effective for social phobia. Often "homework" is assigned for participants to complete between sessions. If a disorder recurs at a later date, the same therapy can be used to treat it successfully a second time.

Medication can be combined with psychotherapy for specific anxiety disorders, and combination treatment has been found to be the best approach for many people.

Some people with anxiety disorders might benefit from joining a self-help or support group and sharing their problems and achievements with others. Internet chat rooms might also be useful in this regard, but any advice received over the Internet should be used with caution, as Internet acquaintances have usually never seen each other and false identities are common. Talking with a trusted friend or member of the clergy can also provide support, but it is not necessarily a sufficient alternative to care from an expert clinician.

Stress management techniques and meditation can help people with anxiety disorders calm themselves and may enhance the effects of therapy. There is preliminary evidence that aerobic exercise may have a calming effect. Since caffeine, certain illicit drugs, and even some over-the-counter cold medications can aggravate the symptoms of anxiety disorders, avoiding them should be considered. Check with your physician or pharmacist before taking any additional medications.

The family can be important in the recovery of a person with an anxiety disorder. Ideally, the family should be supportive but not help perpetuate their loved one's symptoms. Family members should not trivialize the disorder or demand improvement without treatment.

Section 24.2

Psychotherapy

This section includes text excerpted from "Mental Health Information—Psychotherapies," National Institute of Mental Health (NIMH), November 2016.

Psychotherapy (sometimes called "talk therapy") is a term for a variety of treatment techniques that aim to help a person identify and change troubling emotions, thoughts, and behavior. Most psychotherapy takes place with a licensed and trained mental healthcare professional and a patient meeting one on one or with other patients in a group setting.

Someone might seek out psychotherapy for different reasons:

- You might be dealing with severe or long-term stress from a job or family situation, the loss of a loved one, or relationship or other family issues. Or you may have symptoms with no physical explanation: changes in sleep or appetite, low energy, a lack of interest or pleasure in activities that you once enjoyed, persistent irritability, or a sense of discouragement or hopelessness that won't go away.

- A health professional may suspect or have diagnosed a condition such as depression, bipolar disorder, posttraumatic stress or other disorder and recommended psychotherapy as a first treatment or to go along with medication.

- You may be seeking treatment for a family member or child who has been diagnosed with a condition affecting mental health and for whom a health professional has recommended treatment.

An exam by your primary care practitioner can ensure there is nothing in your overall health that would explain your or a loved one's symptoms.

What to Consider When Looking for a Therapist

Therapists have different professional backgrounds and specialties. There are resources at the end of this material that can help you find out about the different credentials of therapists and resources for locating therapists.

There are many different types of psychotherapy. Different therapies are often variations on an established approach, such as cognitive behavioral therapy. There is no formal approval process for psychotherapies as there is for the use of medications in medicine. For many therapies, however, research involving large numbers of patients has provided evidence that treatment is effective for specific disorders. These "evidence-based therapies" have been shown in research to reduce symptoms of depression, anxiety, and other disorders.

The particular approach a therapist uses depends on the condition being treated and the training and experience of the therapist. Also, therapists may combine and adapt elements of different approaches.

One goal of establishing an evidence base for psychotherapies is to prevent situations in which a person receives therapy for months or years with no benefit. If you have been in therapy and feel you are not getting better, talk to your therapist, or look into other practitioners or approaches. The object of therapy is to gain relief from symptoms and improve quality of life.

Once you have identified one or more possible therapists, a preliminary conversation with a therapist can help you get an idea of how treatment will proceed and whether you feel comfortable with the therapist. Rapport and trust are important. Discussions in therapy are deeply personal and it's important that you feel comfortable and trusting with the therapist and have confidence in his or her expertise.

Consider asking the following questions:

- What are the credentials and experience of the therapist? Does he or she have a specialty?

- What approach will the therapist take to help you? Does he or she practice a particular type of therapy? What can the therapist tell you about the rationale for the therapy and the evidence base?

- Does the therapist have experience in diagnosing and treating the age group (for example, a child) and the specific condition for which treatment is being sought? If a child is the patient, how will parents be involved in treatment?

- What are the goals of therapy? Does the therapist recommend a specific time frame or number of sessions? How will progress be assessed and what happens if you (or the therapist) feel you aren't starting to feel better?

- Will there be homework?

- Are medications an option? How will medications be prescribed if the therapist is not an M.D.?

- Are our meetings confidential? How can this be assured?

Psychotherapies and Other Treatment Options

Psychotherapy can be an alternative to medication or can be used along with other treatment options, such as medications. Choosing the right treatment plan should be based on a person's individual needs and medical situation and under a mental health professional's care. Even when medications relieve symptoms, psychotherapy and other interventions can help a person address specific issues. These might include self-defeating ways of thinking, fears, problems with interactions with other people, or dealing with situations at home and at school or with employment.

Elements of Psychotherapy

A variety of different kinds of psychotherapies and interventions have been shown to be effective for *specific disorders*. Psychotherapists may use one primary approach, or incorporate different elements depending on their training, the condition being treated, and the needs of the person receiving treatment.

Here are examples of the elements that psychotherapies can include:

- Helping a person become aware of ways of thinking that may be automatic but are inaccurate and harmful. (An example might be someone who has a low opinion of his or her own abilities.) The therapist helps the person find ways to question these thoughts, understand how they affect emotions and behavior, and try ways to change self-defeating patterns. This approach is central to cognitive behavioral therapy (CBT).

- Identifying ways to cope with stress.

- Examining in depth a person's interactions with others and offering guidance with social and communication skills, if needed.

- Relaxation and mindfulness techniques.

- Exposure therapy for people with anxiety disorders. In exposure therapy, a person spends brief periods, in a supportive environment, learning to tolerate the distress certain items, ideas, or imagined scenes cause. Over time the fear associated with these things dissipates.

- Tracking emotions and activities and the impact of each on the other.

- Safety planning can include helping a person recognize warning signs, and thinking about coping strategies, such as contacting friends, family, or emergency personnel.

- Supportive counseling to help a person explore troubling issues and provide emotional support.

Section 24.3

Antianxiety Medications

This section includes text excerpted from "Mental
Health Information—Antianxiety Medications," National
Institute of Mental Health (NIMH), October 2016.

What Are Antianxiety Medications?

Antianxiety medications help reduce the symptoms of anxiety, such
as panic attacks, or extreme fear and worry. The most common antianxiety medications are called benzodiazepines. Benzodiazepines can
treat generalized anxiety disorder. In the case of panic disorder or
social phobia (social anxiety disorder), benzodiazepines are usually
second-line treatments, behind selective serotonin reuptake inhibitors
(SSRIs) or other antidepressants.

Benzodiazepines used to treat anxiety disorders include:

- Clonazepam

- Alprazolam

- Lorazepam

Short half-life (or short-acting) benzodiazepines (such as Lorazepam
) and beta blockers are used to treat the short-term symptoms of anxiety. Beta blockers help manage physical symptoms of anxiety, such
as trembling, rapid heartbeat, and sweating that people with phobias
(an overwhelming and unreasonable fear of an object or situation,
such as public speaking) experience in difficult situations. Taking
these medications for a short period of time can help the person keep
physical symptoms under control and can be used "as needed" to reduce
acute anxiety.

Buspirone (which is unrelated to the benzodiazepines) is sometimes used for the long-term treatment of chronic anxiety. In contrast to the benzodiazepines, buspirone must be taken every day for
a few weeks to reach its full effect. It is not useful on an "as-needed"
basis.

How Do People Respond to Antianxiety Medications?

Antianxiety medications such as benzodiazepines are effective in relieving anxiety and take effect more quickly than the antidepressant medications (or buspirone) often prescribed for anxiety. However, people can build up a tolerance to benzodiazepines if they are taken over a long period of time and may need higher and higher doses to get the same effect. Some people may even become dependent on them. To avoid these problems, doctors usually prescribe benzodiazepines for short periods, a practice that is especially helpful for older adults, people who have substance abuse problems and people who become dependent on medication easily. If people suddenly stop taking benzodiazepines, they may have withdrawal symptoms or their anxiety may return. Therefore, benzodiazepines should be tapered off slowly.

What Are the Possible Side Effects of Antianxiety Medications?

Like other medications, antianxiety medications may cause side effects. Some of these side effects and risks are serious. The most common side effects for benzodiazepines are drowsiness and dizziness. Other possible side effects include:

- Nausea
- Blurred vision
- Headache
- Confusion
- Tiredness
- Nightmares

Tell your doctor if any of these symptoms are severe or do not go away:

- Drowsiness
- Dizziness
- Unsteadiness
- Problems with coordination
- Difficulty thinking or remembering
- Increased saliva

- Muscle or joint pain
- Frequent urination
- Blurred vision
- Changes in sex drive or ability

If you experience any of the symptoms below, call your doctor immediately:

- Rash
- Hives
- Swelling of the eyes, face, lips, tongue, or throat
- Difficulty breathing or swallowing
- Hoarseness
- Seizures
- Yellowing of the skin or eyes
- Depression
- Difficulty speaking
- Yellowing of the skin or eyes
- Thoughts of suicide or harming yourself
- Difficulty breathing

Common side effects of beta blockers include:

- Fatigue
- Cold hands
- Dizziness or light-headedness
- Weakness

Beta blockers generally are not recommended for people with asthma or diabetes because they may worsen symptoms related to both.

Possible side effects from buspirone include:

- Dizziness
- Headaches
- Nausea

- Nervousness
- Lightheadedness
- Excitement
- Trouble sleeping

Antianxiety medications may cause other side effects that are not included in the lists above.

Chapter 25

Complementary and Alternative Approaches for Anxiety

Chapter Contents

Section 25.1

Are You Considering a Complementary Health Approach?

This section includes text excerpted from "Are You Considering a Complementary Health Approach?" National Center for Complementary and Integrative Health (NCCIH), September 6, 2016.

Millions of Americans use complementary health approaches. Like any decision concerning your health, decisions about whether to use complementary approaches are important.

Take Charge of Your Health

- Be an informed consumer. Find out and consider what scientific studies have been done on the safety and effectiveness of any health approach that is recommended to or interests you.

- Discuss the information and your interests with your healthcare providers before making a decision.

- Choose a complementary health practitioner, such as an acupuncturist, as carefully as you would choose a conventional healthcare provider.

- Before using any dietary supplement or herbal product, make sure you find out about potential side effects or interactions with medications you may be taking.

- Only use treatments for your condition that have been proven safe. Do not use a product or practice that has not been proven to be effective to postpone seeing your healthcare provider for your condition.

- Tell all your healthcare providers—complementary and conventional—about all the health approaches you use. Give them a full picture of what you do to manage your health. This will help ensure coordinated and safe care.

What Do "Complementary," "Alternative," and "Integrative" Mean?

"Complementary and alternative medicine," "complementary medicine," "alternative medicine," "integrative medicine"—you may have seen these terms on the Internet and in marketing, but what do they really mean? While the terms are often used to mean the array of healthcare approaches with a history of use or origins outside of mainstream medicine, they are actually hard to define and may mean different things to different people.

The terms complementary and integrative refer to the use of nonmainstream approaches together with conventional medical approaches.

Alternative health approaches refer to the use of nonmainstream products or practices in place of conventional medicine. National Center for Complementary and Integrative Health (NCCIH) advises against using any product or practice that has not been proven safe and effective as a substitute for conventional medical treatment or as a reason to postpone seeing your healthcare provider about any health problem. In some instances, stopping—or not starting—conventional treatment can have serious consequences. Before making a decision not to use a proven conventional treatment, talk to your healthcare providers.

How Can I Get Reliable Information about a Complementary Health Approach?

It's important to learn what scientific studies have discovered about the complementary health approach you're considering. Evidence from research studies is stronger and more reliable than something you've seen in an advertisement or on a website, or something someone told you about that worked for them.

Understanding a product's or practice's potential benefits, risks, and scientific evidence is critical to your health and safety. Scientific research on many complementary health approaches is relatively new, so this kind of information may not be available for each one. However, many studies are under way, including those that NCCIH supports, and knowledge and understanding of complementary approaches are increasing all the time. Here are some ways to find reliable information:

- **Talk with your healthcare providers.** Tell them about the complementary health approach you're considering and ask any

197

questions you may have about safety, effectiveness, or inter-actions with medications (prescription or nonprescription) or dietary supplements.

- **Visit your local library or a medical library.** Ask the reference librarian to help you find scientific journals and trust-worthy books with information on the product or practice that interests you.

Are Complementary Health Approaches Safe?

As with any medical product or treatment, there can be risks with complementary approaches. These risks depend on the specific product or practice. Each needs to be considered on its own. However, if you're considering a specific product or practice, the following general suggestions can help you think about safety and minimize risks.

- Be aware that individuals respond differently to health products and practices, whether conventional or complementary. How you might respond to one depends on many things, including your state of health, how you use it, or your belief in it.

- Keep in mind that "natural" does not necessarily mean "safe." (Think of mushrooms that grow in the wild: some are safe to eat, while others are not).

- Learn about factors that affect safety. For a practice that is administered by a practitioner, such as chiropractic, these factors include the training, skill, and experience of the practitioner. For a product such as a dietary supplement, the specific ingredients and the quality of the manufacturing process are important factors.

- If you decide to use a practice provided by a complementary health practitioner, choose the practitioner as carefully as you would your primary healthcare provider.

- If you decide to use a dietary supplement, such as an herbal product, be aware that some products may interact in harmful ways with medications (prescription or over-the-counter) or other dietary supplements, and some may have side effects on their own.

- Tell all your healthcare providers about any complementary or integrative health approaches you use. Give them a full picture of what you do to manage your health. This will help ensure coordinated and safe care.

How Can I Determine Whether Statements Made about the Effectiveness of a Complementary Health Approach Are True?

Before you begin using a complementary health approach, it's a good idea to ask the following questions:

- Is there scientific evidence (not just personal stories) to back up the statements?

- What is the source? Statements that manufacturers or other promoters of some complementary health approaches may make about effectiveness and benefits can sound reasonable and promising. However, the statements may be based on a biased view of the available scientific evidence.

- How does the provider or manufacturer describe the approach?

- Beware of terms like "scientific breakthrough," "miracle cure," "secret ingredient," or "ancient remedy."

- If you encounter claims of a "quick fix" that depart from previous research, keep in mind that science usually advances over time by small steps, slowly building an evidence base.

- Remember: If it sounds too good to be true—for example, claims that a product or practice can cure a disease or works for a variety of ailments—it usually is.

Are Complementary Health Approaches Tested to See If They Work?

While scientific evidence now exists regarding the effectiveness and safety of some complementary health approaches, there remain many yet-to-be-answered questions about whether others are safe, whether they work for the diseases or medical conditions for which they are promoted, and how those approaches with health benefits may work. As the Federal Government's lead agency for scientific research on health interventions, practices, products, and disciplines that originate from outside mainstream medicine, NCCIH supports scientific research to answer these questions and determine who might benefit most from the use of specific approaches.

I'm Interested in an Approach That Involves Seeing a Complementary Health Practitioner. How Do I Go about Selecting a Practitioner?

- Your primary healthcare provider or local hospital may be able to recommend a complementary health practitioner.

- The professional organization for the type of practitioner you're seeking may have helpful information, such as licensing and training requirements. Many states have regulatory agencies or licensing boards for certain types of complementary health practitioners; they may be able to help you locate practitioners in your area.

- Make sure any practitioner you're considering is willing to work in collaboration with your other healthcare providers.

Section 25.2

Anxiety and Complementary Health Approaches: What the Science Says

This section includes text excerpted from "Anxiety and Complementary Health Approaches: What the Science Says" National Center for Complementary and Integrative Health (NCCIH), December 12, 2016.

Mind and Body Approaches

Acupuncture

Although some studies of acupuncture for anxiety have had positive outcomes, in general, many of the studies on acupuncture for anxiety have been of poor methodological quality or not of statistical significance. In addition, because the research is extremely variable (e.g., number and variety of acupuncture points, frequency of sessions, and duration of treatment), it is difficult to draw firm conclusions about potential benefits.

The Evidence Base

- The evidence base on efficacy of acupuncture for anxiety consists of several reviews, but sample size, variability, and methodological issues make it difficult to draw firm conclusions.

Efficacy

- A 2012 review of 32 studies of acupuncture for anxiety found that although there have been some positive outcomes, the generally poor methodological quality, combined with the wide range of outcome measures used, number and variety of points, frequency of sessions, and duration of treatment makes drawing firm conclusions difficult.

- A 2014 meta-analysis of 14 studies involving 1,034 participants on the efficacy of acupuncture in reducing preoperative anxiety found that acupuncture has a statistically significant effect relative to placebo or nontreatment controls, but the sample size was small. The meta-analysis supports the possibility that acupuncture is superior to placebo for preoperative anxiety.

Safety

- Acupuncture is generally considered safe when performed by an experienced practitioner using sterile needles. Reports of serious adverse events related to acupuncture are rare, but include infections and punctured organs.

Massage Therapy

In some studies massage therapy helped to reduce anxiety for people with cancer or other comorbid medical conditions; however, other studies did not find a statistically significant beneficial effect.

The Evidence Base

The evidence base on efficacy of massage therapy consists of several randomized controlled trials, mostly involving anxiety associated with medical procedures or conditions.

Efficacy

- A 2014 systematic review and meta-analysis of 18 randomized controlled trials involving 950 women with breast cancer did not find any significant effect of massage on anxiety.

- A 2013 randomized controlled trial of 60 cancer patients examined massage therapy for perioperative pain and anxiety in placement of vascular access devices and found that both massage therapy and structured attention proved beneficial for alleviating preoperative anxiety in these patients.

- A 2012 randomized trial involving 152 cardiac surgery patients found that massage therapy significantly reduced the pain, anxiety, and muscular tension and improved relaxation after cardiac surgery.

- Findings from a 2012 randomized controlled trial of 120 primiparous women with term pregnancy suggest that massage is an effective alternative intervention, decreasing pain and anxiety during labor.

Safety

- Massage therapy appears to have few risks if it is used appropriately and provided by a trained massage professional.

Mindfulness Meditation

Meditation therapy is commonly used and has been shown to be of small to modest benefit for people with anxiety-related symptoms. However, there is a lack of studies with adequate statistical power in patients with clinically diagnosed anxiety disorders, which makes it difficult to draw firm conclusions about its efficacy for anxiety disorders.

The Evidence Base

- The evidence base on efficacy of mindfulness meditation consists of several randomized controlled trials, most of which examine the efficacy of meditation programs on anxiety symptoms and not on clinically diagnosed anxiety disorders.

Efficacy

- A 2014 systematic review and meta-analysis of 47 trials with 3,515 participants found that mindfulness meditation programs had moderate evidence of improved anxiety. The reviewers concluded that clinicians should be aware that meditation programs can result in small to moderate reductions of multiple negative dimensions of psychological stress.

- A 2012 systematic review and meta-analysis of 36 randomized controlled trials found evidence of some efficacy of meditative therapies in reducing anxiety symptoms; however, most studies included in the analysis measured only improvement in anxiety symptoms, but not anxiety disorders as clinically diagnosed.

- A Cochrane review of two randomized controlled trials concluded that because of the small number of studies, conclusions could not be drawn about the efficacy of meditation therapy for anxiety disorders.

Safety

- Meditation is generally considered to be safe for healthy people. However, people with physical limitations may not be able to participate in certain meditative practices involving movement.

Relaxation Techniques

Relaxation techniques may reduce anxiety in individuals with chronic medical problems and those who are having medical procedures. However, evidence demonstrates that conventional psychotherapy, for individuals with generalized anxiety disorder, may be more effective than relaxation techniques.

The Evidence Base

- The evidence base on efficacy of relaxation techniques for anxiety consists of several randomized controlled trials and a meta-analysis.

Efficacy

- A 2014 meta-analysis of a total of 41 studies involving 2,132 participants with generalized anxiety disorder found some indications that cognitive behavioral therapy (CBT) was more effective than relaxation techniques over the long term.

- A 2016 randomized trial of 236 women undergoing large core breast biopsy found that adjunctive self-hypnotic relaxation decreased procedural pain and anxiety.

- A 2012 randomized controlled trial of 39 participants with inflammatory bowel disease found that those who received the relaxation-training intervention showed a statistically significant improvement in anxiety levels as compared to the control group.

Safety

- Relaxation techniques are generally considered safe for healthy people. People with serious physical or mental health problems should discuss relaxation techniques with their healthcare providers.

Natural Products

Kava

Kava extract may produce moderately beneficial effects on anxiety symptoms; however, the use of kava supplements has been linked to a risk of severe liver damage.

The Evidence Base

- The evidence base on efficacy of kava for anxiety consists of several randomized controlled trials and a Cochrane review.

Efficacy

- A 2013 randomized controlled trial involving 75 participants with generalized anxiety disorder concluded that standardized kava extract may be a moderately effective short-term option for the treatment of generalized anxiety disorder.
- A 2011 review of 66 studies of herbal medicine for depression, anxiety, and insomnia found some evidence that kava may produce beneficial effects for anxiety disorders.
- A 2003 Cochrane review of 12 randomized controlled trials found that compared with placebo, kava extract may be an effective symptomatic treatment for anxiety, although the effect size appears small.

Safety

The use of kava supplements has been linked to a risk of severe liver damage, according to the U.S. Food and Drug Administration (FDA).

Kava has been associated with several cases of dystonia and may interact with several drugs, including drugs used for Parkinson's disease.

However, a 2013 randomized controlled trial of 75 participants who received kava extract over a 6-week period found no significant differences across groups for liver function tests, nor any significant adverse reactions associated with kava administration. Long-term safety studies of kava are needed.

Melatonin

There is some evidence that suggests melatonin may help reduce anxiety in patients who are about to have surgery and may be as effective as standard treatment with midazolam in reducing preoperative anxiety.

The Evidence Base

- The evidence base on efficacy of melatonin for anxiety consists of a Cochrane review of several studies comparing melatonin, placebo, and midazolam.

Efficacy

- A 2015 Cochrane review of 12 studies involving 774 participants found that melatonin compared to placebo, given as premedication, reduced preoperative anxiety (measured 50 to 100 minutes after administration) and may reduce postoperative anxiety (6 hours after surgery). The reviewers also found that melatonin may be equally as effective as standard treatment with midazolam in reducing preoperative anxiety.

Safety

- Melatonin supplements appear to be safe when used short term; less is known about long-term safety.

Lavender

Although some studies of oral lavender supplementation for anxiety have shown some therapeutic effects, in general, many of these studies have been of poor methodological quality.

205

The Evidence Base

- The evidence base on efficacy of oral lavender supplementation for anxiety consists of a systematic review of several small randomized controlled trials, many of which have methodological issues.

Efficacy

- A 2012 systematic review of 15 randomized controlled trials concluded that methodological issues limit the extent to which any conclusions can be drawn regarding the efficacy of lavender for anxiety.

Safety

- When lavender teas and extracts are taken by mouth, they may cause headache, changes in appetite, and constipation.

- Using lavender supplements with sedative medications may increase drowsiness.

Section 25.3

Things to Know about Complementary Health Approaches for Anxiety

This section includes text excerpted from "Things to Know about Complementary Health Approaches for Anxiety," National Center for Complementary and Integrative Health (NCCIH), April 13, 2017.

Occasional anxiety is a normal part of life. You might feel anxious when faced with a problem at work, before taking a test, or making an important decision. But for some people, anxiety becomes a severe, persistent problem that's hard to control and can interfere with daily activities; this is called an anxiety disorder. Effective conventional treatments for anxiety disorders, including psychotherapy and medication, are available.

Some people turn to complementary health approaches to help them reduce anxiety and cope with stressful situations, such as medical procedures. Certain complementary health approaches may help relieve this type of anxiety; however, complementary approaches have not been proven effective in treating anxiety disorders. Here are seven things to know about complementary health approaches for anxiety:

1. Although some studies suggest that acupuncture might reduce anxiety, the research is too limited to allow definite conclusions to be reached.

2. In some studies in people with cancer or other medical conditions, massage therapy helped to reduce anxiety; however, other studies did not find a significant beneficial effect. Massage has not been shown to be effective in treating generalized anxiety disorder.

3. Mindfulness meditation may have a small to modest beneficial effect on anxiety-related symptoms. However, meditation has not been shown to be effective in treating anxiety disorders.

4. Relaxation techniques may reduce anxiety in people with chronic medical problems and those who are having medical procedures. However, conventional psychotherapy (cognitive behavioral therapy) may be more effective than relaxation techniques in treating anxiety disorders.

5. Kava extract may produce moderately beneficial effects on anxiety symptoms; however, the use of kava supplements has been linked to a risk of severe liver damage.

6. There is some evidence that suggests melatonin may help reduce anxiety in patients who are about to have surgery.

7. Take charge of your health—talk with your healthcare providers about any complementary health approaches you use. Together, you can make shared, well-informed decisions.

Section 25.4

Abdominal Breathing

This section includes text excerpted from "Abdominal Breathing," Mental Illness Research, Education, and Clinical Centers (MIRECC), July 2013. Reviewed September 2017.

What Is Abdominal Breathing?

The goal of breath-focused relaxation is to shift from quick, shallow chest breathing to deeper, more relaxed abdominal breathing. During times of stress, our natural tendency is to either hold our breath, or to breathe in a shallow, rapid manner. When we are relaxed our breathing is naturally slower and deeper. When stress is chronic, we may habitually breathe shallowly, never really discharging the stale air from our lungs. Holding in your stomach for reasons of vanity also restricts breathing. In order to take a full deep breath, we must allow our diaphragm (the muscle separating our chest cavity from the abdominal cavity below the lungs) to drop down and our abdomen to expand. If we keep our stomach muscles held in tight when we breathe, we restrict the expansion of our lungs and rob our bodies of optimal oxygen. This puts our bodies in a state of alarm that creates the sensation of anxiety. Taking a few slow, deep breaths sends the signal to our body to relax. Deep breathing is also referred to as abdominal breathing, diaphragmatic breathing, or belly breathing. Abdominal breathing is a form of relaxation that you can use any time to help you to calm yourself physically and mentally and in turn, decrease stress.

Instructions for Learning Abdominal Breathing

1. Place one hand, palm side down, on your chest. Place the other hand, palm side down, on your stomach.

2. Breathe in through your nose to a slow count of 3 or 4 (one ... two ...three... four...). Notice the motion of each hand. When you breathe in, does the hand on your chest move? If so, which way does it move (out/up or in/down) and how much does it

move? Does the hand on your stomach move? If so, which way (out or in) and how much?

3. Now exhale through your nose, again to a slow count of 3 or 4. Notice again how each of your hands moves.

For the most relaxing breath, the hand on your chest should move very little while the hand on your stomach pushes out significantly on the inhale (in breath) and goes back in on the exhale (out breath). A common problem is for the chest to inflate on the in breath while the stomach stays still or even sucks in. When this happens, only the upper part of the lungs (the part behind the upper chest) is being used. When a full deep breath is properly taken, the diaphragm muscle drops down into the abdominal cavity to make room for the lungs to expand. As the diaphragm muscle drops down, it pushes the organs in the abdomen forward to make more room for the lungs. That is why the stomach goes out when you take the most relaxing type of breath.

Learning to take abdominal breaths versus chest breathing is a challenge for some people. The following tips can make it easier.

- Imagine yourself filling a medium-sized balloon in your stomach each time you inhale and releasing the air in the balloon when you exhale.

- Breathe in the same amount of air you breathe out.

- It is sometimes easier to first learn abdominal breathing while lying on your back with your hand on your stomach. It is easier to feel the stomach motion in this position versus sitting or standing.

- It is best to only practice a few deep breaths at a time at first. This is because deep breathing can make you feel light headed if you aren't used to it. If you begin to feel light headed, it is just your body's signal that it has had enough practice for now. Return to your normal breathing and practice again later. With practice, you will be able to take a greater number of deep breaths without becoming light headed.

- Start practicing this deep breathing technique when you are calm so you have mastered it and are ready to use it when you are stressed.

Key Points

- Abdominal breathing can help you achieve a state of relaxation because it has both meditative (mentally calming) and sedating (physically calming) qualities.

- Try not to get frustrated by "Worry" or "To-Do" thoughts that enter your head while you're relaxing. Gently let these thoughts pass and return to the task at hand. Focusing on your deep breathing will help you. Sometimes, it also helps to "place" busy thoughts on an imaginary conveyor belt like those found at the airport—eventually your thought luggage will come back round where you can pick it up after your relaxation trip. Or, mentally set your concerns on a shelf until you are ready to address them.

- Practice this type of breathing for about 5 minutes, one or more times a day, most days of the week.

- Learning to focus on one of the most calming processes in the body, namely your breathing, is one of the most reliable ways to achieve a relaxed state!

- This is a great relaxation exercise to learn because you can do it anywhere, anytime you want to take the edge off your anxiety stress level.

- It is normal for this new method of breathing to feel awkward at first. With practice it will feel more natural.

Longer Relaxation Exercises

Deep breathing can be expanded into a longer relaxation exercise as well. Two examples are given below:

Three-Part Rhythmic Breathing

Inhale ... hold the breath ... and then exhale ... with the inhale, hold, and exhale each being of equal length. Inhale and exhale completely using the entire length of the lungs. Keep your shoulders and face relaxed while you hold your breath. Use a count that is comfortable for you. Repeat five times.

Breathing with Imagery

For about 30 seconds, simply relax with your eyes closed. Then start to pay attention to your breathing. Let your breathing become slow and relaxed, like a person sleeping. Feel the air entering thorough your nose with each inhalation, and feel your breath leave as you exhale. Imagine the tension is leaving your body with each out breath.

Now imagine that, as you breathe in, the air comes into your nose and caresses your face like a gentle breeze. As you breathe out, the exhalation carries away the tension from your face. As you breathe slowly in and out, tension gradually leaves your body and you become more and more relaxed.

Now imagine that, as you breathe in, the gentle air enters your nose and spreads relaxation up over the top of your head. As you exhale, imagine the tension leaving this area and passing out of our body. Then imagine the next breath carrying relaxation over your face, your scalp, and both sides of your head. As you exhale, let any tension flow out easily.

If other thoughts come to mind, simply return to paying attention to your breathing. Your breathing is slow and easy, with no effort at all. Let your body relax.

Now let your breath carry relaxation to your neck. As you exhale, tension passes out of your neck and out of your body with the exhaled air. Feel a breath carry relaxation into your shoulders. As you exhale, any tension leaves your shoulders and passes out of your body.

Now one breath at a time, focus your attention on each part of your body from the top down: your upper arms, forearms, hands, chest, back, stomach, hips, thighs, knees, calves, ankles, and feet. Imagine each breath of air carrying relaxation into each part of your body. As you breathe out, let any tension pass out through your nostrils.

This exercise takes several minutes. Do it at your own pace. When you have finished, sit quietly for a minute or two more.

Section 25.5

Chamomile Capsules Ease Anxiety

This section contains text excerpted from the following sources:
Text beginning with the heading "Chamomile" is excerpted from
"Chamomile," National Center for Complementary and Integrative
Health (NCCIH), November 29, 2016; Text under the heading
"Study Shows Chamomile Capsules Ease Anxiety Symptoms" is
excerpted from "Study Shows Chamomile Capsules Ease Anxiety
Symptoms," National Center for Complementary and Integrative
Health (NCCIH), October 21, 2015.

Chamomile

Chamomile was described in ancient medical writings and was
an important medicinal herb in ancient Egypt, Greece, and Rome.
Chamomile is used as a dietary supplement for sleeplessness, anxiety,
and gastrointestinal conditions such as upset stomach, gas, and diarrhea. It is also used topically for skin conditions and for mouth sores
resulting from cancer treatment. There are two types of chamomile:
German chamomile and Roman chamomile. This section focuses on
German chamomile. The flowering tops of the chamomile plant are
used to make teas, liquid extracts, capsules, or tablets. The herb can
also be applied to the skin as a cream or an ointment, or used as a
mouth rinse.

How Much Do We Know?

Not much is known about the health effects of chamomile because
it has not been well studied in people.

What Have We Learned?

- Some preliminary studies suggest that a chamomile dietary
  supplement might be helpful for generalized anxiety disorder
  (GAD).

- Some research has found that products containing certain combinations of herbs that include chamomile may be of benefit for

212

upset stomach, for diarrhea in children, and for infants with colic. But chamomile alone has not been shown to be helpful for these conditions.

What Do We Know about Safety?

- There have been reports of allergic reactions, including rare cases of anaphylaxis (a life-threatening allergic reaction), in people who have consumed or come into contact with chamomile products.

- People are more likely to experience allergic reactions to chamomile if they're allergic to related plants such as ragweed, chrysanthemums, marigolds, or daisies.

- Interactions between chamomile and cyclosporine (a drug used to prevent rejection of organ transplants) and warfarin (a blood thinner) have been reported, and there are theoretical reasons to suspect that chamomile might interact with other drugs as well. Talk to your healthcare provider before taking chamomile if you're taking any type of medicine.

Keep in Mind

- Tell all your healthcare providers about any complementary or integrative health approaches you use. Give them a full picture of what you do to manage your health. This will help to ensure coordinated and safe care.

Study Shows Chamomile Capsules Ease Anxiety Symptoms

Generalized anxiety disorder (GAD) has a wide array of psychological and physical symptoms. Although prescription drugs can help, they often have undesirable side effects. Many people experiencing symptoms of anxiety do not seek medical attention, turning instead to alternatives. One traditional remedy in widespread use is the herb chamomile. However, scientific evidence to support the use of chamomile for anxiety has been lacking.

National Center for Complementary and Alternative Medicine (NCCAM) funded researchers at the University of Pennsylvania recently conducted a randomized, double-blind, placebo-controlled trial to test the effects of chamomile extract in patients diagnosed

213

with mild to moderate GAD. For 8 weeks, the 57 participants received either chamomile capsules containing 220 mg of pharmaceutical-grade extract from Matricaria recutita (German chamomile), standardized to 1.2 percent of the constituent apigenin; or chamomile-scented placebo capsules containing lactose. The initial dose of one capsule daily was increased to two capsules daily at week 2; dosages were then adjusted incrementally (up to five capsules) in some participants. Researchers used the Hamilton Anxiety Rating (HAM-A) and other tests to measure changes in anxiety symptoms over the course of the study; dosage adjustments were based on HAM-A scores.

Compared with placebo, chamomile was associated with a greater reduction in mean HAM-A scores—the study's primary outcome measure. The difference was clinically meaningful and statistically significant. Chamomile also compared favorably with placebo on other outcome measures (although the differences were not statistically significant), and was well tolerated by participants.

These results suggest that chamomile may have modest benefits for some people with mild to moderate GAD. As this was the first controlled trial of chamomile extract for anxiety, the researchers note that additional studies using larger samples and studying effects for longer periods of time would be helpful. They also point out that other chamomile species, preparations (e.g., extracts standardized to constituents other than apigenin), and formulations (e.g., oil or tea) might produce different results.

Section 25.6

Meditation for Treating Anxiety

This section includes text excerpted from "Meditation: In Depth," National Center for Complementary and Integrative Health (NCCIH), September 7, 2017.

What Is Meditation?

Meditation is a mind and body practice that has a long history of use for increasing calmness and physical relaxation, improving psychological balance, coping with illness, and enhancing overall health and well-being. Mind and body practices focus on the interactions among the brain, mind, body, and behavior.

There are many types of meditation, but most have four elements in common:

1. A quiet location with as few distractions as possible;

2. A specific, comfortable posture (sitting, lying down, walking, or in other positions);

3. A focus of attention (a specially chosen word or set of words, an object, or the sensations of the breath); and

4. An open attitude (letting distractions come and go naturally without judging them).

Meditation and the Brain

Some research suggests that meditation may physically change the brain and body and could potentially help to improve many health problems and promote healthy behaviors.

What the Science Says about the Effectiveness of Meditation

Many studies have investigated meditation for different conditions, and there's evidence that it may reduce blood pressure as well as symptoms of irritable bowel syndrome and flare-ups in people who have had ulcerative colitis. It may ease symptoms of anxiety and depression, and may help people with insomnia.

For Anxiety, Depression, and Insomnia

- A 2014 literature review of 47 trials in 3,515 participants suggests that mindfulness meditation programs show moderate evidence of improving anxiety and depression. But the researchers found no evidence that meditation changed health-related behaviors affected by stress, such as substance abuse and sleep.

- A 2012 review of 36 trials found that 25 of them reported better outcomes for symptoms of anxiety in the meditation groups compared to control groups.

- In a small, National Center for Complementary and Integrative Health (NCCIH)-funded study, 54 adults with chronic insomnia learned mindfulness-based stress reduction (MBSR), a form of MBSR specially adapted to deal with insomnia (mindfulness-based therapy for insomnia, or MBTI), or a self-monitoring program. Both meditation-based programs aided sleep, with MBTI providing a significantly greater reduction in insomnia severity compared with MBSR.

What the Science Says about Safety and Side Effects of Meditation

- Meditation is generally considered to be safe for healthy people.

- People with physical limitations may not be able to participate in certain meditative practices involving movement. People with physical health conditions should speak with their healthcare providers before starting a meditative practice, and make their meditation instructor aware of their condition.

- There have been rare reports that meditation could cause or worsen symptoms in people with certain psychiatric problems like anxiety and depression. People with existing mental health conditions should speak with their healthcare providers before starting a meditative practice, and make their meditation instructor aware of their condition.

Section 25.7

Mindfulness Practice in the Treatment of Anxiety

This section includes text excerpted from "Mindfulness Practice in the Treatment of Traumatic Stress," U.S. Department of Veterans Affairs (VA), August 14, 2015.

What Is Mindfulness?

Mindfulness is a way of thinking and focusing that can help you become more aware of your present experiences. Practicing mindfulness can be as simple as noticing the taste of a mint on your tongue.

There are some things you might do every day without even thinking about them, like brushing your teeth in the morning. Mindfulness involves paying attention to the feelings and sensations of these experiences.

While researchers have not yet studied the effects of mindfulness practice in helping trauma survivors diagnosed with posttraumatic stress disorder (PTSD), research has shown mindfulness to be helpful with other anxiety problems. It has also been shown to help with symptoms of PTSD, such as avoidance and hyperarousal. If you have gone through trauma, you may want to learn what mindfulness is and how it might be helpful to you.

Mindfulness practice has two key parts:

- Paying attention to and being aware of the present moment

- Accepting or being willing to experience your thoughts and feelings without judging them

For example, focusing on the inhale and exhale of your breathing is one way to concentrate on the present moment. Mindfulness involves allowing your thoughts and feelings to pass without either clinging to them or pushing them away. You just let them take their natural course. While practicing mindfulness, you may become distracted by your thoughts and that is okay. The process is about being willing to notice where your thoughts take you, and then bringing your attention back to the present.

How Can Mindfulness Help Reduce Trauma Reactions?

Mindfulness might increase your ability to cope with difficult emotions, such as anxiety and depression. Practicing mindfulness can help you to be more focused and aware of the present moment while also being more willing to experience the difficult emotions that sometimes come up after trauma. For example, mindfulness practice might help you to notice your thoughts and feelings more and to be able to just let them go, without labeling them as "good" or "bad" and without acting on them by avoiding or behaving impulsively.

Mindfulness is a practice, a continual process. Although it may be hard to do at first, regular mindfulness practice can help you notice your thoughts and learn to take a step back from them. Mindfulness practice can also help you develop more compassion toward yourself and others. You may be less likely to sit in judgment of your thoughts, feelings, and actions. You may become less critical of yourself. Using mindfulness can help you become more aware and gentle in response to your trauma reactions. This is an important step in recovery.

Cognitive processing therapy (CPT) and prolonged exposure (PE) have been shown to be the most effective treatments for PTSD. In both of these treatments, you are asked to write or talk about trauma with the guidance of your therapist. Mindfulness can prepare you for these treatments by giving you skills and confidence that you can handle your feelings. As you learn to be mindful, you learn to observe what is happening in your body and your mind. You can learn to be more willing to cope with difficult thoughts and feelings in a healthy way. This will help you keep going when you are asked to think and talk about your trauma in treatment. In this way you may get even more out of the PTSD treatment.

There are several types of therapy that use mindfulness practices. These therapies have been used to treat problems that often affect people with PTSD, such as anxiety, depression, and substance use. The therapies may target specific problems such as:

- Difficult feelings and stress in daily living

- The stress of physical health problems, such as chronic pain

- Negative thinking patterns that can lead to repeated episodes of depression

- Trouble working towards your goals in life

- Urges to use drugs or alcohol

Mindfulness practices may be of benefit to trauma survivors. Research findings show that mindfulness can help with problems and symptoms often experienced by survivors. Mindfulness could be used by itself or together with standard treatments proven effective for PTSD.

Section 25.8

Relaxation Therapy

This section includes text excerpted from "Relaxation Techniques for Health," National Center for Complementary and Integrative Health (NCCIH), April 20, 2017.

What Are Relaxation Techniques?

Relaxation techniques include a number of practices such as progressive relaxation, guided imagery, biofeedback, self-hypnosis, and deep breathing exercises. The goal is similar in all: to produce the body's natural relaxation response, characterized by slower breathing, lower blood pressure, and a feeling of increased well-being.

Meditation and practices that include meditation with movement, such as yoga and tai chi, can also promote relaxation. Stress management programs commonly include relaxation techniques. Relaxation techniques have also been studied to see whether they might be of value in managing various health problems.

The Importance of Practice

Relaxation techniques are skills, and like other skills, they need practice. People who use relaxation techniques frequently are more likely to benefit from them. Regular, frequent practice is particularly important if you're using relaxation techniques to help manage a chronic health problem. Continuing use of relaxation techniques is more effective than short-term use.

Relaxation techniques include the following:

- Autogenic training
- Biofeedback-assisted relaxation
- Deep breathing or breathing exercises
- Guided imagery
- Progressive relaxation
- Self-hypnosis

What the Science Says about the Effectiveness of Relaxation Techniques

Researchers have evaluated relaxation techniques to see whether they could play a role in managing a variety of health conditions, including the following:

Anxiety

Studies have shown relaxation techniques may reduce anxiety in people with ongoing health problems such as heart disease or inflammatory bowel disease, and in those who are having medical procedures such as breast biopsies or dental treatment. Relaxation techniques have also been shown to be useful for older adults with anxiety.

On the other hand, relaxation techniques may not be the best way to help people with generalized anxiety disorder. Generalized anxiety disorder is a mental health condition, lasting for months or longer, in which a person is often worried or anxious about many things and finds it hard to control the anxiety. Studies indicate that long-term results are better in people with generalized anxiety disorder who receive a type of psychotherapy called cognitive behavioral therapy (CBT) than in those who are taught relaxation techniques.

Depression

An evaluation of 15 studies concluded that relaxation techniques are better than no treatment in reducing symptoms of depression but are not as beneficial as psychological therapies such as cognitive behavioral therapy.

What the Science Says about the Safety and Side Effects of Relaxation Techniques?

- Relaxation techniques are generally considered safe for healthy people. However, occasionally, people report negative experiences such as increased anxiety, intrusive thoughts, or fear of losing control.

- There have been rare reports that certain relaxation techniques might cause or worsen symptoms in people with epilepsy or certain psychiatric conditions, or with a history of abuse or trauma. People with heart disease should talk to their healthcare provider before doing progressive muscle relaxation.

Who Teaches Relaxation Techniques?

A variety of professionals, including physicians, psychologists, social workers, nurses, and complementary health practitioners, may teach relaxation techniques. Also, people sometimes learn the simpler relaxation techniques on their own.

More to Consider

- If you have severe or long-lasting symptoms of any kind, see your healthcare provider. You might have a condition that needs to be treated promptly. For example, if depression or anxiety persists, it's important to seek help from a qualified healthcare professional.

- Tell all your healthcare providers about any complementary or integrative health approaches you use. Give them a full picture of what you do to manage your health. This will help ensure coordinated and safe care.

Section 25.9

Yoga

This section includes text excerpted from "Yoga: In Depth"
National Center for Complementary and Integrative
Health (NCCIH), September 19, 2017.

Yoga is a mind and body practice with historical origins in ancient Indian philosophy. Like other meditative movement practices used for health purposes, various styles of yoga typically combine physical postures, breathing techniques, and meditation or relaxation. This section provides basic information about yoga, summarizes scientific research on effectiveness and safety.

About Yoga

Yoga in its full form combines physical postures, breathing exercises, meditation, and a distinct philosophy. There are numerous styles of yoga. Hatha yoga, commonly practiced in the United States and Europe, emphasizes postures, breathing exercises, and meditation. Hatha yoga styles include Ananda, Anusara, Ashtanga, Bikram, Iyengar, Kripalu, Kundalini, Viniyoga, and others.

Key Facts

- Recent studies in people with chronic low-back pain suggest that a carefully adapted set of yoga poses may help reduce pain and improve function (the ability to walk and move). Studies also suggest that practicing yoga (as well as other forms of regular exercise) might have other health benefits such as reducing heart rate and blood pressure, and may also help relieve anxiety and depression. Other research suggests yoga is not helpful for asthma, and studies looking at yoga and arthritis have had mixed results.

- People with high blood pressure, glaucoma, or sciatica, and women who are pregnant should modify or avoid some yoga poses.

- Ask a trusted source (such as a healthcare provider or local hospital) to recommend a yoga practitioner. Contact professional organizations for the names of practitioners who have completed an acceptable training program.

- Tell all your healthcare providers about any complementary health approaches you use. Give them a full picture of what you do to manage your health. This will help ensure coordinated and safe care.

What the Science Says about Yoga

Research suggests that a carefully adapted set of yoga poses may reduce low-back pain and improve function. Other studies also suggest that practicing yoga (as well as other forms of regular exercise) might improve quality of life; reduce stress; lower heart rate and blood pressure; help relieve anxiety, depression, and insomnia; and improve overall physical fitness, strength, and flexibility. But some research suggests yoga may not improve asthma, and studies looking at yoga and arthritis have had mixed results.

- One National Center for Complementary and Integrative Health (NCCIH)-funded study of 90 people with chronic low-back pain found that participants who practiced Iyengar yoga had significantly less disability, pain, and depression after 6 months.

- In a study funded by NCCIH, researchers compared yoga with conventional stretching exercises or a self-care book in 228 adults with chronic low-back pain. The results showed that both yoga and stretching were more effective than a self-care book for improving function and reducing symptoms due to chronic low-back pain.

- Conclusions from another study of 313 adults with chronic or recurring low-back pain suggested that 12 weekly yoga classes resulted in better function than usual medical care.

However, studies show that certain health conditions may not benefit from yoga.

- A systematic review of clinical studies suggests that there is no sound evidence that yoga improves asthma.

- A review of the literature reports that few published studies have looked at yoga and arthritis, and of those that have, results are inconclusive. The two main types of arthritis—osteoarthritis and rheumatoid arthritis—are different conditions, and the effects of yoga may not be the same for each. In addition, the reviewers suggested that even if a study showed that yoga helped osteoarthritic finger joints, it may not help osteoarthritic knee joints.

Use of Yoga for Health in the United States

- According to the National Health Interview Survey (NHIS), which included a comprehensive survey on the use of complementary health approaches by Americans, yoga is the sixth most commonly used complementary health practice among adults. According to the survey more than 13 million adults practiced yoga. The survey also found that more than 1.5 million children practiced yoga in the previous year.

- Many people who practice yoga do so to maintain their health and well-being, improve physical fitness, relieve stress, and enhance quality of life. In addition, they may be addressing specific health conditions, such as back pain, neck pain, arthritis, and anxiety.

Side Effects and Risks

- Yoga is generally low-impact and safe for healthy people when practiced appropriately under the guidance of a well-trained instructor.

- Overall, those who practice yoga have a low rate of side effects, and the risk of serious injury from yoga is quite low. However, certain types of stroke as well as pain from nerve damage are among the rare possible side effects of practicing yoga.

- Women who are pregnant and people with certain medical conditions, such as high blood pressure, glaucoma (a condition in which fluid pressure within the eye slowly increases and may damage the eye's optic nerve), and sciatica (pain, weakness, numbing, or tingling that may extend from the lower back to the calf, foot, or even the toes), should modify or avoid some yoga poses.

If You Are Considering Practicing Yoga

- Do not use yoga to replace conventional medical care or to postpone seeing a healthcare provider about pain or any other medical condition.

- If you have a medical condition, talk to your healthcare provider before starting yoga.

- Ask a trusted source (such as your healthcare provider or a nearby hospital) to recommend a yoga practitioner. Find out about the training and experience of any practitioner you are considering.

- Everyone's body is different, and yoga postures should be modified based on individual abilities. Carefully selecting an instructor who is experienced with and attentive to your needs is an important step toward helping you practice yoga safely. Ask about the physical demands of the type of yoga in which you are interested and inform your yoga instructor about any medical issues you have.

- Carefully think about the type of yoga you are interested in. For example, hot yoga (such as Bikram yoga) may involve standing and moving in humid environments with temperatures as high as 105°F. Because such settings may be physically stressful, people who practice hot yoga should take certain precautions. These include drinking water before, during, and after a hot yoga practice and wearing suitable clothing. People with conditions that may be affected by excessive heat, such as heart disease, lung disease, and a prior history of heatstroke may want to avoid this form of yoga. Women who are pregnant may want to check with their healthcare providers before starting hot yoga.

• Tell all your healthcare providers about any complementary health approaches you use. Give them a full picture of what you do to manage your health. This will help ensure coordinated and safe care.

Chapter 26

Technology and the Future of Mental Health Treatment

Technology has opened a new frontier in mental health support and data collection. Mobile devices like cell phones, smartphones, and tablets are giving the public, doctors, and researchers new ways to access help, monitor progress, and increase understanding of mental wellbeing.

Mobile mental health support can be very simple but effective. For example, anyone with the ability to send a text message can contact a crisis center (www.crisistextline.org/textline). New technology can also be packaged into an extremely sophisticated app for smartphones or tablets. Such apps might use the device's built-in sensors to collect information on a user's typical behavior patterns. If the app detects a change in behavior, it may provide a signal that help is needed before a crisis occurs. Some apps are stand-alone programs that promise to improve memory or thinking skills. Others help the user connect to a peer counselor or to a healthcare professional.

Excitement about the huge range of opportunities has led to a burst of app development. There are thousands of mental health apps

This chapter contains text excerpted from the following sources: Text in this chapter begins with excerpts from "Technology and the Future of Mental Health Treatment," National Institute of Mental Health (NIMH), February 2017; Text under the heading "Tweeting, Posting, and Downloading Health Information" is excerpted from "Health Information on the Web," U.S. Food and Drug Administration (FDA), December 16, 2016.

227

available in iTunes and Android app stores, and the number is grow-ing every year. However, this new technology frontier includes a lot of uncertainty. There is very little industry regulation and very little information on app effectiveness, which can lead consumers to wonder which apps they should trust.

Before focusing on the state of the science and where it may lead, it's important to look at the advantages and disadvantages of expanding mental health treatment and research into a mobile world.

The Pros and Cons of Mental Health Apps

Experts believe that technology has a lot of potential for clients and clinicians alike. A few of the advantages of mobile care include:

- **Convenience:** Treatment can take place anytime and any-where (e.g., at home in the middle of the night or on a bus on the way to work) and may be ideal for those who have trouble with in-person appointments.

- **Anonymity:** Clients can seek treatment options without involv-ing other people.

- **An introduction to care:** Technology may be a good first step for those who have avoided mental healthcare in the past.

- **Lower cost:** Some apps are free or cost less than traditional care.

- **Service to more people:** Technology can help mental health providers offer treatment to people in remote areas or to many people in times of sudden need (for example, following a natural disaster or terror attack).

- **Interest:** Some technologies might be more appealing than traditional treatment methods, which may encourage clients to continue therapy.

- **24-hour service:** Technology can provide round-the-clock moni-toring or intervention support.

- **Consistency:** Technology can offer the same treatment program to all users.

- **Support:** Technology can complement traditional therapy by extending an in-person session, reinforcing new skills, and pro-viding support and monitoring.

This new era of mental health technology offers great opportunities but also raises a number of concerns. Tackling potential problems will be an important part of making sure new apps provide benefits without causing harm. That is why the mental health community and software developers are focusing on:

- **Effectiveness:** The biggest concern with technological interventions is obtaining scientific evidence that they work and that they work as well as traditional methods.

- **For whom and for what:** Another concern is understanding if apps work for all people and for all mental health conditions.

- **Guidance:** There are no industry-wide standards to help consumers know if an app or other mobile technology is proven effective.

- **Privacy:** Apps deal with very sensitive personal information so app makers need to be able to guarantee privacy for app users.

- **Regulation:** The question of who will or should regulate mental health technology and the data it generates needs to be answered.

- **Overselling:** There is some concern that if an app or program promises more than it delivers, consumers may turn away from other, more effective therapies.

Current Trends in App Development

Creative research and engineering teams are combining their skills to address a wide range of mental health concerns. Some popular areas of app development include:

Self-Management Apps

"Self-management" means that the user puts information into the app so that the app can provide feedback. For example, the user might set up medication reminders, or use the app to develop tools for managing stress, anxiety, or sleep problems. Some software can use additional equipment to track heart rate, breathing patterns, blood pressure, etc., and may help the user track progress and receive feedback.

Apps for Improving Thinking Skills

Apps that help the user with cognitive remediation (improved thinking skills) are promising. These apps are often targeted toward people with serious mental illnesses.

Skill-Training Apps

Skill-training apps may feel more like games than other mental health apps as they help users learn new coping or thinking skills. The user might watch an educational video about anxiety management or the importance of social support. Next, the user might pick some new strategies to try and then use the app to track how often those new skills are practiced.

Illness Management, Supported Care

This type of app technology adds additional support by allowing the user to interact with another human being. The app may help the user connect with peer support or may send information to a trained health-care provider who can offer guidance and therapy options. Researchers are working to learn how much human interaction people need for app-based treatments to be effective.

Passive Symptom Tracking

A lot of effort is going into developing apps that can collect data using the sensors built into smartphones. These sensors can record movement patterns, social interactions (such as the number of text messages and phone calls), behavior at different times of the day, vocal tone and speed, and more. In the future, apps may be able to analyze these data to determine the user's real-time state of mind. Such apps may be able to recognize changes in behavior patterns that signal a mood episode such as mania, depression, or psychosis before it occurs. An app may not replace a mental health professional, but it may be able to alert caregivers when a client needs additional attention. The goal is to create apps that support a range of users, including those with serious mental illnesses.

Data Collection

Data collection apps can gather data without any help from the user. Receiving information from a large number of individuals at the same time can increase researchers' understanding of mental health and help them develop better interventions.

Research via Smartphone?

Dr. Patricia Areán's pioneering BRIGHTEN study, showed that research via smartphone app is already a reality. The BRIGHTEN study was remarkable because it used technology to both deliver treatment interventions and also to actually conduct the research trial. In other words, the research team used technology to recruit, screen, enroll, treat, and assess participants. BRIGHTEN was especially exciting because the study showed that technology can be an efficient way to pilot test promising new treatments, and that those treatments need to be engaging.

A New Partnership: Clinicians and Engineers

Researchers have found that interventions are most effective when people like them, are engaged, and want to continue using them. Behavioral health apps will need to combine the engineers' skills for making an app easy to use and entertaining with the clinician's skills for providing effective treatment options.

Researchers and software engineers are developing and testing apps that do everything from managing medications to teaching coping skills to predicting when someone may need more emotional help. Intervention apps may help someone give up smoking, manage symptoms, or overcome anxiety, depression, posttraumatic stress disorder (PTSD), or insomnia. While the apps are becoming more appealing and user-friendly, there still isn't a lot of information on their effectiveness.

Evaluating Apps

There are no review boards, checklists, or widely accepted rules for choosing a mental health app. Most apps do not have peer-reviewed research to support their claims, and it is unlikely that every mental health app will go through a randomized, controlled research trial to test effectiveness. One reason is that testing is a slow process and technology evolves quickly. By the time an app has been put through rigorous scientific testing, the original technology may be outdated.

Currently, there are no national standards for evaluating the effectiveness of the hundreds of mental health apps that are available. Consumers should be cautious about trusting a program. However, there are a few suggestions for finding an app that may work for you:

- Ask a trusted healthcare provider for a recommendation. Some larger providers may offer several apps and collect data on their use.

- Check to see if the app offers recommendations for what to do if symptoms get worse or if there is a psychiatric emergency.

- Decide if you want an app that is completely automated or an app that offers opportunities for contact with a trained person.

- Search for information on the app developer. Can you find helpful information about his or her credentials and experience?

- Beware of misleading logos. The National Institute of Mental Health (NIMH) has not developed and does not endorse any apps. However, some app developers have unlawfully used the NIMH logo to market their products.

- Search the PubMed database offered by National Library of Medicine (www.ncbi.nlm.nih.gov/pubmed). This resource contains articles on a wide range of research topics, including mental health app development.

- If there is no information about a particular app, check to see if it is based on a treatment that has been tested. For example, research has shown that Internet-based cognitive behavior therapy (CBT) is as effective as conventional CBT for disorders that respond well to CBT, like depression, anxiety, social phobia, and panic disorder.

- Try it. If you're interested in an app, test it for a few days and decide if it's easy to use, holds your attention, and if you want to continue using it. An app is only effective if keeps users engaged for weeks or months.

Tweeting, Posting, and Downloading Health Information

The use of social media for health communication is on the rise—both as a resource for consumers and as an outreach tool for healthcare providers.

Facebook, YouTube, Twitter, and other forms of social media provide an opportunity for consumers to share information about personal health experiences and seek information from others. Mobile apps provide a convenient way for users to track health-related information and activities; including when and what medications to take, blood sugar levels, and blood pressure, for example.

According to the Albert Einstein College of Medicine, social networks can benefit patients and caregivers in providing, among other things:

- support

- specialized knowledge from peers

- improved outcomes

However, like websites, not all social media outlets are safe and reliable. Many of the steps that should be taken to evaluate the safety and reliability of a website should also be used when using social media. For example: Is a product being offered for sale? Is the discussion about a new "miracle" treatment? Or is the source of the discussion or information unclear? Users also must be careful of medical misinformation—information that is outdated or based on word of mouth. Personal blogs and Twitter sites that discuss health matters are seldom, if ever, regulated.

Use caution when using websites and social media as a tool in your healthcare and always contact your healthcare provider before following medical advice or taking products promoted on the Internet.

Part Four

Anxiety and Other Chronic Illnesses

Chapter 27

Attention Deficit Hyperactive Disorder (ADHD)

Attention deficit hyperactivity disorder (ADHD) is a brain disorder marked by an ongoing pattern of inattention and/or hyperactivity-impulsivity that interferes with functioning or development.

- **Inattention** means a person wanders off task, lacks persistence, has difficulty sustaining focus, and is disorganized; and these problems are not due to defiance or lack of comprehension.

- **Hyperactivity** means a person seems to move about constantly, including in situations in which it is not appropriate; or excessively fidgets, taps, or talks. In adults, it may be extreme restlessness or wearing others out with constant activity.

- **Impulsivity** means a person makes hasty actions that occur in the moment without first thinking about them and that may have high potential for harm; or a desire for immediate rewards or inability to delay gratification. An impulsive person may be socially intrusive and excessively interrupt others or make important decisions without considering the long-term consequences.

This chapter contains text excerpted from the following sources: Text in this chapter begins with excerpts from "Attention Deficit Hyperactivity Disorder," National Institute of Mental Health (NIMH), March 2016; Text under the heading "Other Concerns and Conditions" is excerpted from "Attention-Deficit/Hyperactivity Disorder (ADHD)," Centers for Disease Control and Prevention (CDC), August 31, 2017.

Signs and Symptoms

Inattention and hyperactivity/impulsivity are the key behaviors of ADHD. Some people with ADHD only have problems with one of the behaviors, while others have both inattention and hyperactivity-impulsivity. Most children have the combined type of ADHD.

In preschool, the most common ADHD symptom is hyperactivity.

It is normal to have some inattention, unfocused motor activity and impulsivity, but for people with ADHD, these behaviors:

- are more severe

- occur more often

- interfere with or reduce the quality of how they functions socially, at school, or in a job

Inattention

People with symptoms of inattention may often:

- Overlook or miss details, make careless mistakes in schoolwork, at work, or during other activities

- Have problems sustaining attention in tasks or play, including conversations, lectures, or lengthy reading

- Not seem to listen when spoken to directly

- Not follow through on instructions and fail to finish schoolwork, chores, or duties in the workplace or start tasks but quickly lose focus and get easily sidetracked

- Have problems organizing tasks and activities, such as what to do in sequence, keeping materials and belongings in order, having messy work and poor time management, and failing to meet deadlines

- Avoid or dislike tasks that require sustained mental effort, such as schoolwork or homework, or for teens and older adults, preparing reports, completing forms or reviewing lengthy papers

- Lose things necessary for tasks or activities, such as school supplies, pencils, books, tools, wallets, keys, paperwork, eyeglasses, and cell phones

- Be easily distracted by unrelated thoughts or stimuli

- Be forgetful in daily activities, such as chores, errands, returning calls, and keeping appointments

Hyperactivity-Impulsivity

People with symptoms of hyperactivity-impulsivity may often:

- Fidget and squirm in their seats

- Leave their seats in situations when staying seated is expected, such as in the classroom or in the office

- Run or dash around or climb in situations where it is inappropriate or, in teens and adults, often feel restless

- Be unable to play or engage in hobbies quietly

- Be constantly in motion or "on the go," or act as if "driven by a motor"

- Talk nonstop

- Blurt out an answer before a question has been completed, finish other people's sentences, or speak without waiting for a turn in conversation

- Have trouble waiting his or her turn

- Interrupt or intrude on others, for example in conversations, games, or activities

Diagnosis of ADHD requires a comprehensive evaluation by a licensed clinician, such as a pediatrician, psychologist, or psychiatrist with expertise in ADHD. For a person to receive a diagnosis of ADHD, the symptoms of inattention and/or hyperactivity-impulsivity must be chronic or long-lasting, impair the person's functioning, and cause the person to fall behind normal development for his or her age. The doctor will also ensure that any ADHD symptoms are not due to another medical or psychiatric condition. Most children with ADHD receive a diagnosis during the elementary school years. For an adolescent or adult to receive a diagnosis of ADHD, the symptoms need to have been present prior to age 12.

ADHD symptoms can appear as early as between the ages of 3 and 6 and can continue through adolescence and adulthood. Symptoms of ADHD can be mistaken for emotional or disciplinary problems or missed entirely in quiet, well-behaved children, leading to a delay in diagnosis. Adults with undiagnosed ADHD may have a history of poor academic performance, problems at work, or difficult or failed relationships.

ADHD symptoms can change over time as a person ages. In young children with ADHD, hyperactivity-impulsivity is the most predominant symptom. As a child reaches elementary school, the symptom of inattention may become more prominent and cause the child to struggle academically. In adolescence, hyperactivity seems to lessen and may show more often as feelings of restlessness or fidgeting, but inattention and impulsivity may remain. Many adolescents with ADHD also struggle with relationships and antisocial behaviors. Inattention, restlessness, and impulsivity tend to persist into adulthood.

Risk Factors

Scientists are not sure what causes ADHD. Like many other illnesses, a number of factors can contribute to ADHD, such as:

- Genes

- Cigarette smoking, alcohol use, or drug use during pregnancy

- Exposure to environmental toxins during pregnancy

- Exposure to environmental toxins, such as high levels of lead, at a young age

- Low birth weight

- Brain injuries

ADHD is more common in males than females, and females with ADHD are more likely to have problems primarily with inattention. Other conditions, such as learning disabilities, anxiety disorder, conduct disorder, depression, and substance abuse, are common in people with ADHD.

Treatment and Therapies

While there is no cure for ADHD, currently available treatments can help reduce symptoms and improve functioning. Treatments include medication, psychotherapy, education or training, or a combination of treatments.

Medication

For many people, ADHD medications reduce hyperactivity and impulsivity and improve their ability to focus, work, and learn. Medication also may improve physical coordination. Sometimes several different medications or dosages must be tried before finding the right one that works for a particular person. Anyone taking medications must be monitored closely and carefully by their prescribing doctor.

Stimulants

The most common type of medication used for treating ADHD is called a "stimulant." Although it may seem unusual to treat ADHD with a medication that is considered a stimulant, it works because it increases the brain chemicals dopamine and norepinephrine, which play essential roles in thinking and attention.

Under medical supervision, stimulant medications are considered safe. However, there are risks and side effects, especially when misused or taken in excess of the prescribed dose. For example, stimulants can raise blood pressure and heart rate and increase anxiety. Therefore, a person with other health problems, including high blood pressure, seizures, heart disease, glaucoma, liver or kidney disease, or an anxiety disorder should tell their doctor before taking a stimulant.

Talk with a doctor if you see any of these side effects while taking stimulants:

- decreased appetite
- sleep problems
- tics (sudden, repetitive movements or sounds);
- personality changes
- increased anxiety and irritability
- stomachaches
- headaches

Nonstimulants

A few other ADHD medications are nonstimulants. These medications take longer to start working than stimulants, but can also improve focus, attention, and impulsivity in a person with ADHD. Doctors may prescribe a nonstimulant: when a person has bothersome side effects from stimulants; when a stimulant was not effective; or in combination with a stimulant to increase effectiveness.

Although not approved by the U.S. Food and Drug Administration (FDA) specifically for the treatment of ADHD, some antidepressants are sometimes used alone or in combination with a stimulant to treat ADHD. Antidepressants may help all of the symptoms of ADHD and can be prescribed if a patient has bothersome side effects from stimulants. Antidepressants can be helpful in combination with stimulants if a patient also has another condition, such as an anxiety disorder, depression, or another mood disorder.

Doctors and patients can work together to find the best medication, dose, or medication combination.

Psychotherapy

Adding psychotherapy to treat ADHD can help patients and their families to better cope with everyday problems.

Behavioral therapy is a type of psychotherapy that aims to help a person change his or her behavior. It might involve practical assistance, such as help organizing tasks or completing schoolwork, or working through emotionally difficult events. Behavioral therapy also teaches a person how to:

- monitor his or her own behavior

- give oneself praise or rewards for acting in a desired way, such as controlling anger or thinking before acting

Parents, teachers, and family members also can give positive or negative feedback for certain behaviors and help establish clear rules, chore lists, and other structured routines to help a person control his or her behavior. Therapists may also teach children social skills, such as how to wait their turn, share toys, ask for help, or respond to teasing. Learning to read facial expressions and the tone of voice in others, and how to respond appropriately can also be part of social skills training.

Cognitive behavioral therapy (CBT) can also teach a person mindfulness techniques, or meditation. A person learns how to be aware and accepting of one's own thoughts and feelings to improve focus and concentration. The therapist also encourages the person with ADHD to adjust to the life changes that come with treatment, such as thinking before acting, or resisting the urge to take unnecessary risks.

Family and marital therapy can help family members and spouses find better ways to handle disruptive behaviors, to encourage behavior changes, and improve interactions with the patient.

Education and Training

Children and adults with ADHD need guidance and understanding from their parents, families, and teachers to reach their full potential and to succeed. For school-age children, frustration, blame, and anger may have built up within a family before a child is diagnosed. Parents and children may need special help to overcome negative feelings. Mental health professionals can educate parents about ADHD and how it affects a family. They also will help the child and his or her parents develop new skills, attitudes, and ways of relating to each other.

Parenting skills training (behavioral parent management training) teaches parents the skills they need to encourage and reward positive behaviors in their children. It helps parents learn how to use a system of rewards and consequences to change a child's behavior. Parents are taught to give immediate and positive feedback for behaviors they want to encourage, and ignore or redirect behaviors that they want to discourage. They may also learn to structure situations in ways that support desired behavior.

Stress management techniques can benefit parents of children with ADHD by increasing their ability to deal with frustration so that they can respond calmly to their child's behavior.

Support groups can help parents and families connect with others who have similar problems and concerns. Groups often meet regularly to share frustrations and successes, to exchange information about recommended specialists and strategies, and to talk with experts.

Tips to Help Kids and Adults with ADHD Stay Organized

For Kids

Parents and teachers can help kids with ADHD stay organized and follow directions with tools such as:

- **Keeping a routine and a schedule.** Keep the same routine every day, from wake-up time to bedtime. Include times for homework, outdoor play, and indoor activities. Keep the schedule on the refrigerator or on a bulletin board in the kitchen. Write changes on the schedule as far in advance as possible.

- **Organizing everyday items.** Have a place for everything, and keep everything in its place. This includes clothing, backpacks, and toys.

- **Using homework and notebook organizers.** Use organizers for school material and supplies. Stress to your child the importance of writing down assignments and bringing home the necessary books.

- **Being clear and consistent.** Children with ADHD need consistent rules they can understand and follow.

- **Giving praise or rewards when rules are followed.** Children with ADHD often receive and expect criticism. Look for good behavior, and praise it.

For Adults

A professional counselor or therapist can help an adult with ADHD learn how to organize his or her life with tools such as:

- Keeping routines

- Making lists for different tasks and activities

- Using a calendar for scheduling events

- Using reminder notes

- Assigning a special place for keys, bills, and paperwork

- Breaking down large tasks into more manageable, smaller steps so that completing each part of the task provides a sense of accomplishment.

Other Concerns and Conditions

Attention deficit hyperactivity disorder (ADHD) often occurs with other disorders. About half of children with ADHD referred to clinics have other disorders as well as ADHD.

The combination of ADHD with other disorders often presents extra challenges for children, parents, educators, and healthcare providers. Therefore, it is important for doctors to screen every child with ADHD for other disorders and problems.

- Behavior or conduct problems

- Learning disorder

- Anxiety and depression

- Difficult peer relationships

- Risk of injuries

Chapter 28

Bipolar Disorder

Bipolar disorder, also known as manic-depressive illness, is a brain disorder that causes unusual shifts in mood, energy, activity levels, and the ability to carry out day-to-day tasks.

There are four basic types of bipolar disorder; all of them involve clear changes in mood, energy, and activity levels. These moods range from periods of extremely "up," elated, and energized behavior (known as manic episodes) to very sad, "down," or hopeless periods (known as depressive episodes). Less severe manic periods are known as hypomanic episodes.

- **Bipolar I disorder**—defined by manic episodes that last at least 7 days, or by manic symptoms that are so severe that the person needs immediate hospital care. Usually, depressive episodes occur as well, typically lasting at least 2 weeks. Episodes of depression with mixed features (having depression and manic symptoms at the same time) are also possible.

- **Bipolar II disorder**—defined by a pattern of depressive episodes and hypomanic episodes, but not the full-blown manic episodes described above.

This chapter contains text excerpted from the following sources: Text in this chapter begins with excerpts from "Bipolar Disorder," National Institute of Mental Health (NIMH), April 2016; Text under the heading "How Does Bipolar Disorder Affect Parents and Family?" is excerpted from "Bipolar Disorders in Children and Teens," National Institute of Mental Health (NIMH), 2015.

- **Cyclothymic disorder (also called cyclothymia)**—defined by numerous periods of hypomanic symptoms as well numerous periods of depressive symptoms lasting for at least 2 years (1 year in children and adolescents). However, the symptoms do not meet the diagnostic requirements for a hypomanic episode and a depressive episode.

- **Other specified and unspecified bipolar and related disorders**—defined by bipolar disorder symptoms that do not match the three categories listed above.

Signs and Symptoms

People with bipolar disorder experience periods of unusually intense emotion, changes in sleep patterns and activity levels, and unusual behaviors. These distinct periods are called "mood episodes." Mood episodes are drastically different from the moods and behaviors that are typical for the person. Extreme changes in energy, activity, and sleep go along with mood episodes.

Table 28.1. Manic Symptoms versus Depressive Symptoms

People Having a Manic Episode May:	People Having a Depressive Episode May:
Feel very "up," "high," or related	Feel very sad, down, empty, or hopeless
Have a lot of energy	Have very little energy
Have increased activity levels	Have decreased activity levels
Feel "jumpy" or "wired"	Have trouble sleeping, they may sleep too little or too much
Have trouble sleeping	Feel like they can't enjoy anything
Become more active than usual	Feel worried and empty
Talk really fast about a lot of different things	Have trouble concentrating
Be agitated, irritable, or "touchy"	Forget things a lot
Feel like their thoughts are going very fast	Eat too much or too little
Think they can do a lot of things at once	Feel tired or "slowed down"
Do risky things, like spend a lot of money or have reckless sex	Think about death or suicide

Bipolar disorder can be present even when mood swings are less extreme. For example, some people with bipolar disorder experience hypomania, a less severe form of mania. During a hypomanic episode, an individual may feel very good, be highly productive, and function well. The person may not feel that anything is wrong, but family and friends may recognize the mood swings and/or changes in activity levels as possible bipolar disorder. Without proper treatment, people with hypomania may develop severe mania or depression. Sometimes a mood episode includes symptoms of both manic and depressive symptoms. This is called an episode with mixed features. People experiencing an episode with mixed features may feel very sad, empty, or hopeless, while at the same time feeling extremely energized.

Diagnosis

Proper diagnosis and treatment help people with bipolar disorder lead healthy and productive lives. Talking with a doctor or other licensed mental health professional is the first step for anyone who thinks he or she may have bipolar disorder. The doctor can complete a physical exam to rule out other conditions. If the problems are not caused by other illnesses, the doctor may conduct a mental health evaluation or provide a referral to a trained mental health professional, such as a psychiatrist, who is experienced in diagnosing and treating bipolar disorder.

Bipolar Disorder and Other Illnesses

Some bipolar disorder symptoms are similar to other illnesses, which can make it hard for a doctor to make a diagnosis. In addition, many people have bipolar disorder along with another illness such as anxiety disorder, substance abuse, or an eating disorder. People with bipolar disorder are also at higher risk for thyroid disease, migraine headaches, heart disease, diabetes, obesity, and other physical illnesses.

Psychosis: Sometimes, a person with severe episodes of mania or depression also has psychotic symptoms, such as hallucinations or delusions. The psychotic symptoms tend to match the person's extreme mood. For example:

- Someone having psychotic symptoms during a manic episode may believe she is famous, has a lot of money, or has special powers.

- Someone having psychotic symptoms during a depressive episode may believe he is ruined and penniless, or that he has committed a crime.

As a result, people with bipolar disorder who also have psychotic symptoms are sometimes misdiagnosed with schizophrenia.

Anxiety and ADHD: Anxiety disorders and attention deficit hyperactivity disorder (ADHD) are often diagnosed among people with bipolar disorder.

Substance abuse: People with bipolar disorder may also misuse alcohol or drugs, have relationship problems, or perform poorly in school or at work. Family, friends, and people experiencing symptoms may not recognize these problems as signs of a major mental illness such as bipolar disorder.

Risk Factors

Scientists are studying the possible causes of bipolar disorder. Most agree that there is no single cause. Instead, it is likely that many factors contribute to the illness or increase risk.

Brain Structure and Functioning

Some studies show how the brains of people with bipolar disorder may differ from the brains of healthy people or people with other mental disorders. Learning more about these differences, along with new information from genetic studies, helps scientists better understand bipolar disorder and predict which types of treatment will work most effectively.

Genetics

Some research suggests that people with certain genes are more likely to develop bipolar disorder than others. But genes are not the only risk factor for bipolar disorder. Studies of identical twins have shown that even if one twin develops bipolar disorder, the other twin does not always develop the disorder, despite the fact that identical twins share all of the same genes.

Family History

Bipolar disorder tends to run in families. Children with a parent or sibling who has bipolar disorder are much more likely to develop the illness, compared with children who do not have a family history of the disorder. However, it is important to note that most people with a family history of bipolar disorder will not develop the illness.

Treatments and Therapies

Treatment helps many people—even those with the most severe forms of bipolar disorder—gain better control of their mood swings and other bipolar symptoms. An effective treatment plan usually includes a combination of medication and psychotherapy (also called "talk therapy"). Bipolar disorder is a lifelong illness. Episodes of mania and depression typically come back over time. Between episodes, many people with bipolar disorder are free of mood changes, but some people may have lingering symptoms. Long-term, continuous treatment helps to control these symptoms.

Medications

Different types of medications can help control symptoms of bipolar disorder. An individual may need to try several different medications before finding ones that work best.

Medications generally used to treat bipolar disorder include:

- Mood stabilizers

- Atypical antipsychotics

- Antidepressants

Anyone taking a medication should:

- Talk with a doctor or a pharmacist to understand the risks and benefits of the medication

- Report any concerns about side effects to a doctor right away. The doctor may need to change the dose or try a different medication.

- Avoid stopping a medication without talking to a doctor first. Suddenly stopping a medication may lead to "rebound" or worsening of bipolar disorder symptoms. Other uncomfortable or potentially dangerous withdrawal effects are also possible.

Psychotherapy

When done in combination with medication, psychotherapy (also called "talk therapy") can be an effective treatment for bipolar disorder. It can provide support, education, and guidance to people with bipolar disorder and their families. Some psychotherapy treatments used to treat bipolar disorder include:

- Cognitive behavioral therapy (CBT)
- Family-focused therapy
- Interpersonal and social rhythm therapy
- Psychoeducation

Other Treatment Options

Electroconvulsive Therapy (ECT)

ECT can provide relief for people with severe bipolar disorder who have not been able to recover with other treatments. Sometimes ECT is used for bipolar symptoms when other medical conditions, including pregnancy, make taking medications too risky. ECT may cause some short-term side effects, including confusion, disorientation, and memory loss. People with bipolar disorder should discuss possible benefits and risks of ECT with a qualified health professional.

Sleep Medications

People with bipolar disorder who have trouble sleeping usually find that treatment is helpful. However, if sleeplessness does not improve, a doctor may suggest a change in medications. If the problem continues, the doctor may prescribe sedatives or other sleep medications.

Supplements

Not much research has been conducted on herbal or natural supplements and how they may affect bipolar disorder.

It is important for a doctor to know about all prescription drugs, over-the-counter medications, and supplements a client is taking. Certain medications and supplements taken together may cause unwanted or dangerous effects.

Keeping a Life Chart

Even with proper treatment, mood changes can occur. Treatment is more effective when a client and doctor work closely together and talk openly about concerns and choices. Keeping a life chart that records daily mood symptoms, treatments, sleep patterns, and life events can help clients and doctors track and treat bipolar disorder most effectively.

How Does Bipolar Disorder Affect Family?

Taking care of a child or teenager with bipolar disorder can be stressful for you, too. You have to cope with the mood swings and other problems, such as short tempers and risky activities. This can challenge any parent. Sometimes the stress can strain your relationships with other people, and you may miss work or lose free time.

If you are taking care of a child with bipolar disorder, take care of yourself too. Find someone you can talk to about your feelings. Talk with the doctor about support groups for caregivers. If you keep your stress level down, you will do a better job. It might help your child get better too.

How Does Regular Exercise Affect Family?

Chapter 29

Body Dysmorphic Disorder (BDD)

What Is Body Dysmorphic Disorder (BDD)?

BDD is a severe, often chronic, and common disorder consisting of distressing or impairing preoccupation with perceived defects in one's physical appearance. Individuals with BDD have very poor psychosocial functioning and high rates of hospitalization and suicidality. Because BDD differs in important ways from other disorders, psychotherapies for other disorders are not adequate for BDD. Despite BDD's severity, there is no adequately tested psychosocial treatment (psychotherapy) of any type for this disorder.

Symptoms of BDD

- Being preoccupied with minor or imaginary physical flaws, usually of the skin, hair, and nose, such as acne, scarring, facial

This chapter contains text excerpted from the following sources: Text under the heading "What Is Body Dysmorphic Disorder (BDD)?" is excerpted from "Cognitive Behavioral Therapy and Supportive Psychotherapy for Body Dysmorphic Disorder," ClinicalTrials.gov, National Institutes of Health (NIH), March 15, 2016; Text beginning with the heading "Symptoms of BDD" is excerpted from "Body Image—Cosmetic Surgery," Office on Women's Health (OWH), U.S. Department of Health and Human Services (HHS), September 22, 2009. Reviewed September 2017.

lines, marks, pale skin, thinning hair, excessive body hair, large nose, or crooked nose.

- Having a lot of anxiety and stress about the perceived flaw and spending a lot of time focusing on it, such as frequently picking at skin, excessively checking appearance in a mirror, hiding the imperfection, comparing appearance with others, excessively grooming, seeking reassurance from others about how they look, and getting cosmetic surgery.

Getting cosmetic surgery can make BDD worse. They are often not happy with the outcome of the surgery. If they are, they may start to focus attention on another body area and become preoccupied trying to fix the new "defect." In this case, some patients with BDD become angry at the surgeon for making their appearance worse and may even become violent towards the surgeon.

Treatment for BDD

- **Medications.** Serotonin reuptake inhibitors or SSRIs are antidepressants that decrease the obsessive and compulsive behaviors.
- **Cognitive behavioral therapy.** This is a type of therapy with several steps:
  - The therapist asks the patient to enter social situations without covering up her "defect."
  - The therapist helps the patient stop doing the compulsive behaviors to check the defect or cover it up. This may include removing mirrors, covering skin areas that the patient picks, or not using make-up.
  - The therapist helps the patient change their false beliefs about their appearance.

Chapter 30

Borderline Personality Disorder

Borderline personality disorder (BPD) is a serious mental disorder marked by a pattern of ongoing instability in moods, behavior, self-image, and functioning. These experiences often result in impulsive actions and unstable relationships. A person with BPD may experience intense episodes of anger, depression, and anxiety that may last from only a few hours to days.

Some people with BPD also have high rates of co-occurring mental disorders, such as mood disorders, anxiety disorders, and eating disorders, along with substance abuse, self-harm, suicidal thinking and behaviors, and suicide.

While mental health experts now generally agree that the label "borderline personality disorder" is very misleading, a more accurate term does not exist yet.

Signs and Symptoms

People with BPD may experience extreme mood swings and can display uncertainty about who they are. As a result, their interests and values can change rapidly.

Other symptoms include:

- Frantic efforts to avoid real or imagined abandonment

This chapter includes text excerpted from "Borderline Personality Disorder," National Institute of Mental Health (NIMH), August 2016.

- A pattern of intense and unstable relationships with family, friends, and loved ones, often swinging from extreme closeness and love (idealization) to extreme dislike or anger (devaluation)

- Distorted and unstable self-image or sense of self

- Impulsive and often dangerous behaviors, such as spending sprees, unsafe sex, substance abuse, reckless driving, and binge eating

- Recurring suicidal behaviors or threats or self-harming behavior, such as cutting

- Intense and highly changeable moods, with each episode lasting from a few hours to a few days

- Chronic feelings of emptiness

- Inappropriate, intense anger or problems controlling anger

- Having stress-related paranoid thoughts

- Having severe dissociative symptoms, such as feeling cut off from oneself, observing oneself from outside the body, or losing touch with reality

Seemingly ordinary events may trigger symptoms. For example, people with BPD may feel angry and distressed over minor separations—such as vacations, business trips, or sudden changes of plans—from people to whom they feel close. Studies show that people with this disorder may see anger in an emotionally neutral face and have a stronger reaction to words with negative meanings than people who do not have the disorder.

Some of these signs and symptoms may be experienced by people with other mental health problems—and even by people without mental illness—and do not necessarily mean that they have BPD. It is important that a qualified and licensed mental health professional conduct a thorough assessment to determine whether or not a diagnosis of BPD or other mental disorder is warranted, and to help guide treatment options when appropriate.

Risk Factors

The causes of BPD are not yet clear, but research suggests that genetic, brain, environmental and social factors are likely to be involved.

- **Genetics.** BPD is about five times more likely to occur if a person has a close family member (first-degree biological relatives) with the disorder.

- **Environmental and Social Factors.** Many people with BPD report experiencing traumatic life events, such as abuse or abandonment during childhood. Others may have been exposed to unstable relationships and hostile conflicts. However, some people with BPD do not have a history of trauma. And, many people with a history of traumatic life events do not have BPD.

- **Brain Factors.** Studies show that people with BPD have structural and functional changes in the brain, especially in the areas that control impulses and emotional regulation. However, some people with similar changes in the brain do not have BPD. More research is needed to understand the relationship between brain structure and function and BPD.

Research on BPD is focused on examining biological and environmental risk factors, with special attention on whether early symptoms may emerge at a younger age than previously thought. Scientists are also studying ways to identify the disorder earlier in adolescents.

Tests and Diagnosis

Unfortunately, BPD is often underdiagnosed or misdiagnosed.

A licensed mental health professional experienced in diagnosing and treating mental disorders—such as a psychiatrist, psychologist, or clinical social worker—can diagnose BPD based on a thorough interview and a comprehensive medical exam, which can help rule out other possible causes of symptoms.

The licensed mental health professional may ask about symptoms and personal and family medical histories, including any history of mental illnesses. This information can help the mental health professional decide on the best treatment. In some cases, co-occurring mental illnesses may have symptoms that overlap with BPD, making it difficult to distinguish BPD from other mental illnesses. For example, a person may describe feelings of depression but may not bring other symptoms to the mental health professional's attention.

Treatments and Therapies

BPD has historically been viewed as difficult to treat. However, with newer and proper treatment, many people with BPD experience fewer or less severe symptoms and an improved quality of life. Many factors affect the length of time it takes for symptoms to improve once treatment begins, so it is important for people with BPD and their loved ones to be patient and to receive appropriate support during treatment. People with BPD can recover.

If You Think You Have BPD, It Is Important to Seek Treatment.

NIMH-funded studies indicate that BPD patients who never recovered may be more likely to develop other chronic medical conditions and are less likely to make healthy lifestyle choices. BPD is also associated with a high rate of self-harm and suicidal behavior.

If you are thinking about harming yourself or attempting suicide, tell someone who can help right away. Call your licensed mental health professional if you are already working with one. If you are not already working with a licensed mental health professional, call your personal physician or go to the nearest hospital emergency room.

If a loved one is considering suicide, do not leave him or her alone. Try to get your loved one to seek immediate help from his or her doctor or the nearest hospital emergency room, or call 911. Remove any access he or she may have to firearms or other potential tools for suicide, including medications, sharp edges such as knives, ropes, or belts.

If you or a loved one are in crisis: Call the toll-free National Suicide Prevention Lifeline (NSPL) at 800-273-TALK (800-273-8255), available 24 hours a day, 7 days a week. The service is available to anyone. All calls are confidential.

The treatments described below are just some of the options that may be available to a person with BPD. However, the research on treatments is still in very early stages. More research is needed to determine the effectiveness of these treatments, who may benefit the most, and how best to deliver treatments.

Psychotherapy

Psychotherapy (or "talk therapy") is the main treatment for people with BPD. Current research suggests psychotherapy can relieve some symptoms, but further studies are needed to better understand how well psychotherapy works.

Psychotherapy can be provided one-on-one between the therapist and the patient or in a group setting. Therapist-led group sessions may help teach people with BPD how to interact with others and how to express themselves effectively. It is important that people in therapy get along with and trust their therapist. The very nature of BPD can make it difficult for people with this disorder to maintain a comfortable and trusting bond with their therapist.

Types of psychotherapy used to treat BPD include:

- **Cognitive behavioral therapy (CBT):** CBT can help people with BPD identify and change core beliefs and/or behaviors that underlie inaccurate perceptions of themselves and others and problems interacting with others. CBT may help reduce a range of mood and anxiety symptoms and reduce the number of suicidal or self-harming behaviors.

- **Dialectical behavior therapy (DBT):** This type of therapy utilizes the concept of mindfulness, or being aware of and attentive to the current situation and moods. DBT also teaches skills to control intense emotions, reduce self-destructive behaviors, and improve relationships. DBT differs from CBT in that it integrates traditional CBT elements with mindfulness, acceptance, and techniques to improve a person's ability to tolerate stress and control his or her emotions. DBT recognizes the dialectical tension between the need for acceptance and the need for change.

- **Schema-focused therapy:** This type of therapy combines elements of CBT with other forms of psychotherapy that focus on reframing schemas, or the ways people view themselves. This approach is based on the idea that BPD stems from a dysfunctional self-image—possibly brought on by negative childhood experiences—that affects how people react to their environment, interact with others, and cope with problems or stress.

- **Systems training for emotional predictability and problem solving (STEPPS)** is a type of group therapy that aims to educate family members, significant others, and healthcare professionals about BPD and gives them guidance on how to interact consistently with the person with the disorder using the STEPPS approach and terminology. STEPPS is designed to supplement other treatments the patient may be receiving, such as medication or individual psychotherapy.

Families of people with BPD may also benefit from therapy. The challenges of dealing with a loved one with BPD on a daily basis can be very stressful, and family members may unknowingly act in ways that worsen their relative's symptoms. Some therapies include family members in treatment sessions. These types of programs help families develop skills to better understand and support a relative with BPD. Other therapies focus on the needs of family members and help them understand the obstacles and strategies for caring for a loved one with BPD. Although more research is needed to determine the effectiveness of family therapy in BPD, studies on other mental disorders suggest that including family members can help in a person's treatment.

Other types of psychotherapy may be helpful for some people with BPD. Therapists often adapt psychotherapy to better meet a person's needs. Therapists may also switch from one type of psychotherapy to another, mix techniques from different therapies, or use a combination of psychotherapies.

Medications

Medications should not be used as the primary treatment for BPD as the benefits are unclear. However, in some cases, a mental health professional may recommend medications to treat specific symptoms, such as mood swings, depression, or other disorders that may occur with BPD. Treatment with medications may require care from more than one medical professional.

Because of the high risk of suicide among people with BPD, health-care providers should exercise caution when prescribing medications that may be lethal in the event of an overdose.

Certain medications can cause different side effects in different people. Talk to your doctor about what to expect from a particular medication.

Other Treatments

Some people with BPD experience severe symptoms and require intensive, often inpatient, care. Others may use some outpatient treatments but never need hospitalization or emergency care. Although in rare cases, some people who develop this disorder may improve without any treatment, most people benefit from and improve their quality of life by seeking treatment.

How Can I Help a Friend or Relative Who Has BPD?

If you know someone who has BPD, it affects you too. The first and most important thing you can do is help your friend or relative get the right diagnosis and treatment. You may need to make an appointment and go with your friend or relative to see the doctor. Encourage him or her to stay in treatment or to seek different treatment if symptoms do not appear to improve with the current treatment.

To help a friend or relative you can:

- Offer emotional support, understanding, patience, and encouragement—change can be difficult and frightening to people with BPD, but it is possible for them to get better over time.

- Learn about mental disorders, including BPD, so you can understand what your friend or relative is experiencing.

- With written permission from your friend or loved one, talk with his or her therapist to learn about therapies that may involve family members. Alternatively, you can encourage your loved one who is in treatment for BPD to ask about family therapy.

- Seek counseling from your own therapist about helping a loved one with BPD. It should not be the same therapist that your loved one with BPD is seeing.

Never ignore comments about someone's intent or plan to harm himself or herself or someone else. Report such comments to the person's therapist or doctor. In urgent or potentially life-threatening situations, you may need to call the police or dial 911.

How Can I Help Myself If I Have BPD?

Although it may take some time, you can get better with treatment. To help yourself:

- Talk to your doctor about treatment options and stick with treatment.

- Try to maintain a stable schedule of meals and sleep times.

- Engage in mild activity or exercise to help reduce stress.

- Set realistic goals for yourself.

- Break up large tasks into small ones, set some priorities, and do what you can, as you can.

- Try to spend time with other people and confide in a trusted friend or family member.

- Tell others about events or situations that may trigger symptoms.

- Expect your symptoms to improve gradually over time, not immediately. Be patient.

- Identify and seek out comforting situations, places, and people.

- Continue to educate yourself about this disorder.

- Don't drink alcohol or use illicit drugs—they will likely make things worse.

Chapter 31

Cancer

Anxiety disorders are very strong fears that may be caused by physical or psychological stress. Studies show that almost half of all patients with cancer say they feel some anxiety and about one-fourth of all patients with cancer say they feel a great deal of anxiety. Patients living with cancer find that they feel more or less anxiety at different times. A patient may become more anxious as cancer spreads or treatment becomes more intense. For some patients, feelings of anxiety may become overwhelming and affect cancer treatment. This is especially true for patients who had periods of intense anxiety before their cancer diagnosis. Most patients who did not have an anxiety condition before their cancer diagnosis will not have an anxiety disorder related to the cancer.

Anxiety during Cancer Treatment

Patients are more likely to have anxiety disorders during cancer treatment if they have any of the following:

- A history of an anxiety disorder.

- A history of physical or emotional trauma.

- Anxiety at the time of diagnosis.

This chapter includes text excerpted from "Adjustment to Cancer: Anxiety and Distress (PDQ®)—Patient Version," National Cancer Institute (NCI), January 7, 2015.

- Few family members or friends to give them emotional support.

- Pain that is not controlled well.

- Cancer that is not getting better with treatment.

- Trouble taking care of their personal needs such as bathing or eating.

- Anxiety disorders may be hard to diagnose.

Symptoms of Anxiety during Cancer Treatment

It may be hard to tell the difference between normal fears related to cancer and abnormally severe fears that can be described as an anxiety disorder. The diagnosis is based on how symptoms of anxiety affect the patient's quality of life, what kinds of symptoms began since the cancer diagnosis or treatment, when the symptoms occur, and how long they last.

Anxiety disorders cause serious symptoms that affect day-to-day life, including:

- Feeling worried all the time.

- Not being able to focus.

- Not being able to "turn off thoughts" most of the time.

- Trouble sleeping most nights.

- Frequent crying spells.

- Feeling afraid most of the time.

- Having symptoms such as fast heartbeat, dry mouth, shaky hands, restlessness, or feeling on edge.

- Anxiety that is not relieved by the usual ways to lessen anxiety such as distraction by staying busy.

Causes of Anxiety Disorders in Cancer Patients

There are different causes of anxiety disorders in cancer patients.

In addition to anxiety caused by a cancer diagnosis, the following may cause anxiety in patients with cancer:

- **Pain:** Patients whose pain is not well controlled with medicine feel anxious, and anxiety can increase pain.

- **Other medical problems:** Anxiety may be a warning sign of a change in metabolism (such as low blood sugar), a heart attack, severe infection, pneumonia, or a blood clot in the lung. Sepsis and electrolyte imbalances can also cause anxiety.

- **Certain types of tumors:** Certain hormone-releasing tumors can cause symptoms of anxiety and panic attacks. Tumors that have spread to the brain and spinal cord and tumors in the lungs can cause other health problems with symptoms of anxiety.

- **Taking certain drugs:** Certain types of drugs, including corticosteroids, thyroxine, bronchodilators, and antihistamines, can cause restlessness, agitation, or anxiety.

- **Withdrawing from habit-forming drugs:** Withdrawal from alcohol, nicotine, opioids, or antidepressant medicine can cause agitation or anxiety.

Anxiety from these causes is usually managed by treating the cause itself. A cancer diagnosis may cause anxiety disorders to come back in patients with a history of them. When patients who had an anxiety disorder in the past are diagnosed with cancer, then the anxiety disorder may come back. These patients may feel extreme fear, be unable to remember information given to them by caregivers, or be unable to follow through with medical tests and procedures. They may have symptoms including:

- Shortness of breath

- Sweating

- Feeling faint

- Fast heart beat

Anxiety Types Prevalent among Cancer Patients

Patients with cancer may have the following types of anxiety disorders:

Phobia

Phobias are fears about a situation or an object that lasts over time. People with phobias usually feel intense anxiety and avoid the situation or object they are afraid of. For example, patients with a phobia of small spaces may avoid having tests in small spaces, such as magnetic resonance imaging (MRI) scans.

Phobias may make it hard for patients to follow through with tests and procedures or treatment. Phobias are treated by professionals and include different kinds of therapy.

Panic Disorder

Patients with panic disorder feel sudden intense anxiety, known as panic attacks. Symptoms of panic disorder include the following:

- Shortness of breath

- Feeling dizzy

- Fast heart beat

- Shaking

- Heavy sweating

- Feeling sick to the stomach

- Tingling of the skin

- Being afraid they are having a heart attack

- Being afraid they are "going crazy"

A panic attack may last for several minutes or longer. There may be feelings of discomfort that last for several hours after the attack. Panic attacks are treated with medicine and talk therapy.

Obsessive-Compulsive Disorder (OCD)

Obsessive-compulsive disorder is rare in patients with cancer who did not have the disorder before being diagnosed with cancer. Obsessive-compulsive disorder is diagnosed when a person uses persistent (obsessive) thoughts, ideas, or images and compulsions (repetitive behaviors) to manage feelings of distress. The obsessions and compulsions affect the person's ability to work, go to school, or be in social situations. Examples of compulsions include frequent hand washing or constantly checking to make sure a door is locked. Patients with obsessive-compulsive disorder may be unable to follow through with cancer treatment because of these thoughts and behaviors. Obsessive-compulsive disorder is treated with medicine and individual (one-to-one) counseling.

Generalized Anxiety Disorder (GAD)

Patients with generalized anxiety disorder may feel extreme and constant anxiety or worry. For example, patients with supportive family and friends may fear that no one will care for them. Patients may worry that they cannot pay for their treatment, even though they have enough money and insurance.

A person who has generalized anxiety may feel irritable, restless, or dizzy, have tense muscles, shortness of breath, fast heartbeat, sweating, or get tired quickly. Generalized anxiety disorder sometimes begins after a patient has been very depressed.

Treatment for Anxiety Disorders

There are different types of treatment for patients with anxiety disorders, including methods to manage stress. Ways to manage stress include the following:

- Deal with the problem directly.
- See the situation as a problem to solve or a challenge.
- Get all of the information and support needed to solve the problem.
- Break big problems or events into smaller problems or tasks.
- Be flexible. Take situations as they come.

Patients with anxiety disorders need information and support to understand their cancer and treatment choices.

Psychological Treatments

Psychological treatments for anxiety can also be helpful. These include the following:

- Individual (one-to-one) counseling
- Couple and family counseling
- Crisis counseling
- Group therapy
- Self-help groups

Other Treatments

Other treatments used to lessen the symptoms of anxiety include the following:

- Hypnosis
- Meditation
- Relaxation training
- Guided imagery
- Biofeedback

Using different methods together may be helpful for some patients.

Medicines

Medicine may be used alone or combined with other types of treatment for anxiety disorders. Antianxiety medicines may be used if the patient doesn't want counseling or if it's not available. These medicines relieve symptoms of anxiety, such as feelings of fear, dread, uneasiness, and muscle tightness. They may relieve daytime distress and reduce insomnia. These medicines may be used alone or combined with other therapies. Although some patients are afraid they may become addicted to antianxiety medicines, this is not a common problem in cancer patients. Enough medicine is given to relieve symptoms and then the dose is slowly lowered as symptoms begin to get better. Studies show that antidepressants are useful in treating anxiety disorders. Children and teenagers being treated with antidepressants have an increased risk of suicidal thinking and behavior and must be watched closely.

Chapter 32

Depression

What Is Depression?

Depression is more than just feeling down or having a bad day. When a sad mood lasts for a long time and interferes with normal, everyday functioning, you may be depressed. Symptoms of depression include:

- Feeling sad or anxious often or all the time
- Not wanting to do activities that used to be fun
- Feeling irritable' easily frustrated' or restless
- Having trouble falling asleep or staying asleep
- Waking up too early or sleeping too much
- Eating more or less than usual or having no appetite
- Experiencing aches, pains, headaches, or stomach problems that do not improve with treatment
- Having trouble concentrating, remembering details, or making decisions
- Feeling tired' even after sleeping well

This chapter includes text excerpted from "Mental Health Conditions: Depression and Anxiety," Centers for Disease Control and Prevention (CDC), January 23, 2017.

- Feeling guilty, worthless, or helpless
- Thinking about suicide or hurting yourself

If you think you are depressed' talk with your doctor or a mental health professional immediately. This is especially important if your symptoms are getting worse or affecting your daily activities.

What Causes Depression?

The exact cause of depression is unknown. It may be caused by a combination of genetic, biological, environmental, and psychological factors. Everyone is different' but the following factors may increase a person's chances of becoming depressed:

- Having blood relatives who have had depression
- Experiencing traumatic or stressful events, such as physical or sexual abuse, the death of a loved one, or financial problems
- Going through a major life change' even if it was planned
- Having a medical problem, such as cancer, stroke, or chronic pain
- Taking certain medications. Talk to your doctor if you have questions about whether your medications might be making you feel depressed.
- Using alcohol or drugs

Who Gets Depression?

In general' about 1 out of every 6 adults will have depression at some time in their life. Depression affects about 16 million American adults every year. Anyone can get depressed, and depression can happen at any age and in any type of person. Many people who experience depression also have other mental health conditions. Anxiety disorders often go hand in hand with depression. People who have anxiety disorders struggle with intense and uncontrollable feelings of anxiety, fear, worry, and/or panic. These feelings can interfere with daily activities and may last for a long time.

What Is the Link between Smoking and Mental Health Conditions?

Smoking is much more common among adults with mental health conditions, such as depression and anxiety, than in the general population. About 3 out of every 10 cigarettes smoked by adults in the U.S. are smoked by persons with mental health conditions. Why smokers are more likely than nonsmokers to experience depression, anxiety, and other mental health conditions is uncertain. More research is needed to determine this. No matter the cause' smoking is not a treatment for depression or anxiety. Getting help for your depression and anxiety and quitting smoking is the best way to feel better.

What Are the Treatments for Depression?

Many helpful treatments for depression are available. Treatment for depression can help reduce symptoms and shorten how long the depression lasts. Treatment can include getting therapy and/or taking medications. Your doctor or a qualified mental health professional can help you determine what treatment is best for you.

- **Therapy.** Many people benefit from psychotherapy—also called therapy or counseling. Most therapy lasts for a short time and focuses on thoughts' feelings' and issues that are happening in your life now. In some cases' understanding your past can help' but finding ways to address what is happening in your life now can help you cope and prepare you for challenges in the future. With therapy, you'll work with your therapist to learn skills to help you cope with life, change behaviors that are causing problems' and find solutions. Do not feel shy or embarrassed about talking openly and honestly about your feelings and concerns. This is an important part of getting better. Some common goals of therapy include:

  - Getting healthier

  - Quitting smoking and stopping drug and alcohol use

  - Overcoming fears or insecurities

  - Coping with stress

  - Making sense of past painful events

  - Identifying things that worsen your depression

  - Having better relationships with family and friends

  - Understanding why something bothers you and creating a plan to deal with it

- **Medication.** Many people with depression find that taking prescribed medications called antidepressants can help improve their mood and coping skills. Talk to your doctor about whether they are right for you. If your doctor writes you a prescription for an antidepressant' ask exactly how you should take the medication. If you are already using nicotine replacement therapy or another medication to help you quit smoking, be sure to let your doctor know. Several antidepressant medications are available' so you and your doctor have options to choose from. Sometimes it takes several tries to find the best medication and the right dose for you, so be patient. Also be aware of the following important information:

  - When taking these medications' it is important to follow the instructions on how much to take. Some people start to feel better a few days after starting the medication' but it can take up to 4 weeks to feel the most benefit. Antidepressants work well and are safe for most people' but it is still important to talk with your doctor if you have side effects. Side effects usually do not get in the way of daily life' and they often go away as your body adjusts to the medication.

  - Don't stop taking an antidepressant without first talking to your doctor. Stopping your medicine suddenly can cause symptoms or worsen depression. Work with your doctor to safely adjust how much you take.

  - Some antidepressants may cause risks during pregnancy. Talk with your doctor if you are pregnant or might be pregnant, or if you are planning to become pregnant.

  - Antidepressants cannot solve all of your problems. If you notice that your mood is getting worse or if you have thoughts about hurting yourself' it is important to call your doctor right away.

Quitting smoking will not interfere with your mental health treatment or make your depression worse. In fact, research shows that quitting smoking can actually improve your mental health in the long run.

Depression and Suicide: Getting Help in a Crisis

Some people who are depressed may think about hurting themselves or committing suicide (taking their own life). If you or someone you know is having thoughts about hurting themselves or committing suicide' please seek immediate help. The following resources can help:

- Call 800-273-TALK (800-273-8255) to reach a 24–hour crisis center or dial 911. 800-273-TALK is the National Suicide Prevention Lifeline (NSPL), which provides free' confidential help to people in crisis. The Substance Abuse and Mental Health Services Administration (SAMHSA) runs this lifeline.

- Call your mental health provider.

- Get help from your primary doctor or other healthcare provider.

- Reach out to a close friend or loved one.

- Contact a minister, spiritual leader, or someone else in your faith community.

Chapter 33

Eating Disorders

There is a commonly held view that eating disorders are a lifestyle choice. Eating disorders are actually serious and often fatal illnesses that cause severe disturbances to a person's eating behaviors. Obsessions with food, body weight, and shape may also signal an eating disorder. Common eating disorders include anorexia nervosa, bulimia nervosa, and binge-eating disorder.

Signs and Symptoms

Anorexia Nervosa

People with anorexia nervosa may see themselves as overweight, even when they are dangerously underweight. People with anorexia nervosa typically weigh themselves repeatedly, severely restrict the amount of food they eat, and eat very small quantities of only certain foods. Anorexia nervosa has the highest mortality rate of any mental disorder. While many young women and men with this disorder die from complications associated with starvation, others die of suicide. In women, suicide is much more common in those with anorexia than with most other mental disorders.

Symptoms include:

- Extremely restricted eating

This chapter includes text excerpted from "Eating Disorders," National Institute of Mental Health (NIMH), February 2016.

275

- Extreme thinness (emaciation)
- A relentless pursuit of thinness and unwillingness to maintain a normal or healthy weight
- Intense fear of gaining weight
- Distorted body image, a self-esteem that is heavily influenced by perceptions of body weight and shape, or a denial of the seriousness of low body weight

Other symptoms may develop over time, including:

- Thinning of the bones (osteopenia or osteoporosis)
- Mild anemia and muscle wasting and weakness
- Brittle hair and nails
- Dry and yellowish skin
- Growth of fine hair all over the body (lanugo)
- Severe constipation
- Low blood pressure, slowed breathing and pulse
- Damage to the structure and function of the heart
- Brain damage
- Multiorgan failure
- Drop in internal body temperature, causing a person to feel cold all the time
- Lethargy, sluggishness, or feeling tired all the time
- Infertility

Bulimia Nervosa

People with bulimia nervosa have recurrent and frequent episodes of eating unusually large amounts of food and feeling a lack of control over these episodes. This binge-eating is followed by behavior that compensates for the overeating such as forced vomiting, excessive use of laxatives or diuretics, fasting, excessive exercise, or a combination of these behaviors. Unlike anorexia nervosa, people with bulimia nervosa usually maintain what is considered a healthy or relatively normal weight.

Symptoms include:

- Chronically inflamed and sore throat

- Swollen salivary glands in the neck and jaw area

- Worn tooth enamel and increasingly sensitive and decaying teeth as a result of exposure to stomach acid

- Acid reflux disorder and other gastrointestinal problems

- Intestinal distress and irritation from laxative abuse

- Severe dehydration from purging of fluids

- Electrolyte imbalance (too low or too high levels of sodium, calcium, potassium and other minerals) which can lead to stroke or heart attack

Binge-Eating Disorder

People with binge-eating disorder lose control over his or her eating. Unlike bulimia nervosa, periods of binge-eating are not followed by purging, excessive exercise, or fasting. As a result, people with binge-eating disorder often are overweight or obese. Binge-eating disorder is the most common eating disorder in the United States.

Symptoms include:

- Eating unusually large amounts of food in a specific amount of time

- Eating even when you're full or not hungry

- Eating fast during binge episodes

- Eating until you're uncomfortably full

- Eating alone or in secret to avoid embarrassment

- Feeling distressed, ashamed, or guilty about your eating

- Frequently dieting, possibly without weight loss

Risk Factors

Eating disorders frequently appear during the teen years or young adulthood but may also develop during childhood or later in life. These disorders affect both genders, although rates among women are 2½ times greater than among men. Like women who have eating disorders, men also have a distorted sense of body image. For example, men may have muscle dysmorphia, a type of disorder marked by an extreme concern with becoming more muscular.

Researchers are finding that eating disorders are caused by a complex interaction of genetic, biological, behavioral, psychological, and social factors. Researchers are using the latest technology and science to better understand eating disorders.

One approach involves the study of human genes. Eating disorders run in families. Researchers are working to identify deoxyribonucleic acid (DNA) variations that are linked to the increased risk of developing eating disorders.

Brain imaging studies are also providing a better understanding of eating disorders. For example, researchers have found differences in patterns of brain activity in women with eating disorders in comparison with healthy women. This kind of research can help guide the development of new means of diagnosis and treatment of eating disorders.

Treatments and Therapies

Adequate nutrition, reducing excessive exercise, and stopping purging behaviors are the foundations of treatment. Treatment plans are tailored to individual needs and may include one or more of the following:

- Individual, group, and/or family psychotherapy
- Medical care and monitoring
- Nutritional counseling
- Medications

Psychotherapies

Psychotherapies such as a family-based therapy called the Maudsley approach, where parents of adolescents with anorexia nervosa assume responsibility for feeding their child, appear to be very effective in helping people gain weight and improve eating habits and moods.

To reduce or eliminate binge-eating and purging behaviors, people may undergo cognitive behavioral therapy (CBT), which is another type of psychotherapy that helps a person learn how to identify distorted or unhelpful thinking patterns and recognize and change inaccurate beliefs.

Medications

Evidence also suggests that medications such as antidepressants, antipsychotics, or mood stabilizers approved by the U.S. Food and Drug Administration (FDA) may also be helpful for treating eating disorders and other co-occurring illnesses such as anxiety or depression.

Chapter 34

Erectile Dysfunction

What Is Erectile Dysfunction?

Erectile dysfunction (also known as impotence) is the inability to get and keep an erection firm enough for sex. Having erection trouble from time to time isn't necessarily a cause for concern. But if erectile dysfunction is an ongoing problem, it may cause stress, cause relationship problems or affect your self-confidence. Even though it may seem awkward to talk with your doctor about erectile dysfunction, go in for an evaluation. Problems getting or keeping an erection can be a sign of a health condition that needs treatment, such as heart disease or poorly controlled diabetes. Treating an underlying problem may be enough to reverse your erectile dysfunction. If treating an underlying condition doesn't help your erectile dysfunction, medications or other direct treatments may work.

What Are the Causes of Erectile Dysfunction?

Male sexual arousal is a complex process that involves the brain, hormones, emotions, nerves, muscles, and blood vessels. Erectile dysfunction can result from a problem with any of these. Likewise, stress and mental health problems can cause or worsen erectile dysfunction. Sometimes a combination of physical and psychological issues causes erectile dysfunction. For instance, a minor physical problem that slows

This chapter includes text excerpted from "Erectile Dysfunction (ED)," U.S. Department of Veterans Affairs (VA), July 2013. Reviewed September 2017.

your sexual response may cause anxiety about maintaining an erection. The resulting anxiety can lead to or worsen erectile dysfunction.

Physical causes of erectile dysfunction.

In most cases, erectile dysfunction is caused by something physical. Common causes include:

- Heart disease

- Clogged blood vessels (atherosclerosis)

- High blood pressure

- Diabetes

- Obesity

- Metabolic syndrome, a condition involving increased blood pressure, high insulin levels, body fat around the waist and high cholesterol

- Parkinson disease

- Multiple sclerosis

- Low testosterone

- Peyronie disease, development of scar tissue inside the penis

- Certain prescription medications

- Tobacco use

- Alcoholism and other forms of substance abuse

- Treatments for prostate cancer or enlarged prostate

- Surgeries or injuries that affect the pelvic area or spinal cord

Psychological causes of erectile dysfunction.

The brain plays a key role in triggering the series of physical events that cause an erection, starting with feelings of sexual excitement. A number of things can interfere with sexual feelings and cause or worsen erectile dysfunction. These include:

- Depression, anxiety, or other mental health conditions

- Stress

- Fatigue

- Relationship problems due to stress, poor communication, or other concerns

What Are the Risk Factors for Erectile Dysfunction?

As you get older, erections may take longer to develop and may not be as firm. You may need more direct touch to your penis to get and keep an erection. This isn't a direct consequence of getting older. Usually it's a result of underlying health problems or taking medications, which is more common as men age.

A variety of risk factors can contribute to erectile dysfunction. They include:

- Medical conditions, particularly diabetes or heart problems.

- Using tobacco, which restricts blood flow to veins and arteries. Over time tobacco use can cause chronic health problems that lead to erectile dysfunction.

- Being overweight, especially if you're very overweight (obese).

- Certain medical treatments, such as prostate surgery or radiation treatment for cancer.

- Injuries, particularly if they damage the nerves that control erections.

- Medications, including antidepressants, antihistamines, and medications to treat high blood pressure, pain or prostate cancer.

- Psychological conditions, such as stress, anxiety or depression.

- Drug and alcohol use, especially if you're a long-term drug user or heavy drinker.

- Prolonged bicycling, which can compress nerves and affect blood flow to the penis—leading to temporary erectile dysfunction.

What Are the Tests Used to Diagnose Erectile Dysfunction?

For many men, a physical exam and answering questions (medical history) are all that's needed before a doctor is ready to recommend a treatment. If your doctor suspects that underlying problems may be involved, or you have chronic health problems, you may need further tests or you may need to see a specialist.

Tests for underlying problems may include:

- Physical exam. This may include careful examination of your penis and testicles and checking your nerves for feeling.

- Blood tests. A sample of your blood may be sent to a lab to check for signs of heart disease, diabetes, low testosterone levels and other health problems.

- Urine tests (urinalysis). Like blood tests, urine tests are used to look for signs of diabetes and other underlying health conditions.

- Ultrasound. This test can check blood flow to your penis. It involves using a wand-like device (transducer) held over the blood vessels that supply the penis. It creates a video image to let your doctor see if you have blood flow problems. This test is sometimes done in combination with an injection of medications into the penis to determine if blood flow increases normally.

- Overnight erection test. Most men have erections during sleep without remembering them. This simple test involves wrapping special tape around your penis before you go to bed. If the tape is separated in the morning, your penis was erect at some time during the night. This indicates the cause is of your erectile dysfunction is most likely psychological and not physical.

What Are the Treatments and Medications for Erectile Dysfunction?

A variety of options exist for treating erectile dysfunction. The cause and severity of your condition, and underlying health problems, are important factors in your doctor's recommending the best treatment or treatments for you. Your doctor can explain the risks and benefits of each treatment, and will consider your preferences. Your partner's preferences also may play a role in treatment choices.

Oral medications. Oral medications are a successful erectile dysfunction treatment for many men. They include:

- Sildenafil (Viagra)
- Tadalafil (Cialis)
- Vardenafil (Levitra)

All three medications work in much the same way. These drugs enhance the effects of nitric oxide, a natural chemical your body produces that relaxes muscles in the penis. This increases blood flow and allows you to get an erection in response to sexual stimulation. These medications vary in dosage, how long they work and their side effects. Your doctor will take into account your particular situation to determine which medication may work best. Don't expect these medications to fix your erectile dysfunction immediately. You may need to work with your doctor to find the right medication and dose for you. Before taking any prescription erectile dysfunction medication (including over-the-counter supplements or herbal remedies), get your doctor's OK. Although these medications can help many people, not all men should take them to treat erectile dysfunction. These medications may not work or may be dangerous for you if you:

- Take nitrate drugs for angina, such as nitroglycerin (Nitro-Bid, others), isosorbide mononitrate (Imdur) and isosorbide dinitrate (Isordil)

- Take a blood-thinning (anticoagulant) medication, alpha blockers for enlarged prostate (benign prostatic hyperplasia) or high blood pressure medications

- Have heart disease or heart failure

- Have had a stroke

- Have very low blood pressure (hypotension) or uncontrolled high blood pressure (hypertension)

- Have uncontrolled diabetes

Other medications. Other medications for erectile dysfunction include:

- Alprostadil self-injection. With this method, you use a fine needle to inject alprostadil (Alprostadil, Caverject Impulse, Edex) into the base or side of your penis. In some cases, medications generally used for other conditions are used for penile injections on their own or in combination. Examples include papaverine, alprostadil, and phentolamine. Each injection generally produces an erection in five to 20 minutes that lasts about an hour. Because the needle used is very fine, pain from the injection site is usually minor. Side effects can include bleeding from the injection, prolonged erection and formation of fibrous tissue at the injection site.

- Alprostadil penis suppository. Alprostadil intraurethral (MUSE) therapy involves placing a tiny alprostadil suppository inside your penis. You use a special applicator to insert the suppository about two inches down into your penis. Side effects can include pain, minor bleeding in the urethra, dizziness and formation of fibrous tissue inside your penis.

- Testosterone replacement. Some men have erectile dysfunction caused by low levels of the hormone testosterone, and may need testosterone replacement therapy.

Penis pumps, surgery, and implants. Medications may not work or may not be a good choice for you. If this is the case, your doctor may recommend a different treatment. Other treatments include:

- Penis pumps. A penis pump (vacuum constriction device) is a hollow tube with a hand-powered or battery-powered pump. The tube is placed over your penis, and then the pump is used to suck out the air inside the tube. This creates a vacuum that pulls blood into your penis. Once you get an erection, you slip a tension ring around the base of your penis to hold in the blood and keep it firm. You then remove the vacuum device. The erection typically lasts long enough for a couple to have sex. You remove the tension ring after intercourse.

- Penile implants. This treatment involves surgically placing devices into the two sides of the penis. These implants consist of either inflatable or semirigid rods made from silicone or polyurethane. The inflatable devices allow you to control when and how long you have an erection. The semirigid rods keep the penis firm but bendable. This treatment can be expensive and is usually not recommended until other methods have been tried first. As with any surgery, there is a risk of complications such as infection.

- Blood vessel surgery. In rare cases, a leaking blood vessel can cause erectile dysfunction and surgery is necessary to repair it.

Psychological counseling. If your erectile dysfunction is caused by stress, anxiety or depression, your doctor may suggest that you, or you and your partner, visit a psychologist or counselor. Even if it is caused by something physical, erectile dysfunction can create stress and relationship tension.

What Are Some Things I Can Do about Erectile Dysfunction?

For many men, erectile dysfunction is caused or worsened by lifestyle choices. Here are some things you can do that may help:

- If you smoke, quit. If you have trouble quitting, get help. Try nicotine replacement (such as gum or lozenges), available over-the-counter, or ask your doctor about prescription medication that can help you quit.

• Lose weight. Being overweight can cause—or worsen—erectile dysfunction.

• Get regular exercise. This can help with underlying problems that play a part in erectile dysfunction in a number of ways, including reducing stress, helping you lose weight and increasing blood flow.

• Get treatment for alcohol or drug problems. Drinking too much or taking certain illicit drugs can worsen erectile dysfunction directly or by causing long-term health problems.

• Work through relationship issues. Improve communication with your partner and consider couples or marriage counseling if you're having trouble working through problems on your own.

Chapter 35

Fibromyalgia

What Is Fibromyalgia?

Fibromyalgia is a condition that causes pain all over the body (also referred to as widespread pain), sleep problems, fatigue, and often emotional and mental distress. People with fibromyalgia may be more sensitive to pain than people without fibromyalgia. This is called abnormal pain perception processing. Fibromyalgia affects about 4 million U.S. adults, about 2 percent of the adult population. The cause of fibromyalgia is not known, but it can be effectively treated and managed.

How Do I Know I Might Have Fibromyalgia?

The most common symptoms of fibromyalgia are:

- Pain and stiffness all over the body
- Fatigue and tiredness
- Depression and anxiety
- Sleep problems
- Problems with thinking, memory, and concentration
- Headaches, including migraines

This chapter includes text excerpted from "Fibromyalgia Fact Sheet," Centers for Disease Control and Prevention (CDC), May 4, 2017.

Other symptoms may include:

- Tingling or numbness in hands and feet.

- Pain in the face or jaw, including disorders of the jaw known as temporomandibular joint syndrome (TMJ).

- Digestive problems, such as abdominal pain, bloating, constipation, and even irritable bowel syndrome (IBS)

What Are the Risk Factors for Fibromyalgia?

Known risk factors include:

- **Age.** Fibromyalgia can affect people of all ages, including children. However, most people are diagnosed during middle age and you are more likely to have fibromyalgia as you get older.

- **Lupus or rheumatoid arthritis.** If you have lupus or rheumatoid arthritis (RA), you are more likely to develop fibromyalgia.

Some other factors have been weakly associated with onset of fibromyalgia, but more research is needed to see if they are real. These possible risk factors include:

- Sex. Women are twice as likely to have fibromyalgia as men.

- Stressful or traumatic events, such as car accidents, posttraumatic stress disorder (PTSD).

- Repetitive injuries. Injury from repetitive stress on a joint, such as frequent knee bending.

- Illness (such as viral infections).

- Family history.

- Obesity.

How Is Fibromyalgia Diagnosed?

Doctors usually diagnose fibromyalgia using the patient's history, physical examination, X-rays, and blood work.

How Is Fibromyalgia Treated?

Fibromyalgia can be effectively treated and managed with medication and self-management strategies.

Fibromyalgia should be treated by a doctor or team of healthcare professionals who specialize in the treatment of fibromyalgia and other types of arthritis, called rheumatologists. Doctors usually treat fibromyalgia with a combination of treatments, which may include:

- Medications, including prescription drugs and over-the-counter pain relievers.

- Aerobic exercise and muscle strengthening exercise.

- Patient education classes, usually in primary care or community settings.

- Stress management techniques such as meditation, yoga, and massage.

- Good sleep habits to improve the quality of sleep.

- Cognitive behavioral therapy (CBT) to treat underlying depression. CBT is a type of talk therapy meant to change the way people act or think.

In addition to medical treatment, people can manage their fibromyalgia with the self-management strategies described below, which are proven to reduce pain and disability, so they can pursue the activities important to them.

What Are the Complications of Fibromyalgia?

Fibromyalgia can cause pain, disability, and lower quality of life. U.S. adults with fibromyalgia may have complications such as:

- **More hospitalizations.** If you have fibromyalgia you are twice as likely to be hospitalized as someone without fibromyalgia.

- **Lower quality of life.** Women with fibromyalgia have low quality-of-life. If you're a woman with fibromyalgia you may have 40 percent less physical function and 67 percent less mental health.

- **Higher rates of major depression.** Adults with fibromyalgia are more than 3 times more likely to have major depression than adults without fibromyalgia. Screening and treatment for depression is extremely important.

- **Higher death rates from suicide and injuries.** Death rates from suicide and injuries are higher among fibromyalgia patients, but overall mortality among adults with fibromyalgia is similar to the general population.

- **Higher rates of other rheumatic conditions.** Fibromyalgia often co-occurs with other types of arthritis such as osteoarthritis, rheumatoid arthritis, systemic lupus.

How Can I Improve My Quality of Life?

- **Get physically active.** Experts recommend that adults be moderately physically active for 150 minutes per week. Walk, swim, or bike 30 minutes a day for five days a week. These 30 minutes can be broken into three separate ten-minute sessions during the day. Regular physical activity can also reduce the risk of developing other chronic diseases such as heart disease and diabetes.

- **Go to recommended physical activity programs.** Those concerned about how to safely exercise can participate in physical activity programs that are proven effective for reducing pain and disability related to arthritis and improving mood and the ability to move. Classes take place at local Ys, parks, and community centers. These classes can help you feel better.

- **Join a self-management education class,** which helps people with arthritis or other conditions—including fibromyalgia—be more confident in how to control their symptoms, how to live well and understand how the condition affects their lives.

Chapter 36

HIV/AIDS

What Are HIV and AIDS?

HIV, or human immunodeficiency virus, is the virus that causes acquired immunodeficiency syndrome (AIDS). HIV attacks the immune system by destroying CD4 positive (CD4+) T cells, a type of white blood cell that is vital to fighting off infection. The destruction of these cells leaves people infected with HIV vulnerable to other infections, diseases and other complications.

A person infected with HIV is diagnosed with AIDS when he or she has one or more opportunistic infections (which occur when your immune system is damaged by HIV), such as pneumonia or tuberculosis, and has a dangerously low number of CD4+ T cells (less than 200 cells per cubic millimeter of blood).

People with HIV/AIDS and Mental Health Disorders

If you are living with HIV, it is important for you to be aware that you have an increased risk for developing mood, anxiety, and cognitive disorders. For example, people living with HIV are twice as likely to have depression compared to those who are not infected with HIV. These conditions may be treatable. Many people with mental health conditions recover completely.

This chapter includes text excerpted from "HIV/AIDS and Mental Health," National Institute of Mental Health (NIMH), November 2016.

Some forms of stress can contribute to mental health problems for people living with HIV, including:

- Having trouble getting the services you need

- Experiencing a loss of social support, resulting in isolation

- Experiencing a loss of employment or worries about whether you will be able to perform your work as you did before

- Having to tell others you are HIV-positive

- Managing your HIV medicines

- Going through changes in your physical appearance or abilities due to HIV/AIDS

- Dealing with loss, including the loss of relationships or even death

- Facing the stigma and discrimination associated with HIV/AIDS

The HIV virus itself also can contribute to mental health problems because it enters and resides in your brain. Some other opportunistic infections can also affect your nervous system and lead to changes in your behavior and functioning. Similarly, neuropsychological disorders, such as mild cognitive changes or more severe cognitive conditions, such as dementia, are associated with HIV disease.

You can better manage your overall health and well-being if you know how having HIV can affect your mental health and what resources are available to help you if you need them.

*Fear and Anxiety**

Fear and anxiety may be caused by not knowing what to expect now that you've been diagnosed with HIV, or not knowing how others will treat you after they find out you have HIV. You also may be afraid of telling people—friends, family members, and others—that you are HIV positive. Fear can make your heart beat faster or make it hard for you to sleep. Anxiety also can make you feel nervous or agitated. Fear and anxiety might make you sweat, feel dizzy, or feel short of breath.

Ways to control your feelings of fear and anxiety include the following:

- Learn as much as you can about HIV/AIDS.

- Get your questions answered by your VA healthcare provider.

- Talk with your friends, family members, and healthcare providers.

- Join a support group.

- Help others who are in the same situation, such as by volunteering at an HIV/AIDS service organization. This may empower you and lessen your feelings of fear.

- Talk to your doctor about medicines or other treatments for anxiety if the feelings don't lessen with time or if they get worse.

*Text under the heading excerpted from "Coping with HIV/AIDS: Fear and Anxiety," U.S. Department of Veterans Affairs (VA), July 30, 2015.

Treatments and Therapies

Research shows that HIV treatment should be initiated as soon as infection is detected to achieve the best health outcomes. Once diagnosed, HIV infection is treated using a combination of medicines called antiretroviral therapy (ART). Adequate adherence to prescribed treatment regimens, such as taking the medications as prescribed by the healthcare provider, is critical to controlling the virus and to achieving complete viral suppression. Adequate adherence can be difficult but many strategies have been developed to assist individuals living with HIV/AIDS.

Starting antiretroviral therapy also can affect your mental health in different ways. Sometimes antiretroviral therapy can relieve your anxiety because knowing that you are taking care of yourself can give you a sense of security. However, coping with the reality of living with a chronic illness can be challenging. Depression is one of the most common mental health conditions experienced by people living with HIV, just as it is in the general population. In addition, some antiretroviral medications may cause symptoms of depression, anxiety, and sleep disturbance, and may make some mental health issues worse.

For these reasons, it is important to talk to your healthcare provider about your mental health. A conversation about mental health should be part of your complete medical evaluation before starting antiretroviral medications. Continue to discuss your mental health with your healthcare team throughout treatment. Be open and honest with your provider about any changes in the way you are thinking, or how you are feeling about yourself and life in general. Also discuss any alcohol or substance use with your provider so that he or she can help connect you to treatment if necessary.

In addition, tell your healthcare provider about any over-the-counter or prescribed medications you may be taking, including any psychiatric medications, because some of these drugs may interact with antiretroviral medications.

Chapter 37

Irritable Bowel Syndrome

What Is Irritable Bowel Syndrome (IBS)?

Irritable bowel syndrome (IBS) is a group of symptoms—including pain or discomfort in your abdomen and changes in your bowel movement patterns—that occur together. Doctors call IBS a functional gastrointestinal (GI) disorder. Functional GI disorders happen when your GI tract behaves in an abnormal way without evidence of damage due to a disease.

In the past, doctors called IBS colitis, mucous colitis, spastic colon, nervous colon, and spastic bowel. Experts changed the name to reflect the understanding that the disorder has both physical and mental causes and isn't a product of a person's imagination.

What Are the Four Types of IBS?

Doctors often classify IBS into one of four types based on your usual stool consistency. These types are important because they affect the types of treatment that are most likely to improve your symptoms.

The four types of IBS are:

- IBS with constipation, or IBS-C
  - hard or lumpy stools at least 25 percent of the time

This chapter includes text excerpted from "Digestive Diseases—Irritable Bowel Syndrome (IBS)," National Institute of Diabetes and Digestive and Kidney Diseases (NIDDK), February 2015.

- loose or watery stools less than 25 percent of the time
- IBS with diarrhea, or IBS-D
    - loose or watery stools at least 25 percent of the time
    - hard or lumpy stools less than 25 percent of the time
- Mixed IBS, or IBS-M
    - hard or lumpy stools at least 25 percent of the time
    - loose or watery stools at least 25 percent of the time
- Unsubtyped IBS, or IBS-U
    - hard or lumpy stools less than 25 percent of the time
    - loose or watery stools less than 25 percent of the time

What Are the Symptoms of IBS?

The most common symptoms of irritable bowel syndrome (IBS) include pain or discomfort in your abdomen and changes in how often you have bowel movements or how your stools look. The pain or discomfort of IBS may feel like cramping and have at least two of the following:

- Your pain or discomfort improves after a bowel movement.
- You notice a change in how often you have a bowel movement.
- You notice a change in the way your stools look.

IBS is a chronic disorder, meaning it lasts a long time, often years. However, the symptoms may come and go. You may have IBS if:

- You've had symptoms at least three times a month for the past 3 months.
- Your symptoms first started at least 6 months ago.

People with IBS may have diarrhea, constipation, or both. Some people with IBS have only diarrhea or only constipation. Some people have symptoms of both or have diarrhea sometimes and constipation other times. People often have symptoms soon after eating a meal.

Other symptoms of IBS are:

- bloating
- the feeling that you haven't finished a bowel movement

- whitish mucus in your stool

Women with IBS often have more symptoms during their menstrual periods. While IBS can be painful, IBS doesn't lead to other health problems or damage your gastrointestinal (GI) tract.

What Causes IBS?

Doctors aren't sure what causes IBS. Experts think that a combination of problems can lead to IBS.

Physical Problems

Brain-Gut Signal Problems

Signals between your brain and the nerves of your gut, or small and large intestines, control how your gut works. Problems with brain-gut signals may cause IBS symptoms.

GI Motility Problems

If you have IBS, you may not have normal motility in your colon. Slow motility can lead to constipation and fast motility can lead to diarrhea. Spasms can cause abdominal pain. If you have IBS, you may also experience hyperreactivity—a dramatic increase in bowel contractions when you feel stress or after you eat.

Pain Sensitivity

If you have IBS, the nerves in your gut may be extra sensitive, causing you to feel more pain or discomfort than normal when gas or stool is in your gut. Your brain may process pain signals from your bowel differently if you have IBS.

Infections

A bacterial infection in the GI tract may cause some people to develop IBS. Researchers don't know why infections in the GI tract lead to IBS in some people and not others, although abnormalities of the GI tract lining and mental health problems may play a role.

Small Intestinal Bacterial Overgrowth

Normally, few bacteria live in your small intestine. Small intestinal bacterial overgrowth is an increase in the number or a change in the type of bacteria in your small intestine. These bacteria can produce extra gas and may also cause diarrhea and weight loss. Some experts think small intestinal bacterial overgrowth may lead to IBS. Research continues to explore a possible link between the two conditions.

Neurotransmitters (Body Chemicals)

People with IBS have altered levels of neurotransmitters—chemicals in the body that transmit nerve signals—and GI hormones. The role these chemicals play in IBS is unclear.

Younger women with IBS often have more symptoms during their menstrual periods. Postmenopausal women have fewer symptoms compared with women who are still menstruating. These findings suggest that reproductive hormones can worsen IBS problems.

Genetics

Whether IBS has a genetic cause, meaning it runs in families, is unclear. Studies have shown IBS is more common in people with family members who have a history of GI problems.

Food Sensitivity

Many people with IBS report that foods rich in carbohydrates, spicy or fatty foods, coffee, and alcohol trigger their symptoms. However, people with food sensitivity typically don't have signs of a food allergy. Researchers think that poor absorption of sugars or bile acids may cause symptoms.

Mental Health Problems

Psychological, or mental health, problems such as panic disorder, anxiety, depression, and posttraumatic stress disorder are common in people with IBS. The link between mental health and IBS is unclear. GI disorders, including IBS, are sometimes present in people who have reported past physical or sexual abuse. Experts think people who have been abused tend to express psychological stress through physical symptoms.

If you have IBS, your colon may respond too much to even slight conflict or stress. Stress makes your mind more aware of the sensations in your colon. IBS symptoms can also increase your stress level.

How Do Doctors Diagnose IBS?

Your doctor may be able to diagnose irritable bowel syndrome (IBS) based on a review of your medical history, symptoms, and physical exam. Your doctor may also order tests.

To diagnose IBS, your doctor will take a complete medical history and perform a physical exam.

Medical History

The medical history will include questions about:

- your symptoms

- family history of gastrointestinal (GI) tract disorders

- recent infections

- medicines

- stressful events related to the start of your symptoms

- Your doctor will look for a certain pattern in your symptoms. Your doctor may diagnose IBS if:

- your symptoms started at least 6 months ago

- you've had pain or discomfort in your abdomen at least three times a month for the past 3 months

- your abdominal pain or discomfort has two or three of the following features:

  - Your pain or discomfort improves after a bowel movement.

  - You notice a change in how often you have a bowel movement.

  - You notice a change in the way your stools look.

Physical Exam

During a physical exam, your doctor usually:

- checks for abdominal bloating

- listens to sounds within your abdomen using a stethoscope

- taps on your abdomen checking for tenderness or pain

301

How Do Doctors Treat IBS?

Though irritable bowel syndrome (IBS) doesn't have a cure, your doctor can manage the symptoms with a combination of diet, medicines, probiotics, and therapies for mental health problems. You may have to try a few treatments to see what works best for you. Your doctor can help you find the right treatment plan.

Changes in Eating, Diet, and Nutrition

Changes in eating, diet, and nutrition, such as following a FODMAP diet, can help treat your symptoms.

Medicines

Your doctor may recommend medicine to relieve your symptoms.

- Fiber supplements to relieve constipation when increasing fiber in your diet doesn't help.

- Laxatives to help with constipation. Laxatives work in different ways, and your doctor can recommend a laxative that's right for you.

- Loperamide to reduce diarrhea by slowing the movement of stool through your colon. Loperamide is an antidiarrheal that reduces diarrhea in people with IBS, though it doesn't reduce pain, bloating, or other symptoms.

- Antispasmodics, such as hyoscine, cimetropium, and pinaverium, help to control colon muscle spasms and reduce pain in your abdomen.

- Antidepressants, such as low doses of tricyclic antidepressants and selective serotonin reuptake inhibitors, to relieve IBS symptoms, including abdominal pain. In theory, because of their effect on colon transit, tricyclic antidepressants should be better for people with IBS with diarrhea, or IBS-D, and selective serotonin reuptake inhibitors should be better for people with IBS with constipation, or IBS-C, although studies haven't confirmed this theory. Tricyclic antidepressants work in people with IBS by reducing their sensitivity to pain in the gastrointestinal (GI) tract as well as normalizing their GI motility and secretion.

- Lubiprostone (Amitiza) for people who have IBS-C to improve abdominal pain or discomfort and constipation symptoms.

- Linaclotide (Linzess) for people who have IBS-C to relieve abdominal pain and increase how often you have bowel movements.

- The antibiotic rifaximin to reduce bloating by treating small intestinal bacterial overgrowth. However, experts are still debating and researching the use of antibiotics to treat IBS.

- Coated peppermint oil capsules to reduce IBS symptoms.

Follow your doctor's instructions when you use medicine to treat IBS. Talk with your doctor about possible side effects and what to do if you have them.

Some medicines can cause side effects. Ask your doctor and your pharmacist about side effects before taking any medicine. MedlinePlus maintains the latest information about side effects and drug warnings.

Probiotics

Your doctor may also recommend probiotics. Probiotics are live microorganisms—tiny organisms that can be seen only with a microscope. These microorganisms, most often bacteria, are like the microorganisms that are normally present in your GI tract. Studies have found that taking large enough amounts of probiotics, specifically Bifidobacteria and certain probiotic combinations, can improve symptoms of IBS. However, researchers are still studying the use of probiotics to treat IBS.

You can find probiotics in dietary supplements, such as capsules, tablets, and powders, and in some foods, such as yogurt.

Discuss your use of complementary and alternative medical practices, including probiotics and dietary supplements, with your doctor.

Therapies for Mental Health Problems

Psychological therapies may improve your IBS symptoms.

Managing Stress

Learning to reduce stress can help improve IBS. With less stress, you may find you have less cramping and pain. You may also find it easier to manage your symptoms.

Some options for managing stress include:

- taking part in stress reduction and relaxation therapies such as meditation

- getting counseling and support
- taking part in regular exercise such as walking or yoga
- reducing stressful life situations as much as possible
- getting enough sleep

Talk Therapy

Talk therapy may reduce stress and improve your IBS symptoms. Two types of talk therapy that healthcare professionals use to treat IBS are cognitive behavioral therapy and psychodynamic, or interpersonal, therapy. Cognitive behavioral therapy focuses on your thoughts and actions. Psychodynamic therapy focuses on how your emotions affect your IBS symptoms. This type of therapy often involves relaxation and stress management techniques.

Gut-Directed Hypnotherapy

In gut-directed hypnotherapy, a therapist uses hypnosis to help you relax the muscles in the colon.

Mindfulness Training

Mindfulness training can teach you to focus your attention on sensations occurring at the moment and to avoid catastrophizing, or worrying about the meaning of those sensations.

Chapter 38

Insomnia Disorders

Everyone has an occasional sleepless night. Most people at some point in life report having problems falling asleep or staying asleep through the night. A person may have sleep problems for many reasons. Causes include poor sleep environment, drinking caffeinated or alcoholic beverages, facing stress, or taking certain medications. Sleep problems often occur when a person has a physical problem, such as pain or heart disease, or a mental disorder, such as depression or anxiety.

A sleep problem that occurs at least three days a week for three months or longer is called chronic insomnia. Sleep problems that do not last this long are called acute insomnia. Chronic and acute insomnia can be treated, but acute insomnia sometimes gets better without treatment.

Insomnia means a person spends enough time in bed, but can't sleep. In contrast, sleep deprivation means a person has no trouble sleeping, but spends too little time in bed. Sleep deprivation is not a sleep disorder. Insomnia is the most common sleep complaint in the United States. About 10 percent of adults have chronic insomnia.

Signs and Symptoms

Acute insomnia generally lasts from several weeks up to three months. It often results from situations such as stress at home or

This chapter includes text excerpted from "Behavioral Health Treatments and Services—Treatments for Mental Disorders—Insomnia Disorders," Substance Abuse and Mental Health Services Administration (SAMHSA), May 12, 2017.

at work, the loss of a loved one, a change in sleep environment, or short-term physical discomfort. Chronic insomnia lasts three months or longer. In chronic insomnia, sleep problems sometimes come and go, with several days of good sleep followed by a stretch of bad sleep.

People with acute or chronic insomnia face distress or problems with daily functioning (such as work, driving, social activities, and school). The insomnia impairs quality of life. People with insomnia have one or more of these problems:

- Trouble falling asleep—"tired but wired"

- Trouble staying asleep or waking up multiple times during the night

- Waking up too early in the morning and not being able to go back to sleep

- Waking up in the morning feeling unrefreshed

During the day, insomnia may impair a person's life in these ways:

- Increased sleepiness
- Low energy, tiredness, or fatigue
- Increased anxiety or worry
- Mood disturbance such as irritability, sadness, and shortened temper
- Feeling impulsive or aggressive
- Problems focusing and concentrating
- Problems remembering things
- Problems making decisions

Risk Factors

Insomnia affects more women than men. It can occur at any age, but older adults are more likely to have insomnia than younger people. Acute insomnia is a risk factor for chronic insomnia. Insomnia is linked to several factors, including lifestyle, behavioral health or medical conditions, and medications. In some cases, it is unclear if insomnia is related to any risk factor.

Lifestyle Risk Factors

Many lifestyle factors can play a role in insomnia, including:

- Positive stress, such as planning for a wedding or a trip

- Emotional distress, such as divorce or the death of a loved one

- An uncomfortable sleep environment (bedroom or place where the person sleeps)

- Large temperatures changes in the environment

- Sleep schedules that do not match up with the person's natural wake-sleep cycle, caused by factors such as jet lag (time change when traveling) or working night shifts

- Worrying about having sleep problems

- Drinking large amounts of caffeine or alcohol before bedtime

- Excessive napping in the afternoon or evening

- Spending an excessive amount of time in bed

- Not getting up at the same time each morning

- Having an inactive lifestyle

Behavioral Health and Medical Factors

Some researchers think insomnia is a problem when the brain is unable to stop being awake. Your brain has a sleep cycle and a wake cycle—when one is turned on, the other is turned off. Insomnia can be a problem with either cycle.

Insomnia often occurs along with physical and behavioral health conditions. Some disorders linked to insomnia include:

- Mental disorders such as depression, anxiety, and posttraumatic stress disorder (PTSD)

- Use of substances such as caffeine, over-the-counter stimulant medications (including cough and cold remedies containing dextromethorphan), tobacco and other nicotine products, alcohol, and sedatives

- Illnesses that cause ongoing pain, such as arthritis and headache disorders

- Illnesses that make it hard to breathe, such as asthma and heart failure

- An overactive thyroid

- Gastrointestinal disorders, such as heartburn

- Stroke

- Neurodevelopmental and neurological problems, such as autism, Alzheimer disease, and Parkinson disease

- Other sleep disorders, such as restless legs syndrome and sleep-related breathing problems

- Circadian rhythm disorders (timing of internal sleep clock)

- Menopause and hot flashes

Medication as a Factor

Medications may play a role in sleep problems. This is called a medication-induced sleep disorder. Stimulant medications keep a person from sleeping. Sedative medications make a person feel sleepy. If taken at the wrong time of day, medications may contribute to daytime sleepiness or trouble sleeping at night. For example, certain asthma medicines, allergy medications, and cold medicines may be stimulating and lead to insomnia. Beta blockers, which are used to treat heart disease, are also linked to insomnia. Some medications for treating mental disorders, such as antidepressants and Ritalin for attention deficit hyperactivity disorder (ADHD), may lead to insomnia in some people.

Evidence-Based Treatments

When a sleep problem lasts for just a few days, treatment may be unnecessary. For example, after traveling to another time zone, it may be difficult to sleep due to jet lag and a new sleep environment. In this case, the person's body likely will return naturally to a normal sleep-wake schedule.

In other cases, it is important to treat insomnia, especially when lack of sleep causes ongoing problems in daily life.

Insomnia often is linked to medical illnesses, mood disorders, anxiety disorders, and substance use problems. These should be treated at the same time as insomnia disorder. Insomnia can worsen the symptoms of other medical or mental disorders. Similarly, the other disorders may worsen the insomnia. The treatment plan should consider each person's needs and choices. A person should consult a healthcare professional when choosing the right treatment and consider their own gender, race, ethnicity, language, and culture.

Assessment

Most clinicians start treatment by asking about health and lifestyle factors that might be related to sleep problems. These assessments can help a clinician better understand a person's sleep problem.

A clinician determines sleep history by asking questions such as: What time to you go to bed? How long does it take you to fall asleep? How often do you wake up at night? What time to you get up in the morning (on weekdays and on weekends)? The clinician may ask the person to track their sleep patterns using a sleep log or sleep diary.

Activigraphy is a device worn on the wrist that measures movement. This provides an estimate of how long you sleep at night and how often you wake up at night. The device is generally worn for at least seven days, and often 14 days or longer.

A clinician performs a complete physical exam to rule out medical problems that might cause insomnia. A blood test can check for thyroid problems or other disorders that can cause sleep problems. A physical exam may reveal whether insomnia is an early warning sign of another medical problem.

A person may undergo an overnight sleep study, or polysomnography. The person sleeps overnight in a sleep study lab. There, a machine can monitor stages of sleep. But sleep studies are increasingly done in a person's own home. The main goal is to identify sleep-related breathing difficulties. In general, a sleep study is used for insomnia only if there may be another sleep disorder.

Based on the assessment, a clinician is likely to suggest a course of treatment. This might include sleep hygiene changes, psychotherapy, medication, or a combination.

Sleep Hygiene

Sleep hygiene, sometimes called lifestyle changes, can help promote sleep. These changes can make it easier to fall asleep and stay asleep. A person can do them without seeking professional help. Here are examples of sleep hygiene:

- Adopting good bedtime habits, including a routine with relaxing activities before bed, such as reading, listening to music, or taking a bath
- Avoiding heavy meals or drinking a lot of fluids before bedtime
- Up to eight hours before bedtime, avoiding substances that make sleeping difficult, including caffeine, tobacco, and stimulants such as energy drinks or diet pills

- Avoiding, if possible, certain over-the-counter and prescription medicines, such as some cold and allergy medicines that contain pseudoephedrine
- Avoiding alcohol before bedtime, which increases the likelihood of waking up often during the night
- Creating a sleep-friendly environment by reducing light in the bedroom from windows and digital devices that produce
- Limiting distractions, such as a TV, tablet, smartphone, or computer
- Keeping the room temperature cool and comfortable
- Going to bed when feeling sleepy, but getting up at the same time each day

Psychotherapy

There are many forms of psychotherapy, sometimes called "talk therapy," that are effective for insomnia.

Cognitive behavioral therapy for insomnia (CBT-I) is often the initial treatment for chronic insomnia. It targets difficulty falling sleep, maintaining sleep, or both. It is sometimes combined with other psychotherapy approaches. CBT-I usually lasts for four to 10 weeks. Up to 70 percent of people who complete CBT-I improve, and nearly 40 percent have average or good sleep after treatment. For people with insomnia who have another medical or mental disorder such as depression or chronic pain, CBT-I improves overall health and may reduce thoughts of suicide.

Relaxation training or progressive muscle relaxation teaches a person to tense and relax muscles in different parts of the body. This helps calm the body and promote falling sleep.

Stimulus control, sometimes called **reconditioning,** limits the type of activities allowed in the bedroom. The bed is linked to sleep and sex only, not other activities such as eating, working, watching TV, or scanning the Internet.

Sleep restriction involves a strict schedule of bedtimes and wake times, and limits time in bed to sleep time.

Medications

Many prescription medicines are used to treat insomnia. Some are meant for short-term use. Others may be used for a longer length of time.

Nonpharmacological treatments such as therapy are the first line interventions; however, if pharmacological treatment is needed, it is best to consult a professional for an individualized care plan, as some medications can be habit forming.

It is important to consider the effectiveness and side effects of medications. Some insomnia medicines may lose their effectiveness over time.

Some over-the-counter products claim to treat insomnia. For example, medicines that contain antihistamines, typically used to treat allergies, are often sold as sleep aids. Antihistamines are likely to make a person drowsy, but there may be other side effects.

Other over-the-counter products advertised as sleep aids include natural ingredients such as melatonin, L-tryptophan, and valerian. The U.S. Food and Drug Administration (FDA) does not regulate "natural" products, so the dose and purity of these products can vary.

Complementary Therapies and Activities

Complementary therapies and activities, listed below, can help people improve their overall wellbeing, and are meant to be used along with evidence-based treatments.

- Exercise or physical activity.

- Hypnotherapy.

- Melatonin in small doses may help promote sleep in some people.

- Relaxation techniques.

- Yoga and massage therapy.

- Studies of melatonin in children with sleep problems suggest that it may be helpful, both in generally healthy children and in those with conditions such as autism or attention-deficit hyperactivity disorder. However, both the number of studies and the number of children who participated in the studies are small, and all of the studies tested melatonin only for short periods of time.

- Melatonin supplements appear to be relatively safe for short-term use, although the use of melatonin was linked to bad moods in elderly people (most of whom had dementia) in one study.

- The long-term safety of melatonin supplements has not been established.

- Studies of L-tryptophan supplements as an insomnia treatment have had inconsistent results, and the effects of 5-HTP supplements on insomnia have not been established.

- The use of L-tryptophan supplements may be linked to eosinophilia-myalgia syndrome (EMS), a complex, potentially fatal disorder with multiple symptoms including severe muscle pain. It is uncertain whether the risk of EMS associated with L-tryptophan supplements is due to impurities in L-tryptophan preparations or to L-tryptophan itself.

- Mindfulness-based stress reduction is a type of meditation that can help with sleep.

- Other relaxation techniques involve breathing exercises and guided imagery.

- Dietary supplements, including L-tryptophan and 5-hydroxy-tryptophan (5-HTP), are being studied as sleep aids.

Recovery and Social Support Services and Activities

Recovery is a process of change through which people improve their health and wellness, live self-directed lives, and strive to reach their full potential. One of the hallmarks of effective treatment is that it is durable. Good sleep is an important part of good health and recovery. Treating insomnia may help with recovery and improve health. Recovery from insomnia is likely through a combination of treatment and managing the symptoms.

Self-help and support groups can provide people with the knowledge and support to make treatment decisions that work for them.

Here are resources for people with insomnia and other sleep problems:

- American Academy of Sleep Medicine (AASM)

- American Sleep Apnea Association (ASAA)

- American Sleep Association (ASA)

- National Center on Sleep Disorders Research (NCSDR) (part of the National Heart, Lung and Blood Institute)

- National Alliance on Mental Illness (NAMI)

- National Sleep Foundation (NSF)

- Society of Behavioral Sleep Medicine (SBSM)

Future Directions in Research and Treatment

Researchers look at family history and genetic factors that might influence insomnia. Also, brain imaging studies may help show how brain function differs in people with insomnia. Studies examine how people experience insomnia and respond to treatments. These studies focus on insomnia in children, nursing home residents, postmenopausal women, people with chronic insomnia, and those with insomnia combined with medical or mental disorders.

Researchers study delivery of cognitive behavioral therapy for insomnia by telephone or through the Internet.

Other promising areas of focus for research and treatment include:

- **Biomarkers:** testing blood, saliva, or urine to look for factors that relate to risk or severity of insomnia

- **Circadian rhythm disorders:** how patterns of healthy and unhealthy sleep relate to the timing of a person's internal sleep clock

- **Dismantling studies for CBT-I:** studying separate components of CBT-I to determine which work best and for which type of person

- **Natural history studies:** looking at causes of short-term insomnia and determining how short-term problems become chronic problems

- **Prevention:** how to keep insomnia from becoming a chronic problem, and to prevent medical or mental disorders through early treatment of insomnia

- **Effects of sleep loss:** how untreated insomnia increases the risk for medical and mental disorders

Finding Treatment

Consult a healthcare professional who has training and experience working with insomnia. For general information on mental disorders and to locate treatment services in your area, contact Substance Abuse and Mental Health Services Administration (SAMHSA) National Helpline, 800-662-HELP (800-662-4357). SAMHSA's Behavioral Health Treatment Locator and the National Institute of Mental Health (NIMH) Help for Mental Illnesses webpage have more information and resources. If you are having suicidal thoughts or are worried that someone you know might be suicidal, contact the Suicide Prevention Lifeline, 800-273-TALK (800-273-8255).

Chapter 39

Menopause

What Is Menopause?

Menopause is the point in time when a woman's menstrual periods stop. Menopause happens because the ovaries stop producing the hormones estrogen and progesterone. Once you have gone through menopause, you can't get pregnant anymore. Some people call the years leading up to a woman's last period menopause, but that time actually is the menopausal transition, or perimenopause.

Menopause and Mental Health

Midlife is often considered a period of increased risk for depression in women. Some women report mood swings, irritability, tearfulness, anxiety, and feelings of despair in the years leading up to menopause. But the reason for these emotional problems isn't always clear. Research shows that menopausal symptoms such as sleep

This chapter contains text excerpted from the following sources: Text under the heading "What Is Menopause?" is excerpted from "Menopause Basics," Office on Women's Health (OWH), U.S. Department of Health and Human Services (HHS), September 22, 2010. Reviewed September 2017; Text under the heading "Menopause and Mental Health" is excerpted from "Menopause and Mental Health," Office on Women's Health (OWH), U.S. Department of Health and Human Services (HHS), September 29, 2010. Reviewed September 2017; Text under the heading "Menopause and Mood Changes" is excerpted from "Menstruation, Menopause, and Mental Health," Office on Women's Health (OWH), U.S. Department of Health and Human Services (HHS), March 29, 2010. Reviewed September 2017.

problems, hot flashes, night sweats, and fatigue can affect mood and well-being. The drop in estrogen levels during perimenopause and menopause might also affect mood. Or it could be a combination of hormone changes and menopausal symptoms.

But changes in mood also can have causes that are unrelated to menopause. If you are having emotional problems that are interfering with your quality of life, it is important to discuss them with your doctor. Talk openly with your doctor about the other things going on in your life that might be adding to your feelings. Other things that could cause feelings of depression and/or anxiety during menopause include:

- Having depression before menopause

- Feeling negative about menopause and getting older

- Increased stress

- Having severe menopausal symptoms

- Smoking

- Not being physically active

- Not being happy in your relationship or not being in a relationship

- Not having a job

- Not having enough money

- Having low self-esteem (how you feel about yourself)

- Not having the social support you need

- Feeling disappointed that you can't have children anymore

Menopause and Mood Changes

Women may experience a wide range of feelings, from anxiety and discomfort to release and relief, upon menopause. Most adapt to the changes and continue to live well and remain healthy through these transitions.

Some women, although not all, will experience significant depression before perimenopause. Perimenopause marks the time when your body begins the transition to menopause. It includes the years leading up to menopause—anywhere from two to eight years—plus the first year after your final period. There is no way to tell in advance how long it will last or how long it will take you to go through it. It's a natural part of aging that signals the ending of your reproductive years. Because of the intense hormone changes during perimenopause, women are more likely to have menopause-related depression before they reach actual menopause.

When women go through menopause, some may feel badly at the loss of their ability to bear children. However, some women look at menopause as a time to expand their work and social activities, and to dedicate more time to their spouse or partner. Having a positive attitude about this life change may help.

However, depression is not just in your mind. It can also be caused by hormonal factors. If you are feeling depressed and are going through menopause, be sure to discuss these feelings with your doctor or a healthcare professional.

Chapter 40

Substance Abuse

Chapter Contents

Section 40.1

Mental and Substance Use Disorders

This section contains text excerpted from the following sources: Text beginning with the heading "Mental and Substance Use Disorders" is excerpted from "Mental and Substance Use Disorders," Substance Abuse and Mental Health Services Administration (SAMHSA), March 8, 2016; Text under the heading "Severe Mental Illness Tied to Higher Rates of Substance Use" is excerpted from "Severe Mental Illness Tied to Higher Rates of Substance Use," National Institute of Health (NIH), January 3, 2014. Reviewed September 2017.

Mental and substance use disorders affect people from all walks of life and all age groups. These illnesses are common, recurrent, and often serious, but they are treatable and many people do recover. Learning about some of the most common mental and substance use disorders can help people recognize their signs and to seek help.

According to Substance Abuse and Mental Health Services Administration (SAMHSA) National Survey on Drug Use and Health (NSDUH) an estimated 43.6 million (18.1%) Americans ages 18 and up experienced some form of mental illness. In the past year, 20.2 million adults (8.4%) had a substance use disorder. Of these, 7.9 million people had both a mental disorder and substance use disorder, also known as co-occurring mental and substance use disorders. Various mental and substance use disorders have prevalence rates that differ by gender, age, race, and ethnicity.

Mental Disorders

Mental disorders involve changes in thinking, mood, and/or behavior. These disorders can affect how we relate to others and make choices. Mental disorders take many different forms, with some rooted in deep levels of anxiety, extreme changes in mood, or reduced ability to focus or behave appropriately. Others involve unwanted, intrusive thoughts and some may result in auditory and visual hallucinations or false beliefs about basic aspects of reality. Reaching a level that can be formally diagnosed often depends on a reduction in a person's ability to function as a result of the disorder.

Anxiety disorders are the most common type of mental disorders, followed by depressive disorders. Different mental disorders are more likely to begin and occur at different stages in life and are thus more prevalent in certain age groups. Lifetime anxiety disorders generally have the earliest age of first onset, most commonly around age 6. Other disorders emerge in childhood, approximately 11 percent of children 4 to 17 years of age (6.4 million) have been diagnosed with attention deficit hyperactivity disorder (ADHD) as of 2011. Schizophrenia spectrum and psychotic disorders emerge later in life, usually in early adulthood. Not all mental health issues first experienced during childhood or adolescence continue into adulthood, and not all mental health issues are first experienced before adulthood. Mental disorders can occur once, reoccur intermittently, or be more chronic in nature. Mental disorders frequently co-occur with each other and with substance use disorders. Because of this and because of variation in symptoms even within one type of disorder, individual situations and symptoms are extremely varied.

Serious Mental Illness

Serious mental illness among people ages 18 and older is defined at the federal level as having, at any time during the past year, a diagnosable mental, behavior, or emotional disorder that causes serious functional impairment that substantially interferes with or limits one or more major life activities. Serious mental illnesses include major depression, schizophrenia, and bipolar disorder, and other mental disorders that cause serious impairment. In 2014, there were an estimated 9.8 million adults (4.1%) ages 18 and up with a serious mental illness in the past year. People with serious mental illness are more likely to be unemployed, arrested, and/or face inadequate housing compared to those without mental illness.

Serious Emotional Disturbance

The term serious emotional disturbance (SED) is used to refer to children and youth who have had a diagnosable mental, behavioral, or emotional disorder in the past year, which resulted in functional impairment that substantially interferes with or limits the child's role or functioning in family, school, or community activities. A Centers for Disease Control and Prevention (CDC) review of population-level information found that estimates of the number of children with a mental disorder range from 13 to 20 percent, but current national surveys do not have an indicator of SED.

Substance Use Disorders

Substance use disorders occur when the recurrent use of alcohol and/or drugs causes clinically significant impairment, including health problems, disability, and failure to meet major responsibilities at work, school, or home. In 2014, about 21.5 million Americans ages 12 and older (8.1%) were classified with a substance use disorder in the past year. Of those, 2.6 million had problems with both alcohol and drugs, 4.5 million had problems with drugs but not alcohol, and 14.4 million had problems with alcohol only.

Co-Occurring Mental and Substance Use Disorders

The coexistence of both a mental health and a substance use disorder is referred to as co-occurring disorders. According to SAMHSA's 2014 National Survey on Drug Use and Health (NSDUH), approximately 7.9 million adults had co-occurring disorders in 2014. During the past year, for those adults surveyed who experienced substance use disorders and any mental illness, rates were highest among adults ages 26 to 49 (42.7%). For adults with past-year serious mental illness and co-occurring substance use disorders, rates were highest among those ages 18 to 25 (35.3%) in 2014.

Severe Mental Illness Tied to Higher Rates of Substance Use

People with severe mental illness such as schizophrenia or bipolar disorder have a higher risk for substance use, especially cigarette smoking, and protective factors usually associated with lower rates of substance use do not exist in severe mental illness, according to a new study funded by the National Institute on Drug Abuse (NIDA), part of the National Institutes of Health (NIH). Estimates based on past studies suggest that people diagnosed with mood or anxiety disorders are about twice as likely as the general population to also suffer from a substance use disorder. Statistics from the 2012 National Survey on Drug Use and Health indicate close to 8.4 million adults in the United States have both a mental and substance use disorder. However, only 7.9 percent of people receive treatment for both conditions, and 53.7 percent receive no treatment at all, the statistics indicate.

Studies exploring the link between substance use disorders and other mental illnesses have typically not included people with severe psychotic illnesses.

"Drug use impacts many of the same brain circuits that are disrupted in severe mental disorders such as schizophrenia," said NIDA Director Dr. Nora D. Volkow. "While we cannot always prove a connection or causality, we do know that certain mental disorders are risk factors for subsequent substance use disorders, and vice versa." In the current study, 9,142 people diagnosed with schizophrenia, schizoaffective disorder, or bipolar disorder with psychotic features, and 10,195 controls matched to participants according to geographic region, were selected using the Genomic Psychiatry Cohort program. Mental disorder diagnoses were confirmed using the Diagnostic Interview for Psychosis and Affective Disorder (DI-PAD), and controls were screened to verify the absence of schizophrenia or bipolar disorder in themselves or close family members. The DI-PAD was also used for all participants to determine substance use rates.

Compared to controls, people with severe mental illness were about 4 times more likely to be heavy alcohol users (four or more drinks per day); 3.5 times more likely to use marijuana regularly (21 times per year); and 4.6 times more likely to use other drugs at least 10 times in their lives. The greatest increases were seen with tobacco, with patients with severe mental illness 5.1 times more likely to be daily smokers. This is of concern because smoking is the leading cause of preventable death in the United States.

In addition, certain protective factors often associated with belonging to certain racial or ethnic groups—or being female—did not exist in participants with severe mental illness. "In the general population, women have lower substance use rates than men, and Asian-Americans have lower substance use rates than white Americans, but we do not see these differences among people with severe mental illness," said Dr. Sarah Hartz, from the Washington University School of Medicine in St. Louis and first author on the study. "We also saw that among young people with severe mental illness, the smoking rates were as high as smoking rates in middle-aged adults, despite success in lowering smoking rates for young people in the general population."

Previous research has shown that people with schizophrenia have a shorter life expectancy than the general population, and chronic cigarette smoking has been suggested as a major contributing factor to higher morbidity and mortality from malignancy as well as cardiovascular and respiratory diseases. These new findings indicate that the rates of substance use in people with severe psychosis may be underestimated, highlighting the need to improve the understanding of the association between substance use and psychotic disorders so that both conditions can be treated effectively.

Section 40.2

Link between Marijuana Use and Psychiatric Disorders

This section includes text excerpted from "Is There a
Link between Marijuana Use and Psychiatric Disorders?"
National Institute on Drug Abuse (NIDA), March 2016.

Several studies have linked marijuana use to increased risk for
psychiatric disorders, including psychosis (schizophrenia), depression,
anxiety, and substance use disorders, but whether and to what extent
it actually causes these conditions is not always easy to determine.
The amount of drug used, the age at first use, and genetic vulnerability have all been shown to influence this relationship. The strongest
evidence to date concerns links between marijuana use and substance
use disorders and between marijuana use and psychiatric disorders in
those with a preexisting genetic or other vulnerability.

Research using longitudinal data from the National Epidemiologi-
cal Survey on Alcohol and Related Conditions examined associations
between marijuana use and mood and anxiety disorders and substance
use disorders. After adjusting for various confounding factors, no association between marijuana use and mood and anxiety disorders was
found. The only significant associations were increased risk of alcohol
use disorders, nicotine dependence, marijuana use disorder, and other
drug use disorders.

Recent research has found that marijuana users who carry a specific
variant of the *AKT1* gene, which codes for an enzyme that affects dopamine signaling in the *striatum*, are at increased risk of developing psychosis. The striatum is an area of the brain that becomes activated and
flooded with dopamine when certain stimuli are present. One study found
that the risk for psychosis among those with this variant was seven times
higher for daily marijuana users compared with infrequent- or nonusers.

Another study found an increased risk of psychosis among adults
who had used marijuana in adolescence and also carried a specific
variant of the gene for catechol-O-methyltransferase (COMT), an
enzyme that degrades neurotransmitters such as dopamine and norepinephrine. Marijuana use has also been shown to worsen the course

of illness in patients who already have schizophrenia. As mentioned previously, marijuana can also produce an acute psychotic reaction in non-Schizophrenic users, especially at high doses, although this fades as the drug wears off.

Inconsistent and modest associations have been reported between marijuana use and suicidal thoughts and attempted suicide among teens. Marijuana has also been associated with an *amotivational syndrome*, defined as a diminished or absent drive to engage in typically rewarding activities. Because of the role of the endocannabinoid system in regulating mood and reward, it has been hypothesizes that brain changes resulting from early use of marijuana may underlie these associations, but more research is needed to verify that such links exist and better understand them.

Adverse Consequences of Marijuana Use

Acute (Present during Intoxication)

- Impaired short-term memory
- Impaired attention, judgment, and other cognitive functions
- Impaired coordination and balance
- Increased heart rate
- Anxiety, paranoia
- Psychosis (uncommon)

Persistent (Lasting Longer than Intoxication, But May Not Be Permanent)

- Impaired learning and coordination
- Sleep problems

Long Term (Cumulative Effects of Repeated Use)

- Potential for marijuana addiction
- Impairments in learning and memory with potential loss of IQ
- Increased risk of chronic cough, bronchitis
- Increased risk of other drug and alcohol use disorders
- Increased risk of schizophrenia in people with genetic vulnerability

Part Five

Managing Stress and Everyday Anxiety

Chapter 41

Coping with Stress

Common Stress Reactions[1]

Everyone—adults, teens, and even children—experiences stress at times. Stress can be beneficial by helping people develop the skills they need to cope with and adapt to new and potentially threatening situations throughout life. However, the beneficial aspects of stress diminish when it is severe enough to overwhelm a person's ability to take care of themselves and family. Using healthy ways to cope and getting the right care and support can put problems in perspective and help stressful feelings and symptoms subside.

Sometimes after experiencing a traumatic event that is especially frightening—including personal or environmental disasters, or being threatened with an assault—people have a strong and lingering stress reaction to the event. Strong emotions, jitters, sadness, or depression may all be part of this normal and temporary reaction to the stress of an overwhelming event.

Common reactions to a stressful event can include:

• Disbelief, shock, and numbness

This chapter includes text excerpted from documents published by two public domain sources. Text under headings marked 1 are excerpted from "Violence Prevention—Coping with Stress," Centers for Disease Control and Prevention (CDC), October 2, 2015; Text under heading marked 2 is excerpted from "Stress and Your Health," Office on Women's Health (OWH), U.S. Department of Health and Human Services (HHS), June 13, 2017.

- Feeling sad, frustrated, and helpless
- Fear and anxiety about the future
- Feeling guilty
- Anger, tension, and irritability
- Difficulty concentrating and making decisions
- Crying
- Reduced interest in usual activities
- Wanting to be alone
- Loss of appetite
- Sleeping too much or too little
- Nightmares or bad memories
- Reoccurring thoughts of the event
- Headaches, back pains, and stomach problems
- Increased heart rate, difficulty breathing
- Smoking or use of alcohol or drugs

Effects of Stress on Your Body[2]

The body responds to stress by releasing stress hormones. These hormones make blood pressure, heart rate, and blood sugar levels go up. Long-term stress can help cause a variety of health problems, including:

- Mental health disorders, like depression and anxiety
- Obesity
- Heart disease
- High blood pressure
- Abnormal heart beats
- Menstrual problems
- Acne and other skin problems

Healthy Ways to Cope with Stress[1]

Feeling emotional and nervous or having trouble sleeping and eating can all be normal reactions to stress. Engaging in healthy activities and getting the right care and support can put problems in perspective and help stressful feelings subside in a few days or weeks. Some tips for beginning to feel better are:

- Take care of yourself.
    - Eat healthy, well-balanced meals
    - Exercise on a regular basis
    - Get plenty of sleep
    - Give yourself a break if you feel stressed out
- Talk to others. Share your problems and how you are feeling and coping with a parent, friend, counselor, doctor, or pastor.
- Avoid drugs and alcohol. Drugs and alcohol may seem to help with the stress. In the long run, they create additional problems and increase the stress you are already feeling.
- Take a break. If your stress is caused by a national or local event, take breaks from listening to the news stories, which can increase your stress.

Recognize when you need more help. If problems continue or you are thinking about suicide, talk to a psychologist, social worker, or professional counselor.

Helping Youth Cope with Stress[1]

Because of their level of development, children and adolescents often struggle with how to cope well with stress. Youth can be particularly overwhelmed when their stress is connected to a traumatic event—like a natural disaster (earthquakes, tornados, wildfires), family loss, school shootings, or community violence. Parents and educators can take steps to provide stability and support that help young people feel better.

Tips for Parents

It is natural for children to worry, especially when scary or stressful events happen in their lives. Talking with children about these stressful events and monitoring what children watch or hear about the events can help put frightening information into a more balanced context. Some suggestions to help children cope are:

- **Maintain a normal routine.** Helping children wake up, go to sleep, and eat meals at regular times provide them a sense of stability. Going to school and participating in typical after-school activities also provide stability and extra support.

- **Talk, listen, and encourage expression.** Create opportunities to have your children talk, but do not force them. Listen to your child's thoughts and feelings and share some of yours. After a traumatic event, it is important for children to feel like they can share their feelings and to know that their fears and worries are understandable. Keep these conversations going by asking them how they feel in a week, then in a month, and so on.

- **Watch and listen.** Be alert for any change in behavior. Are children sleeping more or less? Are they withdrawing from friends or family? Are they behaving in any way out of the ordinary? Any changes in behavior, even small changes, may be signs that the child is having trouble coming to terms with the event and may support.

- **Reassure.** Stressful events can challenge a child's sense of physical and emotional safety and security. Take opportunities to reassure your child about his or her safety and wellbeing and discuss ways that you, the school, and the community are taking steps to keep them safe.

- **Connect with others.** Make an on-going effort to talk to other parents and your child's teachers about concerns and ways to help your child cope. You do not have to deal with problems alone-it is often helpful for parents, schools, and health professionals to work together to support and ensuring the wellbeing of all children in stressful times.

Tips for Kids and Teen

After a traumatic or violent event, it is normal to feel anxious about your safety and security. Even if you were not directly involved, you may worry about whether this type of event may someday affect you. How can you deal with these fears? Start by looking at the tips below for some ideas.

- **Talk to and stay connected to others.** This connection might be your parent, another relative, a friend, neighbor, teacher, coach, school nurse, counselor, family doctor, or member of your church or temple. Talking with someone can help you make sense out of your experience and figure out ways to feel better.

If you are not sure where to turn, call your local crisis intervention center or a national hotline.

- **Get active.** Go for a walk, play sports, write a play or poem, play a musical instrument, or join an after-school program. Volunteer with a community group that promotes nonviolence or another school or community activity that you care about. Trying any of these can be a positive way to handle your feelings and to see that things are going to get better.

- **Take care of yourself.** As much as possible, try to get enough sleep, eat right, exercise, and keep a normal routine. It may be hard to do, but by keeping yourself healthy you will be better able to handle a tough time.

- **Take information breaks.** Pictures and stories about a disaster can increase worry and other stressful feelings. Taking breaks from the news, Internet, and conversations about the disaster can help calm you down.

Chapter 42

Walking to Wellness

Most adults in the United States today do not spend enough time exercising to get optimal benefits. People with anxiety and depression symptoms tend to be even less active than people who do not experience these emotional symptoms. Although there is substantial scientific evidence showing that exercise can help manage anxiety and depression, there are few intervention materials that are especially designed to help people use exercise for emotional health.

This chapter on *Walking to Wellness* is designed to be used as an adjunct to other interventions in primary care, mental health (MH), and health promotion clinical settings for managing chronic conditions. *Walking to Wellness* can be used along with medication, psychotherapy, supportive counseling for persons seeking treatment for mental health symptoms, or for other wellness education.

Who Can Benefit from Walking to Wellness?

Almost every adult can experience better physical and mental health if he or she engages in regular exercise. In this program researchers consider any physical activity that is done with the purpose of improving or maintaining health to be "exercise."

- Exercise does not need to be strenuous. The kind of exercise that is encouraged should also not be painful. They especially

This chapter includes text excerpted from "Walking to Wellness—Exercise for Physical and Emotional Health," Mental Illness Research, Education, and Clinical Centers (MIRECC), U.S. Department of Veterans Affairs (VA), December 7, 2015.

recommend walking because walking is safe and available for almost everyone. Some people can use other kinds of exercise to achieve the goals of this program.

- *Walking to Wellness* was designed to be used by adults experiencing mild to moderate stress, anxiety, and/or depression symptoms. The materials are written for someone who can walk for at least 10 minutes, but could be adapted for clients who need to start with very brief walks because of their health conditions. It is believed many people who are struggling with anxiety or depression symptoms will be more successful if they try the activities with a group of other participants or in the context of some kind of individual counseling with a facilitator or therapist.

- *Walking to Wellness* is not an exercise training program to be substituted for therapy provided by exercise or rehabilitation specialists. In a medical setting, it is appropriate to have a note from a participant's medical provider stating that it is safe for him or her to engage in light or moderate walking and whether there are any specific limitations to physical activity that your doctor and you need to consider.

Exercise Can Help Treat and Prevent Many Common Health Problems

The benefits of exercise on physical health, including decreased risk of cardiovascular disease, stroke, type 2 diabetes, breast and colon cancer, and osteoporosis are now widely recognized. Additional benefits for older adults include reduced risk of falls and protecting physical and cognitive function. Many scientific reviews support the value of exercise as part of recovery plans for mental illness, treatment for depression, and improved quality of life in varied patient populations. A Cochrane Database review of 39 controlled clinical trials, a meta-analysis of studies that only included patients with clinically significant depression, and a meta-analysis of 90 articles on depressive symptoms in patients with chronic illness all concluded that aerobic exercise reduces depression symptoms. One study found that exercise could be as effective as adding a second antidepressant medication and another found less relapse in patients with depression who exercised. Although the smaller number of trials of exercise for anxiety outcomes requires more cautious conclusions, controlled studies have shown that exercise reduces anxiety sensitivity and anxiety symptoms. Exercise also reduces reactivity to stressful stimuli. Positive effects of exercise on sleep in middle aged and older adults with insomnia were recently confirmed in a meta-analysis. A carefully controlled trial found clear dose-response relationships between exercise and improvements in self-reported mental and physical quality of life (QoL) in sedentary women. Reviews have also shown mental health (MH) benefits for cancer survivors and for osteoarthritis pain. Almost everyone could potentially receive multiple benefits from regular exercise.

Exercise Benefits Occur across a Wide Dose Range Achievable by Almost All Adults

Although the public health exercise recommendations for moderate intensity aerobic exercise for at least 10 minutes at a time, accumulating to at least 30 minutes total on at least 5 days each week also seem optimal for MH, exercise of lower intensity and duration also has meaningful physical and mental health benefits. "Incidental" short bursts of moderate intensity activity of less than 10 minutes are positively associated with cardiorespiratory fitness. Exercising for just 10 minutes improves vigor, fatigue, and overall mood. Easy-paced regular walking protects cognition in aging women. Exercise at only 50 percent of public health recommended levels produces significant improvement in QoL; and even low levels of activity that do not meet recommended guidelines can prevent future depression. Meeting public health guidelines is the ideal, but every step and every minute counts.

There Are Many Biological and Psychosocial Mechanisms for Exercise Effects on MH

Potential physiologic mechanisms that are especially relevant to MH include favorable effects of exercise on inflammation, serotonin metabolism, the hypothalamic-pituitary-adrenal axis, autonomic nervous system, endogenous endorphins, and neurotropic factors that could augment learning and extinction processes in cognitive behavioral therapy (CBT). Another theoretical mechanism for exercise in MH is behavioral activation, increasing opportunities for positive interactions with the environment, and positive reinforcement. Some of these effects take weeks or months, but most people want to feel better quickly.

People with Depression, Anxiety, Stress, and Related Mental Health Problems Can Initiate and Maintain Exercise

A study compared telephone care management that included a pedometer walking program to a control self-help book in depressed type 2 diabetes mellitus patients. After 12 months, counseling patients had lower depression, better QoL scores, and higher weekly step counts than controls. Another study compared two clinic exercise counseling sessions plus phone calls with usual care control in primary care patients with new episodes of depression. This study has been criticized because many patients in both groups were prescribed antidepressants, and there were no differences in depression scores at follow-up; however, 58 percent of exercise patients achieved exercise goals. These studies demonstrate that primary care patients with significant depression who receive motivational counseling can adopt and sustain increases in physical activity for at least a year.

Brief Exercise Interventions Can Produce Clinically Meaningful Behavior Change

Scientific reviews are consistent in finding that interventions using self-regulation behavioral strategies such as goal-setting and self-monitoring produce meaningful increases in physical activity for previously inactive or under-active adults. Reviews specific to interventions that used pedometers also have found significant increases in steps per day and reduced body mass index compared with controls. In addition to the many successful physical activity interventions that involve multiple sessions over several months, a few trials have evaluated very brief interventions and found meaningful changes in physical activity and health. Obese and overweight patients with impaired glucose tolerance who received a single group session based on behavioral strategies and a step counter significantly increased their steps/day and improved glucose tolerance after 6 and 12 months. Overweight and obese men who completed a motivational intervention worksheet as part of a mailed questionnaire significantly increased frequency of physical activity for at least 20 minutes at a time compared with controls who simply reported on their usual activity. Obese, overweight male Veterans with physical function limitations who had two exercise counseling sessions, 1 or 2 phone calls, and kept exercise diaries significantly increased walking and strength exercises, and were more likely to average at least 30 min/day of moderate activity at 10 months. In another trial with primary care patients, 46 percent of aging men who received a single brief counseling by a nurse began walking at least 3 days/week, and 28 percent were still walking at least 1 day/ week after 12 months.

Chapter 43

Becoming More Resilient

Resilience, as a concept and construct, is the context-specific ability to respond to stress, anxiety, trauma, crisis, or disaster. Resilience develops over time and is the culmination of multiple internal and external factors. For those who develop mental and/or substance use disorders, the influence of both internal development and external environments converge to either promote or restrict the development of personal resilience.

The work of enhancing resilience for persons with mental and/ or substance use problems has its greatest impact during the formative stages to prevent more severe conditions and to promote health. Additionally, although more research is needed to fully examine the possible effects, resilience is also critical in the recovery stage where life skills and other supports can be accessed to manage future stress. It is the interaction of risk and protective factors that plays the central role in the development, enhancement, and activation of resilience.

- **Individual factors** such as development of a desirable personal identity; a feeling of power and control over one's life; a feeling of self-worth; a sense of social justice; a sense of cohesion with others; good self-regulation skills; close relationships with competent adults; connections to prosocial organizations; tolerance for delayed gratification; a sense of humor; development of good

This chapter includes text excerpted from "Resilience Annotated Bibliography," Substance Abuse and Mental Health Services Administration (SAMHSA), March 2013. Reviewed September 2017.

coping and problem-solving skills; an ability to see and set long-term goals; and a positive outlook for the future

- **Family factors** such as consistent, appropriate parental involvement, discipline, and supervision; good parenting skills; trusting relationships; a safe environment; well-defined and appropriate family roles and responsibilities; opportunities to learn to deal appropriately with criticism, rejection, and silence; prosocial values and ethics; and good goal-setting and deci-sion-making skills exhibited by parents

- **Community factors** such as participation in school, work, and the community that create an environment in which an individual has opportunities to develop and practice social and cognitive skills, develop a sense of belonging, contribute to the work of the community, This develop a social network of peers, and learn to handle challenges and practice prosocial behavioral skills and self-efficacy

Risk factors come in many different forms, but at their core they are attitudes, beliefs, or environmental circumstances that put an individual in jeopardy of developing a mental and/or substance use disorder. Depending on the source, risk factors may include:

- **Individual temperament characteristics** related to locus of control (external versus internal), poor self-control, negative emotionality, a need for immediate gratification, and even physi-cal activity level.

- **Family-related risk factors**, which may include parental and sibling drug use, poor child-rearing and socialization practices, ineffective parental supervision of the child, ineffective paren-tal discipline skills, negative parent-child relationships, family conflict, marital discord, domestic violence, abuse and neglect, family disorganization, and family social isolation.

- **Community/environmental risk factors** or the social deter-minants of health, e.g., limited resources, low socioeconomic sta-tus, and communities that lack the knowledge, skills, and pro-gramming necessary to reach out to those in need of assistance.

Although the impact of a single protective or risk factor may have little effect on the individual, a combination of risk factors, for exam-ple, can create multilevel stress events that can overwhelm individ-uals who do not have a well-developed resilience to stress and lack the coping, decision-making, and problem-solving skills necessary to bounce back.

Understanding the role of risk and protective factors resonate with current health reforms that focus on prevention and community wellness, which in turn influence the social determinants of health. The risk and protective factors involved in building, enhancing, and activating resilience in persons with or at risk for behavioral health conditions form the foundations of the social determinants of health.

Chapter 44

Coping with Emotions without Smoking

Stress is a normal part of life—in moderation it can help you reach your goals, but too much stress creates more problems. Managing stress is a key part of quitting smoking. You may have learned to deal with stress by smoking. But there are ways to handle stress without smoking. Here are a few ideas you might find helpful. Some of these tips may take practice, but others you can do right away. Try one or more to learn what works for you.

Relax

Our bodies respond to stress by releasing hormones that increase your heart rate and raise your blood pressure. Practicing relaxation techniques, like the ones below, may improve your health and help you handle your stress in positive ways.

Breathe

Take a few slow, deep breaths—in through your nose, out through your mouth. You will feel your body start to relax.

This chapter includes text excerpted from "Coping with Emotions without Smoking," Smokefree.gov, U.S. Department of Health and Human Services (HHS), September 16, 2017.

Locate Your Stress

Take a minute to figure out how stress affects your body. Where do you feel tension in your body? Finding ways to reduce that tension will also help your mental stress. A warm bath, a massage, or stretching can help you release built-up tension.

Visualize

Think of a place where you feel safe, comfortable, and relaxed. Picture it as clearly as you can, including imagining what you would feel, hear, and maybe even smell if you were in that relaxing place. Let yourself enjoy being there for a few minutes.

Exercise

Being active sends out natural chemicals that help your mood and reduce your stress. Sometimes a short walk is all it takes to relieve stress. And walking is free!

Talk

You don't have to deal with stress alone. Share your feelings with friends, family, and other important people in your life who are able to support you in staying smokefree.

Focus

Life can sometimes be overwhelming. Try not to get caught up in worrying about what's next. Instead, try to focus on what is happening now, not what you might have to deal with in the future.

Care

Make an extra effort to take care of yourself. This includes basic things like eating a balanced diet, drinking lots of water, and getting enough sleep.

Do Good

Doing something nice for others can make your day a little better too. Being caring toward others helps you reduce your own stress.

Decaffeinate

Caffeine can help you stay awake, but it also can make you feel tense, jittery, and stressed. Cutting back or even doing away with caffeine can help reduce your feelings of stress. Switching to herbal tea or even hot water with lemon gives you a chance to enjoy a hot beverage but without the caffeine.

Accept

Life is full of twists and turns. You'll always have some stress in your life. It helps to understand that there will be good days and bad days.

Chapter 45

Pets Are Good for Mental Health

Human-Animal Bond

Many people intuitively believe that they and others derive health benefits from relationships with their animal companions, and numerous scientific studies performed over the past 25 years support this belief. Among other benefits, animals have been demonstrated to improve human cardio-vascular health, reduce stress, decrease loneliness and depression, and facilitate social interactions among people who choose to have pets. Additionally, many terminally ill, pregnant, or immunocompromised people are urged to relinquish their animal companions due to concerns about zoonoses (diseases that may be transmitted between humans and nonhuman animals). However, giving up their beloved friends may have a detrimental, rather than beneficial, effect on their overall health. In many instances, human health professionals can contribute to the welfare of their patients by

This chapter contains text excerpted from the following sources: Text beginning with the heading "Human-Animal Bond" is excerpted from "The Health Benefits of Companion Animals," National Park Service (NPS), February 17, 2017; Text beginning with the heading "Mental Well-Being" is excerpted from "Pets Promote Public Health!" U.S. Public Health Service Commissioned Corps (PHSCC), U.S. Department of Health and Human Services (HHS), May 4, 2015.

encouraging them to maintain bonds with their pets, even in the face of serious illnesses and other challenges.

Physiological Benefits

Numerous studies highlight physiologic benefits. Pet interaction, whether active or passive, tends to lower anxiety levels in subjects, and thus decrease the onset, severity, or progression of stress-related conditions. Furthermore, it is thought that the reduction in blood pressure achieved through dog ownership can be equal to the reduction achieved by changing to a low salt diet or cutting down on alcohol. Pet ownership and other animal contact, such as petting animals and watching fish in an aquarium, have specifically been demonstrated to provide cardiovascular benefits. Examples include:

- Increased survival time after myocardial infarction for dog owners.

- Decreased risk factors for cardiovascular disease, particularly lower systolic blood pressure, plasma cholesterol and plasma triglycerides.

- Decreased heart rate from petting a dog or watching fish in an aquarium

These beneficial effects of pets may be mediated by increased exercise associated with pet ownership as well as decreased stress levels.

In addition to providing cardiovascular benefits, decreased physiological stress is associated with animal interaction, contributing to better overall health:

- Greater reduction of cardiovascular stress response in the presence of a dog in comparison to friends or spouses.

- Decreased pulse rate, increased skin temperature, and decreased muscle tension in elderly people watching an aquarium.

- Enhanced hormone levels of dopamine and endorphins associated with happiness and well-being and decreased levels of cortisol, a stress hormone, following a quiet 30-minute session of interacting with a dog.

- Reduced levels of the stress hormone cortisol in healthcare professionals after as little as 5 minutes interacting with a therapy dog.

Other studies document that children exposed to pets in early life experience enhanced immune function:

- Fewer allergies and less wheezing and asthma in children exposed to pets during infancy.

- Protection against adult asthma and allergies in adults at age 28 when exposed to pets before 18.

Several studies document overall general health benefits of pet ownership and animal interaction:

- Less frequent illness and less susceptibility to upper respiratory infection related to a significant increase in 18 IgA (Immunoglobulin A) levels occurred after petting a dog.

- Increased lung function and overall quality of life in lung transplant patients who are allowed to have a pet.

- Perceived pain significantly reduced in children undergoing major operations after participation in pet therapy programs.

- A significant reduction in minor health problems for at least 10 months after acquiring a dog.

- Fewer doctor visits per year for elderly dog owners than nonowners.

Companion animals have been shown to provide valuable physiological, psychological, and social benefits. These benefits are often especially significant in vulnerable individuals. Because many individuals who visit healthcare professionals are especially sensitive due to illness and the effects illness can have on one's quality of life, it is important for healthcare professionals to support the vital role of animal companionship in their patients' lives.

Psychological Benefits

Many studies have addressed the contribution of pets to human psychological well-being. One general study found that Australian cat owners scored better on psychological health ratings than did nonowners. Other studies have been more specific, focusing on groups facing stressful life events such as bereavement, illness, and homelessness. Findings from these studies often indicate that pets play a significant supportive role, reducing depression and loneliness and providing companionship and a need for responsibility.

One group of studies, performed with recently bereaved elderly subjects, demonstrated that:

- Recently widowed women who owned pets experienced significantly fewer symptoms of physical and psychological disease and reported lower medication use than widows who did not own pets.

- In bereaved elderly subjects with few social confidants, pet ownership and strong attachment were associated with less depression.

Another group of studies, looking at acquired immunodeficiency syndrome (AIDS) patients, found that:

- Patients with AIDS reported that their pets provided companionship and support, reduced stress, and provided a sense of purpose.

- Patients with AIDS reported that cats were an important part of a support system to prevent loneliness.

- Patients with AIDS who owned pets, especially those with few confidants, reported less depression and other benefits compared to those who did not have pets.

A third group of studies, carried out using homeless subjects, showed that:

- Homeless pet owners that were attached to their pets, often reported that their relationships with their pets were their only relationships, and most would not live in housing that would not allow pets.

- Over 40 percent of homeless adolescents reported that their dogs were a main means of coping with loneliness.

Studies focused on service dogs have shown overall improved quality of life for their human companions:

- Mobility-impaired individuals indicated increased "freedom to be capable" since receiving an assistance dog. Participants additionally reported increased independence and self-esteem, decreased loneliness, and experienced frequent friendliness from strangers.

- Quality of life improved in families of epileptic children when a dog that responds to seizures is present in the home.

Psychological studies reviewing the relationship between animals and children have revealed:

- The mere presence of animals positively alters children's attitudes about themselves and increases their ability to relate to others.

- Pets help children develop in various areas including love, attachment, and comfort; sensorimotor and nonverbal learning; responsibility, nurturance, and competence; learning about the life cycle; therapeutic benefits; and nurturing humanness, ecological awareness, and ethical responsibilities.

- Children exhibited a more playful mood, were more focused, and were more aware of their social environments when in the presence of a therapy dog.

Additional studies have shown:

- Alzheimer disease patients still living at home with pets had fewer mood disorders and fewer episodes of aggression and anxiety than did nonpet owners.

- Female pet-owners that have suffered physical abuse report their pets are an important source of emotional support.

- Dog owners were found to be as emotionally close to their dogs as they were their closest family members.

- Psychiatric disability patients who participated in a 10 week horseback riding program had increased self-esteem and an augmented sense of self-efficacy.

Social Benefits

Animals often serve to facilitate social interactions between people. For individuals with visible disabilities who may frequently be socially avoided by others, and in settings such as nursing homes, the role of animals as social catalysts is especially important.

- One study found that elderly people who live in mobile homes and walk their dogs in the area had more conversations focused in the present rather than in the past than those people who walked without their dogs.

- Disabled individuals in wheelchairs accompanied by service dogs during shopping trips received a median of eight friendly approaches from strangers, versus only one approach on trips without a dog.

- Observations of passersby encountering persons in wheelchairs revealed that passersby smiled and conversed more when a service dog was present.

In addition to acting as social catalysts, service dogs provide obvious practical benefits such as alerting their owners to visual hazards, auditory warnings, and impending seizures; assisting with mobility; and seeking help in emergencies. However, studies also indicate that they promote improved psychological well-being and reduce the number of assistance hours required by disabled owners.

Mental Well-Being

- Companion animals improve mental and emotional well-being in humans.

- Pet owners are less likely to suffer from stress, anxiety, and depression than nonpet owners.

- Pet therapy improves a wide array of mental health disabilities, including anxiety, panic, posttraumatic stress, mood obsessive compulsive, and other disorders.

Obesity Preventions

- The National Institutes of Health (NIH) found that dog owners who walk their dogs are significantly more likely to meet physical activity guidelines are less likely to be obese than nondog owners or walkers.

- By providing motivation and social support, pets make it easier for owners to adopt long-term behavior changes that lead to weight loss and other positive health outcomes.

- Pet ownership is associated with key indicators of cardiovascular health such as lower blood pressure, cholesterol, and triglycerides.

Tobacco Cessation

- 28.4 percent of smokers said knowing the adverse impact of cigarette smoke on pet health would motivate them to stop smoking. Secondhand smoke exposure is associated with certain cancers in cats and dogs, allergies in dogs, and eye, skin, and respiratory diseases in birds.

Chapter 46

Reducing Anxiety before Any Surgical Procedure

It is natural to feel anxious before surgery no matter how major or minor the procedure is. Even though most of the surgeries occur with relatively few complications, patients tend to feel anxious beforehand. Sometimes, the fear becomes significant, with the patient experiencing physical symptoms including chest pain, racing heart, and nausea.

The source of this anxiety could be an unknown fear, a previous bad experience with surgery, or fear about the outcome of surgery. It is important not to become overwhelmed by anxiety before surgery. While a magic cure for anxiety does not exist, but things such as relaxation techniques and support from family, friends, and hospital staff go a long way in reducing presurgery stress.

What Are the Effects of Anxiety before Surgery?

For many patients, it is hard not to have anxious feeling about the inherent risks of surgery. Anxiety leads to stress and other related symptoms such as a fast pulse, racing heart, nervous stomach, sleeplessness, and shortness of breath. These symptoms might make it difficult for the patient to properly prepare for surgery or to remember postsurgery instructions.

What Can Be Done to Relieve Anxiety before Surgery?

Anxiety is a normal human response. The body is conditioned to protect itself by going into a defensive stance or escaping from danger. This is known as the "fight-or-flight response" And it is responsible for causing the physiological responses in the body when you are anxious. Unfortunately, they are not of much use when no inherent danger exists Most people learn to adapt to frightening situations over time, but surgery can often be a new and anxiety-inducing event.

Taking the following steps may help ease your anxiety.

Share Your Fears

Talking about your fears is the first step in controlling it. Sharing your thoughts lifts the burden from your mind and results in relief. Also, seek information and determine if there is any basis to your fears or if they are simply unfounded. Talk to the hospital clinical counselor or physician assistant or nurse about your fears. They will be able to understand your anxiety and help alleviate it.

Understand the Surgical Procedure

Fear of the unknown is a primary cause of anxiety and the best way to handle it is to understand what you are getting into. Talk to the surgeon and get to know the surgical procedure and what to expect when it is over. If you are searching the Internet for information, be sure you are sourcing it from credible websites. It is the unanswered questions that cause anxiety. Understanding what you will undergo will calm your nerves. Though it may be clear that surgery is essential for you, it is easy to be confused by medical jargon. Make sure you understand why you need surgery and do not be afraid to get a second opinion.

Learn about Anesthesia

Educate yourself about anesthesia. You may not get a chance to meet the anesthesiologist the day before surgery. So, make an appointment with him or her beforehand. Understand what choices will be available to you. Research the kind of anesthesia you will be given using authoritative websites. You may not have much choice in anesthesia because, after an evaluation of all factors involved, the specific kind of anesthesia to be used is decided only shortly before surgery.

Keep Yourself Busy

Prepare yourself to avoid stress. Take care of chores at home before surgery. Clean your house or if possible make a thorough clean up. Take care of your work and apply for leave if needed. If you have kids, make arrangements for their care while you are in recovery. Tell your partner about things to take care at home, such as cooking meals, so that your absence will not be felt.

Distract Yourself

It is easy to dwell on negative thoughts and brood over them. Don't let your imagination get the better of you. Use common distraction techniques such as reading a book, watching a TV show or movie, or listening to your favorite music. This should keep your mind relaxed and delay your thoughts about surgery until much later.

Use Relaxation Techniques

If you are prone to anxiety, then find out about specific techniques to reduce it. Breathing exercises, meditation, and mindfulness help reduce anxiety, stress, and lowers blood pressure. Such techniques have been scientifically proven to reduce stress and anxiety.

Allow Hospital Staff to Help You

Doctors and nurses at the hospital are well aware of patients' potential anxiety. Most staff try to make wait times minimal and your stay as pleasant as possible. Hospitals have counselors and volunteers on call to offer support and assistance. Make use of their services. Personal coping strategies serve the purpose best, but they tend to be different for each individual.

Do Not Smoke before Surgery

Smoking before surgery is linked to complications and is best avoided even though you think it will help relax you. Smoking adversely affects healing of wounds and you should begin nicotine replacement therapy a few months before surgery if possible in order to reduce risk of complications.

Use of Sedatives

If you are admitted to the hospital the night before surgery you might be given a sedative, usually a benzodiazepine, to make you sleep better and to control anxiety. Sedatives make you drowsy and can cause nausea but they also make you relax and reduce anxiety. You may also be given a sedative an hour or two before anesthesia is administered.

Helping Your Child Who Is Anxious about Surgery

It is very important to address concerns about surgery in children because this usually translates to better outcomes after surgery. Children tend to emulate the attitude of parents when it comes to surgery, be it good or bad. If a parent is fearful or anxious, chances are the child becoming fearful too. Children should be told about the surgery in advance and allowed to ask questions. Any anxiety or fearfulness about surgery should be put to rest. It is best not to surprise a child because it could result in a lasting fear of healthcare. Also, it is better to sound positive and upbeat about surgery with your child. He or she should know what the advantages are that will come after surgery.

The approach adopted with children varies with age. Very young children need to be informed just a few days before surgery. Slightly older children may already know what surgery entails and should be given enough opportunities to voice their doubts and fears with doctors and parents. Older children may know the surgical procedure in detail from books, TV, or the Internet. They should meet the surgeon with their parent for a 'reality check' so they understand what the procedure actual entails. Most hospitals offer a presurgery tour and information presentations to relieve anxiety before surgery.

References

1. "What Can Help Relieve Anxiety before Surgery?" PubMed Health, IQWiG (Institute for Quality and Efficiency in Health Care), May 21, 2014.

2. "5 Ways to Calm Your Nerves before Surgery," The Healthcare Management Trust, July 26, 2016.

3. TahoeDoc. "How to Calm Yourself Down before a Day Surgery Procedure," HealDove, April 28, 2017.

4. Whitlock, Jennifer., RN, MSN, FNP-C. "Understanding and Dealing with a Fear of Surgery," VeryWell, April 21, 2016.

Part Six

Looking Ahead

Chapter 47

Living with Anxiety Disorders

If you have an anxiety disorder, you're not alone. Each year, tens of millions of Americans of all ages suffer from long-term anxiety. Among children, anxiety disorders are the most common form of mental illness—one they may carry into adulthood.

Anxiety is an uneasy feeling that something may harm you or a loved one. This feeling can be normal and sometimes even helpful. If you're starting a new job or taking a test, it might make you more alert and ready for action. But sometimes anxiety can linger or become overwhelming. When it gets in the way of good health and peace of mind, it's called an anxiety disorder.

"Everybody has anxiety," says Dr. Daniel Pine, a psychiatrist and an National Institutes of Health (NIH) neuroscientist. "The tricky part is how to tell the difference between normal and abnormal anxiety."

"For those with anxiety disorders, fears, worries, and anxieties can cause so much distress that they interfere with daily life. The anxiety grows out of proportion to the stressful situation or occurs when there is no real danger.

Anxiety activates the body's stress response. Nearly all the cells, tissues, and organs in your body go on high alert. This stress response

---

This chapter includes text excerpted from "Living with Anxiety Disorders, Worried Sick," MedlinePlus, National Institutes of Health (NIH), 2015.

can wear your body down over time. People with chronic (long-term) anxiety have a higher risk of both physical and mental health problems. Some people visit their doctors because of headaches, racing heart, or other physical complaints without realizing that these symptoms may be connected to how anxious they feel.

Treatment for anxiety disorders usually includes both medication and cognitive behavioral therapy (CBT). CBT is a form of talk therapy. It helps people change both the thinking patterns that support their fears and the way they react to anxiety-provoking situations. Current treatments can be highly effective for most people.

If you are troubled by anxiety, the first person to see is your family doctor or nurse practitioner. He or she can check for any underlying physical illness or a related condition. You may be referred to a mental health specialist, who might help to identify the specific type of anxiety disorder and the appropriate treatment. With proper care, most people with anxiety disorders can lead normal, fulfilling lives.

Diagnosis and Treatment

Anxiety disorders are treatable. If you think you have an anxiety disorder, talk to your doctor.

Sometimes a physical evaluation is advisable to determine whether a person's anxiety is associated with a physical illness. If anxiety is diagnosed, the pattern of co-occurring symptoms should be identified, as well as any coexisting conditions, such as depression or substance abuse. Sometimes alcoholism, depression, or other coexisting conditions have such a strong effect on the individual that treating the anxiety should wait until the coexisting conditions are brought under control.

If your doctor thinks you may have an anxiety disorder, the next step is usually seeing a mental health professional. It is advisable to seek help from professionals who have particular expertise in diagnosing and treating anxiety. Certain kinds of cognitive and behavioral therapy and certain medications have been found to be especially helpful for anxiety.

You should feel comfortable talking with the mental health professional you choose. If you do not, you should seek help elsewhere. Once you find a clinician with whom you are comfortable, the two of you should work as a team and make a plan to treat your anxiety disorder together.

In general, anxiety disorders are treated with medication, specific types of psychotherapy, or both. Treatment choices depend on the type of disorder, the person's preference, and the expertise of the clinician.

Most insurance plans, including health maintenance organizations (HMOs), will cover treatment for anxiety disorders. Check with your insurance company and find out.

What Medications Are Used to Treat Anxiety Disorders?

Medication does not necessarily cure anxiety disorders, but it often reduces the symptoms. Medication typically must be prescribed by a doctor. A psychiatrist is a doctor who specializes in mental disorders. Many psychiatrists offer psychotherapy themselves or work as a team with psychologists, social workers, or counselors who provide psychotherapy. The principal medications used for anxiety disorders are antidepressants, antianxiety drugs, and beta blockers. Be aware that some medications are effective only if they are taken regularly and that symptoms may recur if the medication is stopped.

Choosing the right medication, medication dose, and treatment plan should be based on a person's individual needs and medical situation, and done under an expert's care. Only an expert clinician can help you decide whether the medicine's ability to help is worth the risk of a side effect. Your doctor may try several medicines before finding the right one.

Antidepressants

Antidepressants were developed to treat depression, but they also help people with anxiety disorders. They are commonly prescribed for panic disorder, obsessive-compulsive disorder (OCD), posttraumatic stress disorder (PTSD), and social anxiety disorder. Some tricyclic antidepressants work well for anxiety. Monoamine oxidase inhibitors (MAOIs) are also used for anxiety disorders.

Benzodiazepines (Antianxiety Medications)

The antianxiety medications called benzodiazepines can start working more quickly than antidepressants.

Beta Blockers

Beta blockers control some of the physical symptoms of anxiety, such as trembling and sweating.

Cognitive Behavioral Therapy (CBT)

CBT (sometimes called "talk therapy" or psychotherapy) involves talking with a trained clinician, such as a psychiatrist, psychologist, social worker, or counselor, to understand what caused an anxiety disorder and how to deal with it.

CBT can be useful in treating anxiety disorders. It can help people change the thinking patterns that support their fears and change the way they react to anxiety-provoking situations.

For example, CBT can help people with panic disorder learn that their panic attacks are not really heart attacks and help people with social phobia learn how to overcome the belief that others are always watching and judging them. When people are ready to confront their fears, they are shown how to use exposure techniques to desensitize themselves to situations that trigger their anxieties.

Exposure-based treatment has been used for many years to treat specific phobias. The person gradually encounters the object or situation that is feared, perhaps at first only through pictures or tapes, then later face-to-face. Sometimes the therapist will accompany the person to a feared situation to provide support and guidance. Exposure exercises are undertaken once the patient decides he is ready for it and with his cooperation.

To be effective, therapy must be directed at the person's specific anxieties and must be tailored to his or her needs. A typical "side effect" is temporary discomfort involved with thinking about confronting feared situations.

CBT may be conducted individually or with a group of people who have similar problems. Group therapy is particularly effective for social phobia. Often "homework" is assigned for participants to complete between sessions. If a disorder recurs at a later date, the same therapy can be used to treat it successfully a second time.

Medication can be combined with psychotherapy for specific anxiety disorders, and combination treatment has been found to be the best approach for many people.

Some people with anxiety disorders might benefit from joining a self-help or support group and sharing their problems and achievements with others. Internet chat rooms might also be useful in this regard, but any advice received over the Internet should be used with caution, as Internet acquaintances have usually never seen each other and false identities are common. Talking with a trusted friend or member of the clergy can also provide support, but it is not necessarily a sufficient alternative to care from an expert clinician.

Stress management techniques and meditation can help people with anxiety disorders calm themselves and may enhance the effects of therapy. There is preliminary evidence that aerobic exercise may have a calming effect. Since caffeine, certain illicit drugs, and even some over-the-counter (OTC) cold medications can aggravate the symptoms of anxiety disorders, avoiding them should be considered. Check with your physician or pharmacist before taking any additional medications.

The family can be important in the recovery of a person with an anxiety disorder. Ideally, the family should be supportive but not help perpetuate their loved one's symptoms. Family members should not trivialize the disorder or demand improvement without treatment.

Chapter 48

Facing Mental Health Problems: What You Need to Do

For People with Mental Health Problems

If you have, or believe you may have, mental health problem, it can be helpful to talk about these issues with others. It can be scary to reach out for help, but it is often the first step to helping you heal, grow, and recover. Having a good support system and engaging with trustworthy people are key elements to successfully talking about your own mental health.

Build Your Support System

Find someone—such as a parent, family member, teacher, faith leader, healthcare provider or other trusted individual, who:

- Gives good advice when you want and ask for it; assists you in taking action that will help

- Likes, respects, and trusts you and who you like, respect, and trust, too

This chapter includes text excerpted from "For People with Mental Health Problems," MentalHealth.gov, U.S. Department of Health and Human Services (HHS), May 31, 2013. Reviewed September 2017.

- Allows you the space to change, grow, make decisions, and even make mistakes

- Listens to you and shares with you, both the good and bad times

- Respects your need for confidentiality so you can tell him or her anything

- Lets you freely express your feelings and emotions without judging, teasing, or criticizing

- Works with you to figure out what to do the next time a difficult situation comes up

- Has your best interest in mind

Find a Peer Group

Find a group of people with mental health problems similar to yours. Peer support relationships can positively affect individual recovery because:

- People who have common life experiences have a unique ability to help each other based on a shared history and a deep understanding that may go beyond what exists in other relationships

- People offer their experiences, strengths, and hopes to peers, which allows for natural evolution of personal growth, wellness promotion, and recovery

- Peers can be very supportive since they have "been there" and serve as living examples that individuals can and do recover from mental health problems

- Peers also serve as advocates and support others who may experience discrimination and prejudice

You may want to start or join a self-help or peer support group. National organizations across the country have peer support networks and peer advocates.

Participate in Your Treatment Decisions

It's also important for you to be educated, informed, and engaged about your own mental health.

Get involved in your treatment through shared decision making. Participate fully with your mental health provider and make informed treatment decisions together. Participating fully in shared decision making includes:

- Recognizing a decision needs to be made
- Identifying partners in the process as equals
- Stating options as equal
- Exploring understanding and expectations
- Identifying preferences
- Negotiating options/concordance
- Sharing decisions
- Arranging follow-up to evaluate decision-making outcomes

Develop a Recovery Plan

Recovery is a process of change where individuals improve their health and wellness, live a self-directed life, and strive to reach their full potential. Studies show that most people with mental health problems get better, and many recover completely.

You may want to develop a written recovery plan. Recovery plans:

- Enable you to identify goals for achieving wellness
- Specify what you can do to reach those goals
- Can be daily activities as well as longer term goals
- Track your mental health problem
- Identify triggers or other stressful events that can make you feel worse, and help you learn how to manage them

For Young People Looking for Help

Mental health problems don't only affect adults. Children, teens and young adults can have mental health problems, too. In fact, three out of four people with mental health problems showed signs before they were 24 years old.

What Does "Mental Health Problem" Mean?

Are you having trouble doing the things you like to do or need to do because of how you feel—like going to school, work or hanging out with friends?

Are you having a rough day? Have you been feeling down for a while? Everyone goes through tough times, and no matter how long you've had something on your mind, it's important that you talk to someone about it.

Talk to your parents or a trusted adult if you experience any of these things:

- Can't eat or sleep
- Can't perform daily tasks like going to school
- Don't want to hang out with your friends or family
- Don't want to do things you usually enjoy
- Fight a lot with family and friends
- Feel like you can't control your emotions and it's effecting your relationships with your family and friends
- Have low or no energy
- Feel hopeless
- Feel numb or like nothing matters
- Can't stop thinking about certain things or memories
- Feel confused, forgetful, edgy, angry, upset, worried, or scared
- Want to harm yourself or others
- Have random aches and pains
- Smoke, drink, or use drugs
- Hear voices

Where Can I Get Help?

You are not alone. Lots of people have been where you are or are there right now. But there are also lots of people who want to help you. If you're thinking about harming yourself get help immediately. You can call 911 or the National Suicide Prevention Line (NSPL) at 800-273-TALK (800-273-8255).

Another way to get help is by talking to someone you trust. This could be a parent, family member, teacher, school counselor, spiritual leader or another trusted adult, who:

- Gives good advice when you want and ask for it
- Respects your need for privacy so you can tell him or her anything

- Lets you talk freely about your feelings and emotions without judging, teasing, or criticizing

- Helps you figure out what to do the next time a difficult situation comes up

For Parents and Caregivers

As a parent or caregiver, you want the best for your children or other dependents. You may be concerned or have questions about certain behaviors they exhibit and how to ensure they get help.

What to Look for

It is important to be aware of warning signs that your child may be struggling. You can play a critical role in knowing when your child may need help.

Consult with a school counselor, school nurse, mental health provider, or another healthcare professional if your child shows one or more of the following behaviors:

- Feeling very sad or withdrawn for more than two weeks

- Seriously trying to harm or kill himself or herself, or making plans to do so

- Experiencing sudden overwhelming fear for no reason, sometimes with a racing heart or fast breathing

- Getting in many fights or wanting to hurt others

- Showing severe out-of-control behavior that can hurt oneself or others

- Not eating, throwing up, or using laxatives to make himself or herself lose weight

- Having intense worries or fears that get in the way of daily activities

- Experiencing extreme difficulty controlling behavior, putting himself or herself in physical danger or causing problems in school

- Using drugs or alcohol repeatedly

- Having severe mood swings that cause problems in relationships

- Showing drastic changes in behavior or personality

Because children often can't understand difficult situations on their own, you should pay particular attention if they experience:

- Loss of a loved one

- Divorce or separation of their parents

- Any major transition—new home, new school, etc.

- Traumatic life experiences, like living through a natural disaster

- Teasing or bullying

- Difficulties in school or with classmates

What to Do

If you are concerned your child's behaviors, it is important to get appropriate care. You should:

- Talk to your child's doctor, school nurse, or another healthcare provider and seek further information about the behaviors or symptoms that worry you

- Ask your child's primary care physician if your child needs further evaluation by a specialist with experience in child behavioral problems

- Ask if your child's specialist is experienced in treating the problems you are observing

- Talk to your medical provider about any medication and treatment plans

How to Talk about Mental Health

Do you need help starting a conversation with your child about mental health? Try leading with these questions. Make sure you actively listen to your child's response.

- Can you tell me more about what is happening? How you are feeling?

- Have you had feelings like this in the past?

- Sometimes you need to talk to an adult about your feelings. I'm here to listen. How can I help you feel better?

- Do you feel like you want to talk to someone else about your problem?

- I'm worried about your safety. Can you tell me if you have thoughts about harming yourself or others?

When talking about mental health problems with your child you should:

- Communicate in a straightforward manner

- Speak at a level that is appropriate to a child or adolescent's age and development level (preschool children need fewer details than teenagers)

- Discuss the topic when your child feels safe and comfortable

- Watch for reactions during the discussion and slow down or back up if your child becomes confused or looks upset

- Listen openly and let your child tell you about his or her feelings and worries

For Friends and Family Members

Anyone can experience mental health problems. Friends and family can make all the difference in a person's recovery process.

Supporting a Friend or Family Member with Mental Health Problems

You can help your friend or family member by recognizing the signs of mental health problems and connecting them to professional help.

Talking to friends and family about mental health problems can be an opportunity to provide information, support, and guidance. Learning about mental health issues can lead to:

- Improved recognition of early signs of mental health problems

- Earlier treatment

- Greater understanding and compassion

If a friend or family member is showing signs of a mental health problem or reaching out to you for help, offer support by:

- Finding out if the person is getting the care that he or she needs and wants—if not, connect him or her to help

- Expressing your concern and support

- Reminding your friend or family member that help is available and that mental health problems can be treated

- Asking questions, listening to ideas, and being responsive when the topic of mental health problems come up

- Reassuring your friend or family member that you care about him or her

- Offering to help your friend or family member with everyday tasks

- Including your friend or family member in your plans—continue to invite him or her without being overbearing, even if your friend or family member resists your invitations

- Educating other people so they understand the facts about mental health problems and do not discriminate

- Treating people with mental health problems with respect, compassion, and empathy

How to Talk about Mental Health

Do you need help starting a conversation about mental health? Try leading with these questions and make sure to actively listen to your friend or family member's response.

- I've been worried about you. Can we talk about what you are experiencing? If not, who are you comfortable talking to?

- What can I do to help you to talk about issues with your parents or someone else who is responsible and cares about you?

- What else can I help you with?

- I am someone who cares and wants to listen. What do you want me to know about how you are feeling?

- Who or what has helped you deal with similar issues in the past?

- Sometimes talking to someone who has dealt with a similar experience helps. Do you know of others who have experienced these types of problems who you can talk with?

- It seems like you are going through a difficult time. How can I help you to find help?

- How can I help you find more information about mental health problems?

- I'm concerned about your safety. Have you thought about harming yourself or others?

When talking about mental health problems:

- Know how to connect people to help

- Communicate in a straightforward manner

- Speak at a level appropriate to a person's age and development level (preschool children need fewer details as compared to teenagers)

- Discuss the topic when and where the person feels safe and comfortable

- Watch for reactions during the discussion and slow down or backup if the person becomes confused or looks upset

Sometimes it is helpful to make a comparison to a physical illness. For example, many people get sick with a cold or the flu, but only a few get really sick with something serious like pneumonia. People who have a cold are usually able to do their normal activities. However, if they get pneumonia, they will have to take medicine and may have to go to the hospital.

Similarly, feelings of sadness, anxiety, worry, irritability, or sleep problems are common for most people. However, when these feelings get very intense, last for a long period of time, and begin to interfere with school, work, and relationships, it may be a sign of a mental health problem. And just like people need to take medicine and get professional help for physical conditions, someone with a mental health problem may need to take medicine and/or participate in therapy in order to get better.

Chapter 49

Financial Assistance for Treating Mental Health Problems

Health Insurance and Mental Health Services

How Does the Affordable Care Act (ACA) Help People with Mental Health Issues?

The Affordable Care Act (ACA) provides one of the largest expansions of mental health and substance use disorder coverage in a generation, by requiring that most individual and small employer health insurance plans, including all plans offered through the Health Insurance Marketplace cover mental health and substance use disorder services. Also required are rehabilitative and habilitative services that can help support people with behavioral health challenges. These new protections build on the Mental Health Parity and Addiction

---

This chapter contains text excerpted from the following sources: Text under the heading "Health Insurance and Mental Health Services" is excerpted from "Health Insurance and Mental Health Services," MentalHealth.gov, U.S. Department of Health and Human Services (HHS), December 9, 2014. Reviewed September 2017; Text under the heading "Medicare and Mental Healthcare" is excerpted from "Medicare and Your Mental Health Benefits," Centers for Medicare and Medicaid Services (CMS), August 2017.

Equity Act (MHPAEA) of 2008 provisions to expand mental health and substance use disorder benefits and federal parity protections to an estimated 62 million Americans.

Because of the law, most health plans must now cover preventive services, like depression screening for adults and behavioral assessments for children, at no additional cost. And, as of 2014, most plans cannot deny you coverage or charge you more due to preexisting health conditions, including mental illnesses.

Does the ACA Require Insurance Plans to Cover Mental Health Benefits?

As of 2014, most individual and small group health insurance plans, including plans sold on the Marketplace are required to cover mental health and substance use disorder services. Medicaid Alternative Benefit Plans also must cover mental health and substance use disorder services. These plans must have coverage of essential health benefits, which include 10 categories of benefits as defined under the healthcare law. One of those categories is mental health and substance use disorder services. Another is rehabilitative and habilitative services. Additionally, these plans must comply with mental health and substance use parity requirements, as set forth in MHPAEA, meaning coverage for mental health and substance abuse services generally cannot be more restrictive than coverage for medical and surgical services.

How Do I Find out If My Health Insurance Plan Is Supposed to Be Covering Mental Health or Substance Use Disorder Services in Parity with Medical and Surgical Benefits? What Do I Do If I Think My Plan Is Not Meeting Parity Requirements?

In general, for those in large employer plans, if mental health or substance use disorder services are offered, they are subject to the parity protections required under MHPAEA. And, as of 2014, for most small employer and individual plans, mental health and substance use disorder services must meet MHPAEA requirements.

If you have questions about your insurance plan, we recommend you first look at your plan's enrollment materials, or any other information you have on the plan, to see what the coverage levels are for all benefits. Because of the ACA, health insurers are required to provide you with an easy-to-understand summary about your benefits including mental health benefits, which should make it easier to see what your coverage is.

Does Medicaid Cover Mental Health or Substance Use Disorder Services?

All state Medicaid programs provide some mental health services and some offer substance use disorder services to beneficiaries, and Children's Health Insurance Program (CHIP) beneficiaries receive a full service array. These services often include counseling, therapy, medication management, social work services, peer supports, and substance use disorder treatment. While states determine which of these services to cover for adults, Medicaid and CHIP requires that children enrolled in Medicaid receive a wide range of medically necessary services, including mental health services. In addition, coverage for the new Medicaid adult expansion populations is required to include essential health benefits, including mental health and substance use disorder benefits, and must meet mental health and substance abuse parity requirements under MHPAEA in the same manner as health plans.

Does Medicare Cover Mental Health or Substance Use Disorder Services?

Yes, Medicare covers a wide range of mental health services.

- Medicare Part A (Hospital Insurance) covers inpatient mental healthcare services you get in a hospital. Part A covers your room, meals, nursing care, and other related services and supplies.

- Medicare Part B (Medical Insurance) helps cover mental health services that you would generally get outside of a hospital, including visits with a psychiatrist or other doctor, visits with a clinical psychologist or clinical social worker, and lab tests ordered by your doctor.

- Medicare Part D (Prescription Drug) helps cover drugs you may need to treat a mental health condition. Each Part D plan has its own list of covered drugs, known as formulary.

If you get your Medicare benefits through a Medicare Advantage Plan (like an HMO or PPO) or other Medicare health plan, check your plan's membership materials or call the plan for details about how to get your mental health benefits.

What Can I Do If I Think I Need Mental Health or Substance Use Disorder Services for Myself or Family Members?

Here are three steps you can take right now:

1. Learn more about how you, your friends, and your family can obtain health insurance coverage provided by Medicaid or CHIP or the Health Insurance Marketplaces.

2. Share with friends, family, and colleagues about the mental health benefits accessible under the Affordable Care Act so more people know.

3. Learn more about how the law is expanding coverage of mental health and substance use disorder benefits and federal parity protections.

4. Find help with the aid of a Health Center.

What Is the Health Insurance Marketplace?

The Health Insurance Marketplace is designed to make buying health coverage easier and more affordable. The Marketplace allows individuals to compare health plans, get answers to questions, find out if they are eligible for tax credits to help pay for private insurance or health programs like the Children's Health Insurance Program (CHIP), and enroll in a health plan that meets their needs. The Marketplace Can Help You:

- Look for and compare private health plans.
- Get answers to questions about your health coverage options.
- Get reduced costs, if you're eligible.
- Enroll in a health plan that meets your needs.

Medicare and Mental Healthcare

Mental health conditions, like depression or anxiety, can happen to anyone at any time. If you think you may have problems that affect your mental health, you can get help. Talk to your doctor or other healthcare provider if you have:

- Thoughts of ending your life (like a fixation on death or suicidal thoughts or attempts)

- Sad, empty, or hopeless feelings

- Loss of self-worth (like worries about being a burden, feelings of worthlessness, or self-loathing)

- Social withdrawal and isolation (like you don't want to be with friends, engage in activities, or leave home)

- Little interest in things you used to enjoy

- A lack of energy

- Trouble concentrating

- Trouble sleeping (like difficulty falling asleep or staying asleep, oversleeping, or daytime sleepiness)

- Weight loss or loss of appetite

- Increased use of alcohol or other drugs

Mental healthcare includes services and programs to help diagnose and treat mental health conditions. These services and programs may be provided in outpatient and inpatient settings. Medicare helps cover outpatient and inpatient mental healthcare, as well as prescription drugs you may need to treat a mental health condition.

Medicare Helps Cover Mental Health Services

Medicare Part A (Hospital Insurance) helps cover mental healthcare if you're a hospital inpatient. Part A covers your:

- Room

- Meals

- Nursing care

- Therapy or other treatment for your condition

- Lab tests

- Medications

- Other related services and supplies

Medicare Part B (Medical Insurance) helps cover mental health services that you would get from a doctor and services that you generally get outside of a hospital, like:

- Visits with a psychiatrist or other doctor

- Visits with a clinical psychologist or clinical social worker

- Lab tests ordered by your doctor

Part B may also pay for partial hospitalization services if you need intensive coordinated outpatient care.

Medicare prescription drug coverage (Part D) helps cover drugs you may need to treat a mental health condition.

Outpatient Mental Healthcare

What original Medicare covers:

Medicare Part B (Medical Insurance) helps cover mental health services and visits with these types of health professionals (deductibles and coinsurance may apply):

- Psychiatrist or other doctor

- Clinical psychologist

- Clinical social worker

- Clinical nurse specialist

- Nurse practitioner

- Physician assistant

Psychiatrists and other doctors must accept assignment if they participate in Medicare. Ask your doctor or psychiatrist if they accept assignment before you schedule an appointment. The other health professionals listed above must always accept assignment.

Part B covers outpatient mental health services, including services that are usually provided outside a hospital (like in a clinic, doctor's office, or therapist's office) and services provided in a hospital's outpatient department. Part B also covers outpatient mental health services for treatment of inappropriate alcohol and drug use. Part B helps pay for these covered outpatient services (deductibles and coinsurance may apply):

- One depression screening per year. The screening must be done in a primary care doctor's office or primary care clinic that can provide follow-up treatment and referrals. You pay nothing for your yearly depression screening if your doctor or healthcare provider accepts assignment.

- Individual and group psychotherapy with doctors or certain other licensed professionals allowed by the state where you get the services.

- Family counseling, if the main purpose is to help with your treatment.

- Testing to find out if you're getting the services you need and if your current treatment is helping you.

- Psychiatric evaluation.

- Medication management.

- Certain prescription drugs that aren't usually "self administered" (drugs you would normally take on your own), like some injections.

- Diagnostic tests.

- Partial hospitalization.

- A one-time "Welcome to Medicare" preventive visit. This visit includes a review of your potential risk factors for depression. You pay nothing for this visit if your doctor or other healthcare provider accepts assignment. (Note: This visit is only covered if you get it within the first 12 months you have Part B.)

- A yearly "Wellness" visit. Medicare covers a yearly "Wellness" visit once every 12 months (if you've had Part B for longer than 12 months). This is a good time to talk to your doctor or other healthcare provider about changes in your mental health so they can evaluate your changes year to year. You pay nothing for your yearly "Wellness" visit if your doctor or other healthcare provider accepts assignment.

What original Medicare doesn't cover:

- Meals.

- Transportation to or from mental healthcare services.

- Support groups that bring people together to talk and socialize. (Note: This is different from group psychotherapy, which is covered.)

- Testing or training for job skills that isn't part of your mental health treatment.

Inpatient Mental Healthcare

What original Medicare covers:

Medicare Part A (Hospital Insurance) helps pay for mental health services you get in a hospital that require you to be admitted as an

387

inpatient. You can get these services either in a general hospital or in a psychiatric hospital that only cares for people with mental health conditions. No matter which type of hospital you choose, Part A will help cover inpatient mental health services.

If you're in a psychiatric hospital (instead of a general hospital), Part A only pays for up to 190 days of inpatient psychiatric hospital services during your lifetime.

What original Medicare doesn't cover:

- Private duty nursing

- A phone or television in your room

- Personal items (like toothpaste, socks, or razors)

- A private room (unless medically necessary)

Chapter 50

Caregivers and Mental Health

Chapter Contents

Section 50.1

Understanding Anxiety Disorders—From a Caregiver's Perspective

This section includes text excerpted from "Understanding Anxiety Disorders—Caregiver: Get the Facts," Substance Abuse and Mental Health Services Administration (SAMHSA), May 3, 2017.

Hearing a healthcare professional say your youth or young adult has an anxiety disorder can be confusing. The good news is that the emotions and behaviors you have been concerned about are actually symptoms of a treatable disorder. By engaging in treatment and entering recovery, people with an anxiety disorder can manage their symptoms and feel better. Recovery does not necessarily mean a cure. It does mean people are actively moving towards wellness.

What Do We Mean by Recovery?

Recovery is a process of change through which individuals improve their health and wellness, live a self-directed life, and strive to reach their full potential. Recovery focuses on wellness and resilience, encouraging (people) to participate actively in their own care.

What Is an Anxiety Disorder?

People with anxiety disorders worry excessively. These feelings go well beyond the typical kind of worry that is appropriate to life situations and can help people focus and be alert. The apprehensiveness that your youth or young adult feels with an anxiety disorder occurs almost daily and may be overwhelming. Symptoms of an anxiety disorder include restlessness, a heart-pounding sensation, muscle tension and fatigue, irritability, difficulty concentrating, and/or sleep disturbances. These feelings are severe enough to interfere with day-to-day functioning in school, at work, or in social situations.

There are 3 types of anxiety disorders: generalized anxiety disorder (GAD), phobias, and panic disorders. Some youth and young adults have milder forms of anxiety disorders that do not last forever and

390

respond well to treatment. Others with more severe forms of anxiety disorders may experience lifelong symptoms, with the specific type of anxiety changing over time or including mood symptoms. However, treatments for an anxiety disorder that involve medications, psychotherapy, and other elements of an individualized treatment program can help your youth or young adult to be more resilient, manage symptoms, improve everyday functioning, and help them to lead a full, meaningful life. An individualized treatment program can include positive family and peer support.

What Caused This?

Researchers and healthcare professionals do not completely understand what causes anxiety disorders. It is unlikely that a single factor causes an anxiety disorder. It is most likely caused by a combination of things such as genetics (i.e., family history of anxiety disorders), chemical or other changes in the brain, and/or environmental factors. Traumatic experiences can also contribute to the development of psychiatric disorders. If your child has experienced a traumatic incident, it is critical to share that information with their mental health specialist and pediatrician.

Should I Have Known?

It is very difficult for parents and caregivers to know if their youth or young adult is acting like a typical youth or young adult or if their moods and behaviors are actually symptoms of an anxiety disorder. Teenagers may be moody or withdrawn at times and are sometimes reluctant to talk openly about emotions or behaviors. Perhaps you tried to ask questions but were not able to get answers. Working with a trained healthcare professional is important to help you and your youth or young adult understand whether or not they have an anxiety disorder and how to start moving forward.

What Are the Treatment Approaches?

An anxiety disorder can be managed in many ways. This includes the use of psychotherapy or a combination of medications and therapy. You should discuss treatment options with your youth or young adult and their healthcare provider, and make decisions based on individual health goals and priorities. Youth or young adults of consenting age may need to provide written consent for parents or caregivers to participate on the treatment team. Decisions may be made based on many factors, including the severity of symptoms, but should always account for your youth or young adult's health goals, priorities, and ambitions.

It is important to talk to your healthcare providers about other types of treatment, such as complementary medicine, as well as programs that can provide additional support related to education, employment, housing, and vocation and career development. It is also important to encourage good self-care, such as a healthy diet, exercise, sleep, and abstinence from illicit drugs. Understanding how treatment works will help you to play an active role in your youth or young adult's recovery.

Medications

Medications (particularly a class of medications called selective serotonin reuptake inhibitors or SSRIs) can help manage many of the symptoms of an anxiety disorder. Each person reacts differently to these medications. For that reason, the prescribing healthcare professional may try different doses and different kinds of medication before finding the most effective approach for your youth or young adult. Finding the best medication and the most effective dose for your youth or young adult may take time. In milder cases of anxiety disorders, medication may not be necessary. Therapy or lifestyle changes (e.g., smoking cessation, decreased caffeine intake, regular exercise, or mindfulness exercises) may be sufficient to manage symptoms.

Therapy

Healthcare professionals may recommend behavioral therapy, cognitive behavioral therapy, or other forms of psychotherapy as stand-alone treatment or in combination with medications depending on severity of symptoms. Psychotherapy helps your youth or young adult develop behaviors and daily routines that can protect them from experiencing frequent, severe, or prolonged symptoms.

Support

Peer and family support is also an important part of treatment for an anxiety disorder. Positive family members, caregivers, and peers can be part of a comprehensive treatment team. As a partner on this team, you can provide important support and encouragement to help your youth or young adult stay focused on reaching their treatment and recovery goals. Additionally, talking with other caregivers who also have a child diagnosed with an anxiety disorder can help you to learn more and know what to expect. You may benefit from having someone further along in the process with whom to discuss your own questions, thoughts, and feelings.

Is This My Fault?

No, it is not. Decades of medical research provide evidence that anxiety disorders and other mental disorders can be the result of a complex interaction of genetics and biological, environmental, social, physical, and emotional influences. None of the contributing factors alone are sufficient to cause a mental disorder. Your youth or young adult is not to blame and neither are you.

How Common Is This Disorder?

Anxiety disorders represent one of the most common forms of mental disorders among children and adolescents, but they often go undetected or untreated. Data from the Centers for Disease Control and Prevention (CDC) show that the rate of anxiety disorders among 3-17-year-olds is in the range of 3 percent (current symptoms) to 4.7 percent (ever reported having anxiety).

How Can I Help?

Parents, caregivers, and family members can be important partners in treatment and recovery from an anxiety disorder. You can play a major role by monitoring symptoms and responses to medication changes and encouraging your youth or young adult to stick with their treatment and treatment plan. Alert your healthcare providers about your youth or young adult's symptoms, such as any particular fears or phobias, including social situations, insomnia, or persistent low mood, as well as if he or she uses drugs, excessive caffeine, nicotine, or alcohol. Seek help immediately if your youth or young adult has thoughts or plans of harming themselves or others. There is significant evidence that your involvement can improve treatment outcomes. Your own self-care is also an important part of caring for a child with a mental health disorder. Self-care may include talking to your own mental health professional, friends, or family, as well as joining a local support group through the National Federation of Families for Children's Mental Health (FFCMH) or the National Alliance on Mental Illness (NAMI), exercising, getting a good night's sleep, or meditation.

Section 50.2

Self-Care for Family Caregivers

This section includes text excerpted from "Caring for the
Caregiver," National Cancer Institute (NCI), September 2014.
Reviewed September 2017.

Caring for the Caregiver

Who Is a Caregiver?

You may not think of yourself as a caregiver. You may feel you are
doing something natural. You are just caring for someone you love.
Some caregivers are family members. Others are friends.

What Does "Giving Care" Mean?

Giving care can mean helping with daily needs. These include going
to doctor visits, making meals, and picking up medicines. It can also
mean helping your loved one cope with feelings. Like when he or she
feels sad or angry. Sometimes having someone to talk to is what your
loved one needs most.

While giving care, it's normal to put your own needs and feelings
aside. But putting your needs aside for a long time is not good for
your health. You need to take care of yourself, too. If you don't, you
may not be able to care for others. This is why you need to take good
care of you.

A New Role

Whether you're younger or older, you may find yourself in a new
role as a caregiver. For example, you may be taking care of your spouse
who has always been healthy or an adult child taking care of your
parent. Whatever your roles are now, it's normal to feel confused and
stressed at this time.

If caregiving feels new to you, try not to worry. Many caregivers
say that they learn more as they go through their loved one's treatment. And if you need to, try to share your feelings with friends, a

counselor or a support group. Many caregivers say that talking with others helped them. They feel they were able to say things that they couldn't always say to their loved ones.

Your Feelings

It's common to feel stressed and overwhelmed at this time. Like your loved one, you may feel angry, sad, or worried. Try to share your feelings with others who can help you. It can help to talk about how you feel. You could even talk to a counselor or social worker.

Understanding Your Feelings

You probably have many feelings as you take care of your loved one. There is no right way for you to feel. Each person is different.

The first step to understanding your feelings is to know that they're normal. Give yourself some time to think through them. Some feelings that may come and go are:

- **Sadness.** It's okay to feel sad. But if it lasts for more than 2 weeks, and it keeps you from doing what you need to do, you may be depressed.

- **Anger.** You may be angry at yourself or family members. You may be angry at the person you're caring for. Know that anger often comes from fear, panic, or stress. Try to look at what is beneath the anger.

- **Grief.** You may be feeling a loss of what you value most. This may be your loved one's health. Or it may be the loss of the day-to-day life you had before. Let yourself grieve these losses.

- **Guilt.** Feeling guilty is common, too. You may think you aren't helping enough. Or you may feel guilty that you are healthy.

- **Loneliness.** You can feel lonely, even with lots of people around you. You may feel that no one understands your problems. You may also be spending less time with others.

What May Help

Know that you are not alone. Other caregivers share these feelings. Talk with someone if your feelings get in the way of daily life. Maybe you have a family member, friend, priest, pastor, or spiritual leader to talk to. Your doctor may also be able to help.

Here are some other things that may help you:

- **Forgive yourself**. Know that we all make mistakes whenever we have a lot on our minds. No one is perfect, and chances are that you're doing what you can at this moment.

- **Cry or express your feelings**. You don't have to pretend to be cheerful. It's okay to show that you are sad or upset.

- **Focus on things that are worth your time and energy**. Let small things go for now. For example, don't fold clothes if you are tired.

- **Don't take your loved one's anger personally**. It's very common for people to direct their feelings at those who are closest. Their stress, fears, and worries may come out as anger.

- **Be hopeful**. What you hope for may change over time. But you can always hope for comfort, joy, acceptance, and peace.

Asking for Help

Many people who were once caregivers say they did too much on their own. Some wished that they had asked for help sooner.

Accepting help from others isn't always easy. When tough things happen, many people tend to pull away. They think, "We can handle this on our own." But things can get harder as the patient goes through treatment. As a result, many caregivers have said, "There's just too much on my plate."

Take a look at how busy you are now. Be honest with yourself about what you can do. Think about tasks you can give to others. And let go of tasks that aren't as important right now.

Asking for help also helps your loved one.

Don't be afraid to ask for help. Remember, if you get help for yourself:

- You may stay healthier and have more energy.

- Your loved one may feel less guilty about your help.

- Other helpers may offer time and skills that you don't have.

How Can Others Help You?

People may want to help you but don't know what you need. Here are some things you can ask them to do:

- Help with tasks such as:
  - Cooking
  - Cleaning
  - Shopping
  - Yard work
  - Child care
  - Eldercare
- Talk with you and share your feelings.
- Help with driving errands such as:
- Doctor visits
- Picking up your child
- Find information you need.
- Tell others how your loved one is doing.

Know That Some People May Say, "No."

Some people may not be able to help. There could be one or more reasons such as:

- They may be coping with their own problems.
- They may not have time right now.
- They may not know how to help.
- They may feel uneasy around people who are sick.

Caring for Yourself

Make Time for Yourself

You may feel that your needs aren't important right now. Or that you've spent so much time caring for your loved one, there's no time left for yourself.

Taking time for yourself can help you be a better caregiver. Caring for your own needs and desires is important to give you strength to carry on. This is even more true if you have health problems.

You may want to:

- Find nice things you can do for yourself. Even just a few minutes can help. You could watch TV, call a friend, work on a hobby, or do anything that you enjoy.

- Be active. Even light exercise such as walking, stretching, or dancing can make you less tired. Yard work, playing with kids or pets, or gardening are helpful, too.

- Find ways to connect with friends. Are there places you can meet others who are close to you? Or can you chat or get support by phone or email?

- Give yourself more time off. Ask friends or family members to pitch in. Take time to rest.

Do something for yourself each day. It doesn't matter how small it is. Whatever you do, don't neglect yourself.

Joining a Caregiver Support Group

In a support group for caregivers, people may talk about their feelings and trade advice. Others may just want to listen. You can talk things over with other caregivers. This could give you some ideas for coping. It may also help you know you aren't alone.

In many cities, support groups are held in other languages besides English. There are also groups that meet over the Internet. Ask a nurse or a social worker to help you find a support group that meets your needs.

Caring for Your Body

You may feel too busy or worried about your loved one to think about your own health. And yet it's common for caregivers to have sleep problems, headaches, and anxiety, along with other changes. But if you take care of yourself, you can lower your stress. Then you can have the strength to take care of someone else.

Did you have health problems before you became a caregiver? If so, now it's even more important to take care of yourself. Also, adding extra stressors to your life can cause new health problems. Be sure to tell your doctor if you notice any new changes in your body.

Keep up with your own health needs. Try to:

- Go to all your checkups

- Take your medicines

- Eat healthy meals

- Get enough rest

- Exercise

- Make time to relax

These ideas may sound easy. But they can be hard to do for most caregivers. Try to pay attention to how your body and your mind are feeling.

Section 50.3

Caregiver Stress

This section includes text excerpted from "Caregiver Stress," Office on Women's Health (OWH), U.S. Department of Health and Human Services (HHS). January 25, 2015.

Who Are Caregivers?

Most Americans will be informal caregivers at some point during their lives. A survey found that 36 percent of Americans provided unpaid care to another adult with an illness or disability in the past year. That percentage is expected to go up as the proportion of people in the United States who are elderly increases. Also, changes in healthcare mean family caregivers now provide more home-based medical care. Nearly half of family caregivers in the survey said they give injections or manage medicines daily. Also, most caregivers are women. And nearly three in five family caregivers have paid jobs in addition to their caregiving.

What Is Caregiver Stress?

Caregiver stress is due to the emotional and physical strain of caregiving. Caregivers report much higher levels of stress than people who are not caregivers. Many caregivers are providing help or are "on call" almost all day. Sometimes, this means there is little time for work or other family members or friends. Some caregivers may feel overwhelmed by the amount of care their aging, sick or disabled family member needs.

Although caregiving can be very challenging, it also has its rewards. It feels good to be able to care for a loved one. Spending time together can give new meaning to your relationship.

Remember that you need to take care of yourself to be able to care for your loved one.

Who Gets Caregiver Stress?

Anyone can get caregiver stress, but more women caregivers say they have stress and other health problems than men caregivers. And some women have a higher risk for health problems from caregiver stress, including those who:

- **Care for a loved one who needs constant medical care and supervision.** Caregivers of people with Alzheimer disease or dementia are more likely to have health problems and to be depressed than caregivers of people with conditions that do not require constant care.

- **Care for a spouse.** Women who are caregivers of spouses are more likely to have high blood pressure, diabetes, and high cholesterol and are twice as likely to have heart disease as women who provide care for others, such as parents or children.

Women caregivers also may be less likely to get regular screenings, and they may not get enough sleep or regular physical activity.

What Are the Signs and Symptoms of Caregiver Stress?

Caregiver stress can take many forms. For instance, you may feel frustrated and angry one minute and helpless the next. You may make mistakes when giving medicines. Or you may turn to unhealthy behaviors like smoking or drinking too much alcohol.

Other signs and symptoms include:

- Feeling overwhelmed
- Feeling alone, isolated, or deserted by others
- Sleeping too much or too little
- Gaining or losing a lot of weight
- Feeling tired most of the time
- Losing interest in activities you used to enjoy
- Becoming easily irritated or angered

- Feeling worried or sad often

- Having headaches or body aches often

Talk to your doctor about your symptoms and ways to relieve stress. Also, let others give you a break. Reach out to family, friends, or a local resource.

How Does Caregiver Stress Affect My Health?

Some stress can be good for you, as it helps you cope and respond to a change or challenge. But long-term stress of any kind, including caregiver stress, can lead to serious health problems.

Some of the ways stress affects caregivers include:

- **Depression and anxiety.** Women who are caregivers are more likely than men to develop symptoms of anxiety and depression. Anxiety and depression also raise your risk for other health problems, such as heart disease and stroke.

- **Weak immune system.** Stressed caregivers may have weaker immune systems than noncaregivers and spend more days sick with the cold or flu. A weak immune system can also make vaccines such as flu shots less effective. Also, it may take longer to recover from surgery.

- **Obesity.** Stress causes weight gain in more women than men. Obesity raises your risk for other health problems, including heart disease, stroke, and diabetes.

- **Higher risk for chronic diseases.** High levels of stress, especially when combined with depression, can raise your risk for health problems, such as heart disease, cancer, diabetes, or arthritis.

- **Problems with short-term memory or paying attention.** Caregivers of spouses with Alzheimer disease are at higher risk for problems with short-term memory and focusing.

Caregivers also report symptoms of stress more often than people who are not caregivers.

What Can I Do to Prevent or Relieve Caregiver Stress?

Taking steps to relieve caregiver stress helps prevent health problems. Also, taking care of yourself helps you take better care of your loved one and enjoy the rewards of caregiving.

Here are some tips to help you prevent or manage caregiver stress:

- **Learn ways to better help your loved one.** Some hospitals offer classes that can teach you how to care for someone with an injury or illness.

- **Find caregiving resources in your community to help you.** Many communities have adult daycare services or respite services to give primary caregivers a break from their caregiving duties.

- **Ask for and accept help.** Make a list of ways others can help you. Let helpers choose what they would like to do. For instance, someone might sit with the person you care for while you do an errand. Someone else might pick up groceries for you.

- **Join a support group for caregivers.** You can find a general caregiver support group or a group with caregivers who care for someone with the same illness or disability as your loved one. You can share stories, pick up caregiving tips, and get support from others who face the same challenges as you do.

- **Get organized.** Make to-do lists, and set a daily routine.

- **Take time for yourself.** Stay in touch with family and friends, and do things you enjoy with your loved ones.

- **Take care of your health.** Find time to be physically active on most days of the week, choose healthy foods, and get enough sleep.

- **See your doctor for regular checkups.** Make sure to tell your doctor or nurse you are a caregiver. Also, tell her about any symptoms of depression or sickness you may have.

If you work outside the home and are feeling overwhelmed, consider taking a break from your job. Under the federal Family and Medical Leave Act (FMLA), eligible employees can take up to 12 weeks of unpaid leave per year to care for relatives. Ask your human resources office about your options.

What Caregiving Services Can I Find in My Community?

Caregiving services include:

- Meal delivery

- Home healthcare services, such as nursing or physical therapy

- Nonmedical home care services, such as housekeeping, cooking, or companionship

- Making changes to your home, such as installing ramps or modified bathtubs

- Legal and financial counseling

- Respite care, which is substitute caregiving (someone comes to your home, or you may take your loved one to an adult day care center or day hospital)

How Can I Pay for Home Healthcare and Other Caregiving Services?

Medicare, Medicaid, and private insurance companies will cover some costs of home healthcare. Other costs you will have to pay for yourself.

- If the person who needs care has insurance, check with the person's insurance provider to find out what's included in the plan.

- If the person who needs care has Medicare, find out what home health services are covered.

- If the person who needs care has Medicaid, coverage of home health services vary between states.

Chapter 51

Clinical Trials

Chapter Contents

Section 51.1

Importance of Clinical Trials

This section includes text excerpted from "Clinical Research Trials and You: Questions and Answers," National Institute of Mental Health (NIMH), 2016.

What Is a Clinical Trial?

Clinical trials are part of clinical research and at the heart of all medical advances. Clinical trials look at new ways to prevent, detect, or treat diseases. Treatments might be new drugs or new combinations of drugs, new surgical procedures or devices, or new ways to use existing treatments. The goal of clinical trials is to determine if a new test or treatment works and is safe. Clinical trials can also look at other aspects of care, such as improving the quality of life for people with chronic illnesses.

Who Participates in Clinical Trials?

Many different types of people participate in clinical trials. Some are healthy, while others may have illnesses. A healthy volunteer is a person with no known significant health problems who participates in clinical research to test a new drug, device, or intervention. Research procedures with healthy volunteers are designed to develop new knowledge, not to provide direct benefit to study participants.

A patient volunteer has a known health problem and participates in research to better understand, diagnose, treat, or cure that disease or condition. Research procedures with a patient volunteer help develop new knowledge. These procedures may or may not benefit the study participants.

Patient volunteers may be involved in studies similar to those in which healthy volunteers participate. These studies involve drugs, devices, or interventions designed to prevent, treat, or cure a disease. Although these studies may provide direct benefit to patient volunteers, the main aim is to show, by scientific means, the effects and limitations of the experimental treatment. Consequently, some patients serve as controls by not taking the test drug or by receiving test doses of the drug large enough only to show that it is present, but not at a level that can treat the condition. A study's benefits may be indirect for the volunteers but may help others.

People participate in clinical trials for a variety of reasons. Healthy volunteers say they participate to help others and to contribute to moving science forward. Participants with an illness or disease also participate to help others, but also to possibly receive the newest treatment and to have the additional care and attention from the clinical trial staff. Clinical trials offer hope for many people and an opportunity to help researchers find better treatments for others in the future.

All clinical trials have guidelines about who can participate, called inclusion/exclusion criteria. Factors that allow someone to participate in a clinical trial are "inclusion criteria." Those that exclude or do not allow participation are "exclusion criteria." These criteria are based on factors such as age, gender, the type and stage of a disease, previous treatment history, and other medical conditions. Before joining a clinical trial, a participant must qualify for the study. Some research studies seek participants with illnesses or conditions to be studied in the clinical trial, while others need healthy volunteers. Some studies need both types.

Inclusion and exclusion criteria are not used to reject people personally; rather, the criteria are used to identify appropriate participants and keep them safe, and to help ensure that researchers can find new information they need.

What Are the Benefits and Risks of a Clinical Trial?

Clinical trials involve risks, just as routine medical care and the activities of daily living do. When weighing the risks of research, you can consider two important factors:

- the chance of any harm occurring, and

- the degree of harm that could result from participating in the study

Most clinical studies pose the risk of minor discomfort, which lasts only a short time. However, some study participants experience complications that require medical attention. In rare cases, participants have been seriously injured or have died of complications resulting from their participation in trials of experimental therapies. The specific risks associated with a research protocol are described in detail in the informed consent document, which participants are asked to read and sign before participating in research. Also, a member of the research team explains the major risks of participating in a study and will answer any questions you have about the study. Before deciding to participate, carefully consider possible risks and benefits.

Potential Benefits

Well-designed and well-executed clinical trials provide the best approach for participants to:

- Play an active role in their healthcare
- Gain access to new research treatments before they are widely available
- Receive regular and careful medical attention from a research team that includes doctors and other health professionals
- Help others by contributing to medical research

Potential Risks

Risks to participating in clinical trials include the following:

- There may be unpleasant, serious, or even life-threatening side effects to experimental treatment.
- The study may require more time and attention than standard treatment would, including visits to the study site, more blood tests, more treatments, hospital stays, or complex dosage requirements.

If I Choose to Take Part in a Clinical Trial, How Will My Safety Be Protected?

Ethical Guidelines

The goal of clinical research is to develop knowledge that improves human health or increases understanding of human biology. People who participate in clinical research make it possible for this to occur. The path to finding out if a new drug is safe or effective is to test it on patient volunteers. By placing some people at risk of harm for the good of others, clinical research has the potential to exploit patient volunteers. The purpose of ethical guidelines is both to protect patient volunteers and to preserve the integrity of the science.

Ethical guidelines in place today were primarily a response to past research abuses.

Informed Consent

Informed consent is the process of learning the key facts about a clinical trial before deciding whether to participate. The process of providing information to participants continues throughout the study. To help someone decide whether to participate, members of the research team explain the details of the study. The research team provides an informed consent document, which includes such details about the study, as its purpose, duration, required procedures, and whom to contact for various purposes. The informed consent document also explains risks and potential benefits.

If the participant decides to enroll in the trial, the informed consent document will be signed. Informed consent is not a contract. Volunteers are free to withdraw from the study at any time.

IRB Review

Most, but not all, clinical trials in the United States are approved and monitored by an Institutional Review Board (IRB) in order to ensure that the risks are minimal and are worth any potential benefits. An IRB is an independent committee that consists of physicians, statisticians, and members of the community who ensure that clinical trials are ethical and that the rights of participants are protected. Potential research participants should ask the sponsor or research coordinator whether the research they are considering participating in was reviewed by an IRB.

What Questions Should I Ask before Deciding If I Want to Take Part in a Clinical Trial?

If you are offered a clinical trial, feel free to ask any questions or bring up any issues concerning the trial at any time. The following suggestions may give you some ideas as you think about your own questions.

The Study

- What is the purpose of the study?
- Why do researchers think the approach may be effective?

- Who will fund the study?
- Who has reviewed and approved the study?
- How are study results and safety of participants being checked?
- How long will the study last?
- What will my responsibilities be if I participate?

Possible Risks and Benefits

- What are my possible short-term benefits?
- What are my possible long-term benefits?
- What are my short-term risks, such as side effects?
- What are my possible long-term risks?
- What other options do people with my disease have?
- How do the possible risks and benefits of this trial compared with those options?

Participation and Care

- What kinds of therapies, procedures, and/or tests will I have during the trial?
- Will they hurt, and if so, for how long?
- How do the tests in the study compare with those I would have outside of the trial?
- Will I be able to take my regular medications while participating in the clinical trial?
- Where will I have my medical care?
- Who will be in charge of my care?

Personal Issues

- How could being in this study affect my daily life?
- Can I talk to other people in the study?

Cost Issues

- Will I have to pay for any part of the trial, such as tests or the study drug?

- If so, what will the charges likely be?

- What is my health insurance likely to cover?

- Who can help answer any questions from my insurance company or health plan?

- Will there be any travel or child care costs that I need to consider while I am in the trial?

Tips for Asking Your Doctor about Trials

- Consider taking a family member or friend along for support and for help in asking questions or recording answers.

- Plan ahead what to ask, but don't hesitate to ask any new questions you think of while you're there.

- Write down your questions in advance to make sure you remember to ask them all.

- Write down the answers, so that you can review them whenever you want.

- Ask about bringing a tape recorder to record what's said (even if you write down answers).

Where Can I Find a Mental Health Clinical Trial?

Around the Nation and Worldwide

The National Institutes of Health (NIH), the nation's medical research agency, conducts clinical research trials for many diseases and conditions, including a variety of mental disorders.

To search for other diseases and conditions, you can visit Clinical-Trials.gov. This is a searchable registry and results database of federally and privately supported clinical trials conducted in the United States and around the world. ClinicalTrials.gov gives you information about a trial's purpose, who may participate, locations, and phone numbers for more details. This information should be used in conjunction with advice from healthcare professionals.

What Is the Next Step after I Find a Clinical Trial?

Once you find a study that you might want to join, contact the clinical trial or study coordinator. You can usually find this contact information in the description of the study. The next step is a screening appointment to see if you qualify to participate. This appointment also gives you a chance to ask your questions about the study.

Let your doctor know that you are thinking about joining a clinical trial. He or she may want to talk to the research team about your health to make sure the study is safe for you and to coordinate your care while you are in the study.

Section 51.2

Attention Bias Modification Treatment (ABMT) for Anxiety Disorders

This section includes text excerpted from "Attention Bias Modification Treatment (ABMT) for Anxiety Disorders in Youth Who Do Not Respond to CBT," ClinicalTrials.gov, National Institutes of Health (NIH), October 2016.

Purpose

First-line psychosocial treatments for anxiety disorders in children are largely exposure-based cognitive behavioral therapies (CBTs). Despite strong evidence supporting CBT's efficacy, for up to 50 percent of youth patient, symptoms of anxiety persist after a full course of treatment. What are the treatment options for these youth? Unfortunately, there is not a single empirical study in the youth anxiety treatment literature that has systematically examined treatment augmentation for youth who fail to respond to CBT. Empirical efforts to address this issue are important because youth who do not respond to CBT continue to suffer emotional distress and impairment associated with anxiety disorders.

This study will address this gap via double-blind randomized controlled trial of Attention Bias Modification Treatment (ABMT) for anxious 10–18 year-olds who did not respond to standard CBT. Attention biases in threat processing have been assigned a prominent role in the etiology and maintenance of anxiety disorders. ABMT utilizes computer-based protocols to implicitly modify biased attentional patterns in anxious patients. Here, participants will be CBT nonresponders who will be assessed by using clinical interviews and parent- and self-rated questionnaires before and after eight sessions of ABMT or placebo control, and again at an eight-week follow-up. A reduction in anxiety symptoms is expected to be seen in the ABMT group relative to the placebo control group. The findings are also expected to inform pathways to treatments for anxious children who do not respond to current standard first-line therapy, and to provide initial information on mechanisms of ABMT efficacy.

Outcomes

Primary outcome measures:

- The Pediatric Anxiety Rating Scale (PARS) [Time Frame: expected average time frame of 6 weeks.]

The PARS assesses global anxiety severity across different anxiety disorders in youth.

Secondary outcome measures:

- Anxiety Related Emotional Disorders—Child/Parent Version (SCARED-C/P) [Time Frame: expected average time frame of 6 weeks.]

The SCARED is a 41-item self and parent-report instrument designed to assess anxiety in children and adolescents.

- Estimated enrollment: 100

- Study start date: January 2015

- Estimated study completion Date: July 2018

- Estimated primary completion date: July 2018 (Final data collection date for primary outcome measure)

Criteria

To be included all youth must:

1. have received a full course of CBT and were deemed treatment nonresponders.

2. they must still have a primary diagnosis of GAD, SOP, or SAD.

3. if they have comorbid attention deficit hyperactivity disorder (ADHD) or depressive disorders, it must be treated with medication and stable.

413

4. if they have tics or impulse control problems, those problems must be treated with medication and stable and cause minimal or no impairment.

To be excluded youth must:

1. meet diagnostic criteria for Organic Mental Disorders, Psychotic Disorders, Pervasive Developmental Disorders, or Mental Retardation.

2. show high likelihood of hurting themselves or others.

3. have not been living with a primary caregiver who is legally able to give consent for the child's participation.

4. be a victim of previously undisclosed abuse requiring investigation or ongoing supervision.

5. be involved currently in another psychosocial treatment.

6. have a serious vision problem that is not corrected with prescription lenses.

7. have a physical disability that interferes with their ability to click a mouse button rapidly and repeatedly.

Section 51.3

Gaze Contingent Feedback for Anxiety Disorders in Children

This section includes text excerpted from "Gaze Contingent Feedback for Anxiety Disorders in Children," ClinicalTrials.gov, National Institutes of Health (NIH), May 2017.

Purpose

The purpose of this study is to determine whether giving gaze-contingent feedback is an effective attention modification procedure, helping in the treatment of anxiety disorders in children.

Outcomes

Primary outcome measures:

- Change from baseline in anxiety symptoms—the Pediatric Anxiety Rating (PARS) [Time Frame: Post treatment (1 week after treatment completion)]

The PARS assesses global anxiety severity across different anxiety disorders in children
Secondary outcome measures:

- Change from baseline in anxiety related emotional disorders symptoms—Child/Parent (the SCARED 41-item) [Time Frame: Post treatment (1 week after treatment completion)]

The SCARED is a 41-item self and parent-report instrument designed to assess anxiety in children.

- Estimated Enrollment: 12
- Actual Study Start Date: April 1, 2017
- Estimated Study Completion Date: September 2017
- Estimated Primary Completion Date: September 2017 (Final data collection date for primary outcome measure)

Detailed Description

Attention biases in threat processing have been assigned a prominent role in the etiology and maintenance of anxiety disorders. The purpose of this study is to determine whether giving gaze-contingent feedback is an effective treatment for anxiety disorders in clinically anxious 6–10 year-olds children. Participants will be assessed using clinical interviews and parent- and self-rated questionnaires before and after eight training sessions. Outcome measures will be anxiety symptoms and depression as measured by gold standard questionnaires as well as structured clinical interviews with children and their parents. Attentional threat bias and Attentional control will also be measured to explore potential mediators of ABMT's effect on anxiety.

Criteria

To be included youth must:

- Primary diagnosis of GAD, SOP, or SAD.

- Comorbid attention deficit hyperactivity disorder (ADHD) or depressive disorders must be treated with medication and stable.

- Tics or impulse control problems must be treated with medication, stable and cause minimal or no impairment.

To be excluded youth must:

- meet diagnostic criteria for Organic Mental Disorders, Psychotic Disorders, Pervasive Developmental Disorders, or Mental Retardation.

- show high likelihood of hurting themselves or others.

- have not been living with a primary caregiver who is legally able to give consent for the child's participation.

- be a victim of previously undisclosed abuse requiring investigation or ongoing supervision.

- be involved currently in another psycho-social treatment.

- have a serious vision problem that is not corrected with prescription lenses.

- have a physical disability that interferes with their ability to click a mouse button rapidly and repeatedly.

Section 51.4

Elective Coronary Angiography and Anxiety Study (ANGST)

This section includes text excerpted from "Elective Coronary Angiography and Anxiety Study (ANGST)," ClinicalTrials.gov, National Institutes of Health (NIH), June 2016.

Purpose

Anxiety will be assessed from two aspects, the somatic and emotional. ANGST aims to determine how anxiety correlates with psychological parameters (personality traits, coping strategies and depressive symptoms) and with the outcome of elective coronary angiography (CA).

Outcome

Primary outcome measures:

- Change between emotional anxiety in patients without depressive symptoms [Time Frame: Baseline, 2 hours before CA, 24h after CA and 1 month after CA]

  Measured with Spielberger State Anxiety Inventory

- Change between somatic anxiety in patients without depressive symptoms [Time Frame: Baseline, 2 hours before CA, 24h after CA and 1 month after CA]

  Measured with Beck Anxiety Inventory
  Secondary outcome measures:

- Depressive symptoms [Time Frame: Baseline, 1 month after CA]

  Measured with Cardiac Depression Scale

- Personality traits [Time Frame: Baseline]

  Measured with 10-item short version of Big Five Inventory

- Response on stress [Time Frame: Baseline]

  Measured with COPE Inventory

- Trait Anxiety [Time Frame: Baseline]

  Measured with Spielberger Trait Anxiety Inventory

Primary outcome measures:

- Change between emotional anxiety in patients without depressive symptoms [Time Frame: Baseline, 2 hours before CA, 24h after CA and 1 month after CA]

  Measured with Spielberger State Anxiety Inventory

- Change between somatic anxiety in patients without depressive symptoms [Time Frame: Baseline, 2 hours before CA, 24h after CA and 1 month after CA]

  Measured with Beck Anxiety Inventory

Detailed Description

This research is a prospective cross section study of patients undergoing elective CA. Research design will allow studying anxiety at four timepoints and its correlation with CA outcome and psychological parameters. This study will be conducted at the Coronary care unit of the department of Cardiology, General and Teaching Hospital Celje, Slovenia.

Data regarding prior to CA, during hospital stay and after discharge variables will be collected in order to control for confounding variables when testing the association between anxiety and psychological parameters. All the data needed for this study will be collected within one month from the patient enrollment in this study at four occasions:

1. 14 days prior CA—all patients will receive questionnaires by post,

2. on the day of the admission, 2–4 hours before CA,

3. 24 hours after CA, but prior to discharge and

4. 4–6 weeks after discharge.

Clinical and demographical data will be collected from medical records. Data regarding anxiety and other psychological parameters will be assessed using standardized questionnaires. These will be sent to the patient together with covering letter providing instructions to complete the questionnaires 14 days prior CA without help of family members/friends. A month after CA, the questionnaires for anxiety and depressive symptoms will be sent to participants address with reply paid envelope provided.

The Republic of Slovenia National Medical Ethics Committee has approved this study.

Criteria

Inclusion criteria:

- invited to elective CA because of suspected/unknown: coronary artery disease, valvular heart disease, heart failure etiology, unexplained arrhythmia, cardiomyopathy etiology;

- written consent;

- completed first set of questionnaires 14 days prior to coronary angiography.

  Exclusion criteria:

- need for an urgent coronary angiography,

- coronary angiography in last 6 months,

- unable to provide written consent,

- severe physical and/or mental disease/disability,

- help needed in completing the questionnaires,

- unsigned consent form,

- incomplete first set of questionnaires 14 days prior to coronary angiography.

Section 51.5

Stuttering and Anxiety

This section includes text excerpted from "Stuttering and Anxiety," ClinicalTrials.gov, National Institutes of Health (NIH), May 2017.

Purpose

Stuttering was defined as a common neurodevelopmental speech disorder characterized by repetitions, prolongations, and interruptions in the flow of speech. In other words, stuttering is a speech disorder characterized by involuntary disruptions to speech which impede the capacity to communicate effectively.

Physiological and emotional anxiety has been reported in persons who stutter. It has been reported that as high as 44 percent of clients seeking treatment for stuttering could be assigned a co-occurring social phobia or social anxiety diagnosis.

Outcome

Primary outcome measures:

- Stuttering severity index [Time Frame: 30 minutes]

Score of stuttering severity index a ranging from 1 to 40. It grades was divided into (very mild- mild- moderate- severe- very severe) Secondary outcome measures:

- Child Behavior Checklist for age 4-18 [Time Frame: 30 minutes]

Questionnaire for detect presence of anxiety in children

- Estimated Enrollment: 100
- Actual Study Start Date: May 17, 2017
- Estimated Study Completion Date: April 1, 2019
- Estimated Primary Completion Date: April 1, 2018 (Final data collection date for primary outcome measure)

Detailed Description

According to the Diagnostic and Statistical Manual of Mental Disorders, social anxiety disorder is characterized by marked or intense fear of social or performance-based situations where scrutiny or evaluation by others may occur. Feared situations often include speaking in public, meeting new people, and talking with authority figures.

There are several reasons to expect that stuttering may be associated with social anxiety disorder. To begin with, stuttering is accompanied by numerous negative consequences across the lifespan which may increase vulnerability to social and psychological difficulties. These consequences are intensified during the school years when children become more involved in social and speaking situations. As a result, children and adolescents who stutter frequently experience peer victimization, social isolation and rejection, and they may also be less popular than their nonstuttering peers.

Criteria

Inclusion criteria:

- Age ≥ 6 years to 16 years
- Gender: both sex is included in the study

- Intelligence quotient ≥ 85

  Exclusion criteria:

- Intelligence quotient < 85
- Age below 6 years or above 16 years
- Presence of other speech, language or physical disorders

Chapter 52

Research on Anxiety Disorders

Section 52.1

Role of Research in Improving the Understanding and Treatment of Anxiety Disorders

This section includes text excerpted from "Role of Research in Improving the Understanding and Treatment of Anxiety Disorders," National Institute of Mental Health (NIMH), July 31, 2013. Reviewed September 2017.

Scientists are looking at what role genes play in the development of certain mental disorders and are also investigating the effects of environmental factors such as pollution, physical and psychological stress, and diet. In addition, studies are being conducted on the "natural history" (what course the illness takes without treatment) of a variety of individual anxiety disorders, combinations of anxiety disorders, and anxiety disorders that are accompanied by other mental illnesses such as depression.

Scientists currently think that, like heart disease and type 1 diabetes, mental illnesses are complex and probably result from a combination of genetic, environmental, psychological, and developmental factors. For instance, although certain sponsored studies of twins and families suggest that genetics play a role in the development of some anxiety disorders, problems such as posttraumatic stress disorder (PTSD) are triggered by trauma. Genetic studies may help explain why some people exposed to trauma develop PTSD and others do not.

Several parts of the brain are key actors in the production of fear and anxiety. Using brain imaging technology and neurochemical techniques, scientists have discovered that the amygdala and the hippocampus play significant roles in most anxiety disorders.

The amygdala is an almond-shaped structure deep in the brain that is believed to be a communications hub between the parts of the brain that process incoming sensory signals and the parts that interpret these signals. It can alert the rest of the brain that a threat is present and trigger a fear or anxiety response. It appears that emotional memories are stored in the central part of the amygdala and may play a role in anxiety disorders involving very distinct fears, such as fears of dogs, spiders, or flying.

The hippocampus is the part of the brain that encodes threatening events into memories. Studies have shown that the hippocampus appears to be smaller in some people who were victims of child abuse or who served in military combat. Research will determine what causes this reduction in size and what role it plays in the flashbacks, deficits in explicit memory, and fragmented memories of the traumatic event that are common in PTSD.

By learning more about how the brain creates fear and anxiety, scientists may be able to devise better treatments for anxiety disorders. For example, if specific neurotransmitters are found to play an important role in fear, drugs may be developed that will block them and decrease fear responses; if enough is learned about how the brain generates new cells throughout the lifecycle, it may be possible to stimulate the growth of new neurons in the hippocampus in people with PTSD. Current research on anxiety disorders includes studies that address how well medication and behavioral therapies work in the treatment of OCD, and the safety and effectiveness of medications for children and adolescents who have a combination of anxiety disorders and attention deficit hyperactivity disorder.

Section 52.2

Pediatrics-Based Brief Therapy Outdoes Referral for Youths with Anxiety and Depression

This section includes text excerpted from "Pediatrics-Based Brief Therapy Outdoes Referral for Youths with Anxiety and Depression," National Institute of Mental Health (NIMH), May 31, 2017.

A streamlined behavioral therapy delivered in a pediatrics practice offered much greater benefit to youth with anxiety and depression than a more standard referral to mental healthcare with follow-up in a clinical trial comparing the two approaches. The benefit of the former approach in comparison with referral was especially striking in Hispanic youth, a finding that may help inform efforts to address disparities in care.

Depression and anxiety disorders are prevalent among youth; an estimated 25.1 percent of 13 to 18-year-olds have an anxiety disorder. Surveys also suggest that less than a third of youth with anxiety and just over 40 percent with mood disorders receive treatment. These disorders can have serious consequences for affected youth; depression and anxiety can compromise education, employment, and relationships with friends and family.

A clinical trial that was held at the University of Pittsburgh, which enrolled 185 youths, ages 8 to 16, from pediatric clinics in San Diego and Pittsburgh. Participants in the trial met criteria for depression or an anxiety disorder, including separation anxiety, generalized anxiety disorder, or social phobia. Each was randomly assigned to either a brief behavioral therapy (BBT) or to referral to mental healthcare with periodic check-in calls.

The BBT tested in this trial simultaneously addresses both depression and anxiety, rather than targeting one or the other, and it is streamlined in comparison to some standard approaches, with fewer therapeutic components. Of the 95 youths assigned to BBT in the trial, 50 (56.8%) improved on a scale that assesses improvement across anxiety and depression, while 20 (28.2%) of youths in the assisted referral group improved. Raters who evaluated the youth were unaware of which treatment each received. Youth in the BBT group also did better on a scale of overall functioning and had fewer symptoms of anxiety. The contrast in results between the Hispanic youth receiving BBT and those receiving assisted referral was even greater: 13 of 17 (76.5%) responded to BBT, while 1 of 14 (7.1%) assigned to assisted referral did. Hispanic youths receiving BBT also did much better on measures of functioning.

One of the central elements of the BBT was behavioral activation in which a youth is encouraged to engage in activities that he or she finds desirable but difficult, such as social functions. "In these interventions, kids learn not to withdraw from what's upsetting them." Slowly they learn to approach and actively problem solve. Step by step, they re-engage with the tasks that they need to do or want to do—school, social, family-related—but previously struggled to do, because negative emotions were in the way.

Any differences in the number of therapeutic sessions received either with BBT or as a result of referral did not account for the differences measured in benefits to youth. The referral coordinators successfully connected 82 percent of families with specialty mental healthcare, and the youth in that group had an average of 6.5 therapeutic visits (versus an average of 11.2 sessions of BBT). But even the referral group youth with the most therapeutic sessions had worse outcomes than those in BBT.

An important impetus for the development of the therapy tested in this trial was to provide an intervention that is easy to disseminate, and in particular, adaptable for use in primary care settings where many children and adolescents get regular care. "In order to reach the very large number of youth suffering from emotional problems, we need to explore treatment delivery settings, like pediatrics, with a wide reach and low stigma," said Dr. Weersing. "This has great promise for improving access to care, particularly for Latino youth."

Joel Sherrill, Ph.D., deputy director of National Institute of Mental Health's (NIMH) Division of Services and Intervention Research (DSIR), said "This study is remarkable in its attention to testing a brief intervention that lends itself to scale-up in settings readily accessible to youth; and in the deployment-focused approach to matching the intensity of the intervention to the capacity within the primary care setting."

Section 52.3

Estrogen Alters Memory Circuit Function in Women with Gene Variant

This section includes text excerpted from "Estrogen Alters Memory Circuit Function in Women with Gene Variant," National Institute of Mental Health (NIMH), April 19, 2017.

Fluctuations in estrogen can trigger atypical functioning in a key brain memory circuit in women with a common version of a gene, National Institute of Mental Health (NIMH) scientists have discovered. Brain scans revealed altered circuit activity linked to changes in the sex hormone in women with the gene variant while they performed a working memory task.

The findings may help to explain individual differences in menstrual cycle and reproductive-related mental disorders linked to fluctuations in the hormone. They may also shed light on mechanisms underlying sex-related differences in onset, severity, and course of mood and anxiety disorders and schizophrenia. The gene-by-hormone interaction's effect on circuit function was found only with one of two versions of the gene that occurs in about a fourth of white women.

Drs. Karen Berman, Peter Schmidt, Shau-Ming Wei, and colleagues, of the NIMH Intramural Research Program (IRP), report on this first such demonstration in women April 18, 2017 in the journal *Molecular Psychiatry*. Prior to the study, there was little evidence from research on the human brain that might account for individual differences in cognitive and behavioral effects of sex hormones. For example, why do some women develop postpartum depression and others do not—in response to the same hormone changes?

Why do some women report that estrogen replacement improved their memory, whereas large studies of postmenopausal estrogen therapy show no overall improvement in memory performance? Evidence from humans has also been lacking for the neural basis of stark sex differences in prevalence and course of mental disorders that are likely related to sex hormones. For example, why are there higher rates of mood disorders in females and higher rates of attention-deficit hyperactivity disorder (ADHD) in males—or later onset of schizophrenia in females?

In seeking answers to these questions, the researchers focused on working memory, a well-researched brain function often disturbed in many of these disorders. It was known that working memory is mediated by a circuit from the brain's executive hub, the prefrontal cortex, to its memory hub, the hippocampus. Notably, hippocampus activity is typically suppressed during working memory processing. Following-up on a clue from experiments in mice, the NIMH team hypothesized that estrogen tweaks circuit function by interacting with a uniquely human version of the gene that codes for brain derived neurotrophic factor (BDNF), a pivotal chemical messenger operating in this circuit. To find out, the researchers experimentally manipulated estrogen levels in healthy women with one or the other version of the BDNF gene over a period of months. Researchers periodically scanned the women's brain activity while they performed a working memory task to see any effects of the gene-hormone interaction on circuit function.

428

The researchers first scanned 39 women using PET (positron emission tomography) and later confirmed the results in 27 women using fMRI (functional magnetic resonance imaging). Both pegged atypical activity in the hippocampus to the interaction. Turning up the same findings using two types of neuroimaging strengthens the case for the accuracy of their observations, say the researchers. Such gene-hormone interactions affecting thinking and behavior are consistent with findings from animal studies and are suspect mechanisms conferring risk for mental illness, they add.

Section 52.4

Circuitry for Fearful Feelings, Behavior Untangled in Anxiety Disorders

This section includes text excerpted from "Circuitry for Fearful Feelings, Behavior Untangled in Anxiety Disorders," National Institute of Mental Health (NIMH), September 9, 2016.

An "incorrect" assumption that fear and anxiety are mediated in the brain by a single "fear circuit" has stalled progress in developing better treatments for anxiety disorders, argue two leading experts. Designing future research based on a "two-system" framework holds promise for improving treatment outcomes, say Daniel Pine, M.D., a clinical researcher in the National Institute of Mental Health (NIMH) Emotion and Development Branch, and Joseph LeDoux, Ph.D., a basic scientist and NIMH grantee at New York University.

Pine, who conducts brain imaging studies of anxiety disorders in youth, and LeDoux, well-known for discovering circuitry underlying threat processing, offer their "conceptual reframing" September 9, 2016 in the *American Journal of Psychiatry*.

Neuroscience advances in understanding how the brain detects and responds to threat have failed to translate into significantly improved treatments because the field has been led astray by a simplistic notion of a "fear system," contend Pine and LeDoux. For example, hopes that medications that lessen rodents' stress reactivity might help people feel less fearful or anxious often haven't borne out.

Rather, the authors point to mounting evidence that such subjective feeling states are mediated via different circuitry than defensive behaviors. The former via higher order processing in the cortex—and the latter via the amygdala and related centers, mostly deeper in the brain.

For starters, Pine and LeDoux propose more precise use of terminology. Fear and anxiety describe conscious subjective feeling states; defensive reactions refer to rapidly-deployed behaviors or physiological responses. Fear denotes feelings associated with an imminent threat, anxiety feelings associated with an uncertain or more distant source of harm. For example, the amygdala, often colloquially dubbed the brain's "fear center," in fact unconsciously detects and responds to imminent threats and contributes to fear only indirectly. States like fear and anxiety instead arise from areas of the cortex associated with higher order thinking processes and language in people, only some of which occur in other animals.

"If feelings of fear or anxiety are not products of circuits that control defensive behavior, studies of defensive behavior in animals will be of limited value in finding medications that can relieve feelings of fear and anxiety in people," observe the authors, who note that making such distinctions will help in the design of more realistic translational studies.

Meanwhile, the distinctions may also temper expectations for development of specific-acting antianxiety agents. "Existing medications are blunt tools," note Pine and LeDoux. If the experience of fear and anxiety is rooted in cortical changes in thinking, attention and memory, some "anxiolytic" effects might result from "general emotional blunting" or "impaired cognitive processing," they add.

Improving treatments will require a more exact understanding of how treatments work. With this knowledge and the two-systems perspective, existing treatments might be adapted to work better. Brain imaging biomarkers might help tailor treatments to target circuit dysfunctions of specific patients. For example, anxious patients showing altered activity profiles in cortex circuitry underlying working memory might receive psychotherapies that teach them how to regulate emotion through reappraisal or other thinking strategies.

Section 52.5

The Relationship between PTSD and Suicide

This section includes text excerpted from "The Relationship between PTSD and Suicide," U.S. Department of Veterans Affairs (VA), March 28, 2017.

How Common Is Suicide?

It is challenging to determine an exact number of suicides. Many times, suicides are not reported and it can be very difficult to determine whether or not a particular individual's death was intentional. For a suicide to be recognized, examiners must be able to say that the deceased meant to die. Other factors that contribute to the difficulty are differences among states as to who is mandated to report a death, as well as changes over time in the coding of mortality data.

Data from the National Vital Statistics System, a collaboration between the National Center for Health Statistics of the U.S. Department of Health and Human Services (HHS) and each U.S. state, provides the best estimate of suicides. Overall, men have significantly higher rates of suicide than women. This is true whether or not they are Veterans. For comparison:

- From 1999-2010, the suicide rate in the U.S. population among males was 19.4 per 100,000, compared to 4.9 per 100,000 in females.

- Based on the most recent data available, in fiscal year 2009, the suicide rate among male Veteran VA users was 38.3 per 100,000, compared to 12.8 per 100,000 in females.

Does Trauma Increase an Individual's Suicide Risk?

A body of research indicates that there is a correlation between many types of trauma and suicidal behaviors. For example, there is evidence that traumatic events such as childhood abuse may increase a person's suicide risk. A history of military sexual trauma (MST) also increases the risk for suicide and intentional self-harm, suggesting a need to screen for suicide risk in this population.

431

Importance of Combat Exposure in Veterans

Though considerable research has examined the relation between combat or war trauma and suicide, the relationship is not entirely clear. Some studies have shown a relationship while others have not. There is strong evidence, though, that among Veterans who experienced combat trauma, the highest relative suicide risk is observed in those who were wounded multiple times and/or hospitalized for a wound. This suggests that the intensity of the combat trauma, and the number of times it occurred, may influence suicide risk in Veterans. This study assessed only combat trauma, not a diagnosis of PTSD, as a factor in the suicidal behavior.

Does PTSD Increase an Individual's Suicide Risk?

Considerable debate exists about the reason for the heightened risk of suicide in trauma survivors. Whereas some studies suggest that suicide risk is higher among those who experienced trauma due to the symptoms of PTSD, others claim that suicide risk is higher in these individuals because of related psychiatric conditions. However, a study analyzing data from the National Comorbidity Survey, a nationally representative sample, showed that PTSD alone out of six anxiety diagnoses was significantly associated with suicidal ideation or attempts. While the study also found an association between suicidal behaviors and both mood disorders and antisocial personality disorder, the findings pointed to a robust relationship between PTSD and suicide after controlling for comorbid disorders. A later study using the Canadian Community Health Survey data also found that respondents with PTSD were at higher risk for suicide attempts after controlling for physical illness and other mental disorders.

Some studies that point to PTSD as a precipitating factor of suicide suggest that high levels of intrusive memories can predict the relative risk of suicide. Anger and impulsivity have also been shown to predict suicide risk in those with PTSD. Further, some cognitive styles of coping such as using suppression to deal with stress may be additionally predictive of suicide risk in individuals with PTSD.

PTSD and Suicide Risk in Veterans

Other research looking specifically at combat-related PTSD in Vietnam era Veterans suggests that the most significant predictor of both suicide attempts and preoccupation with suicide is combat-related guilt. Many Veterans experience highly intrusive thoughts and extreme guilt about acts committed during times of war. These thoughts can often overpower the emotional coping capacities of Veterans.

With respect to OIF/OEF Veterans, PTSD has been found to be a risk factor for suicidal ideation. Subthreshold PTSD also carries risk. A recent study found that among OIF/OEF Veterans, those with subthreshold PTSD were 3 times more likely to report hopelessness or suicidal ideation than those without PTSD.

Can PTSD Treatment Help?

Current practice guidelines for treatment of PTSD indicate that trauma-focused therapies are not recommended for individuals with "significant suicidality." Because "suicidality" is a vague term and there is no guidance for what significant suicidality means, this recommendation is interpreted to pertain to actively suicidal patients, or those in an acute clinical emergency for whom suicidality should be addressed without delay. Providers must therefore use clinical judgment prior to initiating and throughout trauma-focused therapy.

Individuals with PTSD who present with intermittent but manageable suicidal thoughts may benefit from trauma-focused therapy. Two effective treatments for PTSD, Cognitive Processing Therapy (CPT) and prolonged exposure (PE) have been shown to reduce suicidal ideation. A recent study that randomized women who experienced rape into CPT or PE treatment found that reductions in PTSD symptoms were associated with decreases in suicidal ideation throughout treatment. The reductions were maintained over a 5-10 year follow-up period. The effect of PTSD treatment on suicidal ideation was greater for women who completed CPT. Further research is needed to provide additional evidence in other populations.

Suicide as a Traumatic Event

Researchers have also examined exposure to suicide as a traumatic event. Studies show that trauma from exposure to suicide can contribute to PTSD. In particular, adults and adolescents are more likely to develop PTSD as a result of exposure to suicide if one or more of the following conditions are true: if they witness the suicide, if they are very connected with the person who dies, or if they have a history of psychiatric illness. Studies also show that traumatic grief is more likely to arise after exposure to traumatic death such as suicide. Traumatic grief refers to a syndrome in which individuals experience functional impairment, a decline in physical health, and suicidal ideation. These symptoms occur independently of other conditions such as depression and anxiety.

Part Seven

Additional Help and Information

Chapter 53

Glossary of Terms Related to Anxiety Disorders

abandonment: A situation in which the child has been left by the parent(s), the parent's identity or whereabouts are unknown, the child suffers serious harm, or the parent has failed to maintain contact with the child or to provide reasonable support for a specified period of time.

acupuncture: A family of procedures involving stimulation of anatomical points on the body by a variety of techniques.

acute stress disorder (ASD): A mental disorder that can occur in the first month following a trauma. ASD may involve feelings such as not knowing where you are, or feeling as if you are outside of your body.

addiction: A chronic, relapsing disease characterized by compulsive drug seeking and use and by long-lasting changes in the brain.

adolescence: A human life stage that begins at twelve years of age and continues until twenty-one complete years of age, generally marked by the beginning of puberty and lasting to the beginning of adulthood.

agitation: A condition in which a person is unable to relax and be still. The person may be very tense and irritable, and become easily annoyed by small things.

This glossary contains terms excerpted from documents produced by several sources deemed reliable.

agoraphobia: An intense fear of being in open places or in situations where it may be hard to escape, or where help may not be available.

amygdala: An almond-shaped structure involved in processing and remembering strong emotions such as fear. It is part of the limbic system and located deep inside the brain.

anorexia nervosa: An eating disorder caused by a person having a distorted body image and not consuming the appropriate calorie intake resulting in severe weight loss.

anticonvulsant: A drug or other substance used to prevent or stop seizures or convulsions. Also called antiepileptic.

antidepressant: Medication used to treat depression and other mood and anxiety disorders.

antipsychotic: Medication used to treat psychosis.

anxiety: An abnormal sense of fear, nervousness, and apprehension about something that might happen in the future.

assessment: The ongoing practice of informing decision-making by identifying, considering, and weighing factors that impact children, youth, and their families. Assessment occurs from the time children and families come to the attention of the child welfare system and continues until case closure.

atherosclerosis: A blood vessel disease characterized by the buildup of plaque, or deposits of fatty substances and other matter in the inner lining of an artery.

avoidance: One of the symptoms of posttraumatic stress disorder (PTSD). Those with PTSD avoid situations and reminders of their trauma.

behavior problem: Behavior of the child in the school and/or community that adversely affects socialization, learning, growth, and moral development. May include adjudicated or nonadjudicated behavior problems. Includes running away from home or a placement.

behavioral health: A state of mental/emotional being and/or choices and actions that affect wellness. Substance abuse and misuse, as well as serious psychological distress, suicide, and mental illness, are examples of some behavioral health problems.

behavioral therapy: Behavioral therapy focuses on a person's actions and aims to change unhealthy behavior patterns.

beta blockers: A type of medication that reduces nerve impulses to the heart and blood vessels, which makes the heart beat slower and with less force.

biofeedback: A technique that uses simple electronic devices to teach clients how to consciously regulate bodily functions, such as breathing, heart rate, and blood pressure, to improve overall health. Biofeedback is used to reduce stress, eliminate headaches, recondition injured muscles, control asthma attacks, and relieve pain.

bipolar disorder: A disorder that causes severe and unusually high and low shifts in mood, energy, and activity levels, as well as unusual shifts in the ability to carry out day-to-day tasks. (Also known as Manic Depression)

bonding: The process of developing lasting emotional ties with one's immediate caregivers; seen as the first and primary developmental achievement of a human being and central to a person's ability to relate to others throughout life.

borderline personality disorder: BPD is a serious mental illness marked by unstable moods, behavior, and relationships.

cognition: Conscious mental activities (such as thinking, communicating, understanding, solving problems, processing information and remembering) that are associated with gaining knowledge and understanding.

cognitive behavioral therapy (CBT): Helps people focus on how to solve their current problems. The therapist helps the patient learn how to identify distorted or unhelpful thinking patterns, recognize and change inaccurate beliefs, relate to others in more positive ways, and change behaviors accordingly.

compulsion: Uncontrollable thoughts or impulses to perform an act, often repetitively, as an unconscious mechanism to avoid unacceptable ideas and desires which, by themselves, arouse anxiety; the anxiety becomes fully manifest if performance of the compulsive act is prevented; may be associated with obsessive thoughts.

deep breathing: An active process that involves conscious control over breathing in and out. This may involve controlling the way in which air is drawn in (for example, through the mouth or nostrils), the rate (for example, quickly or over a length of time), the depth (for example, shallow or deep), and the control of other body parts (for example, relaxation of the stomach).

dementia: Loss of brain function that occurs with certain diseases. It affects memory, thinking, language, judgment and behavior.

depression: A group of diseases including major depressive disorder (commonly referred to as depression), dysthymia, and bipolar disorder.

discipline: Training that develops self-control, self-sufficiency, and orderly conduct. Discipline is based on respect for an individual's capability and is not to be confused with punishment.

domestic violence: A pattern of assaultive and/or coercive behaviors, including physical, sexual, and psychological attacks, as well as economic coercion, that adults or adolescents use against their intimate partners. Intimate partners include spouses, sexual partners, parents, children, siblings, extended family members, and dating relationships.

dopamine: A brain chemical, classified as a neurotransmitter, found in regions of the brain that regulate movement, emotion, motivation, and pleasure.

drug abuse: Compulsive use of drugs that is not of a temporary nature. Applies to infants addicted at birth.

eating disorder: Eating disorders, such as anorexia nervosa, bulimia nervosa, and binge-eating disorder, involve serious problems with eating.

electroconvulsive therapy (ECT): A treatment for severe depression that is usually used only when people do not respond to medications and psychotherapy. ECT involves passing a low-voltage electric current through the brain. The person is under anesthesia at the time of treatment.

gene: the basic unit of heredity, composed of a segment of DNA containing the code for a specific trait; see deoxyribonucleic acid (DNA).

hallucinations: Hearing, seeing, touching, smelling or tasting things that are not real.

hormone: A chemical message produced by an endocrine gland which travels through the bloodstream to a target organ.

hypersomnia: A state characterized by subjective report of tiredness and objective evidence of inability to maintain vigilance.

hypertension: High blood pressure has been linked to cognitive decline, stroke, and types of dementia that affect the white matter regions of the brain.

hypnosis: An altered state of consciousness characterized by increased responsiveness to suggestion. The procedure is used to effect positive changes and to treat numerous health conditions including ulcers, chronic pain, respiratory ailments, stress, and headaches.

impulse: An electrical communication signal sent between neurons by which neurons communicate with each other.

insomnia: A chronic or acute sleep disorder characterized by a complaint of difficulty initiating, and/or maintaining sleep, and/or a subjective complaint of poor sleep quality that result in daytime impairment and subjective report of impairment.

isolation: State of being separated from others. Isolation is sometimes used to prevent disease from spreading.

magnetic resonance imaging: An imaging technique that uses magnetic fields to take pictures of the brain's structure.

massage therapy: Massage therapy encompasses many different techniques. In general, therapists press, rub, and otherwise manipulate the muscles and other soft tissues of the body.

meditation: A group of techniques, most of which started in Eastern religious or spiritual traditions. In meditation, individuals learn to focus their attention and suspend the stream of thoughts that normally occupy the mind. This practice is believed to result in a state of greater physical relaxation, mental calmness, and psychological balance. Practicing meditation can change how a person relates to the flow of emotions and thoughts in the mind.

mental illness: A health condition that changes a person's thinking, feelings, or behavior (or all three) and that causes the person distress and difficulty in functioning.

migraine: Headaches that are usually pulsing or throbbing and occur on one or both sides of the head. They are moderate to severe in intensity, associated with nausea, vomiting, sensitivity to light and noise, and worsen with routine physical activity.

mood disorders: Mental disorders primarily affecting a person's mood.

neurotransmitter: A chemical messenger between neurons. These substances are released by the axon on one neuron and excite or inhibit activity in a neighboring neuron.

obsessive-compulsive disorder: An anxiety disorder in which a person suffers from obsessive thoughts and compulsive actions, such as cleaning, checking, counting, or hoarding.

panic disorder: An anxiety disorder in which a person suffers from sudden attacks of fear and panic. The attacks may occur without a known reason, but many times they are triggered by events or thoughts that produce fear in the person, such as taking an elevator or driving.

phobia: An anxiety disorder in which a person suffers from an unusual amount of fear of a certain activity or situation.

postpartum depression: Postpartum depression is when a new mother has a major depressive episode within one month after delivery.

posttraumatic stress disorder: An anxiety disorder that develops in reaction to physical injury or severe mental or emotional distress, such as military combat, violent assault, natural disaster, or other life-threatening events.

psychiatrist: A doctor (M.D.) who treats mental illness. Psychiatrists must receive additional training and serve a supervised residency in their specialty. They can prescribe medications.

psychologist: A clinical psychologist is a professional who treats mental illness, emotional disturbance, and behavior problems. They use talk therapy as treatment, and cannot prescribe medication. A clinical psychologist will have a master's degree (M.A.) or doctorate (Ph.D.) in psychology, and possibly more training in a specific type of therapy.

sedative: Drugs that suppress anxiety and promote sleep; the National Survey on Drug Use and Health (NSDUH) classification includes benzodiazepines, barbiturates, and other types of CNS depressants.

selective serotonin reuptake inhibitors: A group of medications used to treat depression. These medications cause an increase in the amount of the neurotransmitter serotonin in the brain.

serotonin: a neurotransmitter present throughout the body and brain that plays an important role in headache and migraine, mood disorders, regulating body temperature, sleep, vomiting, sexuality, and appetite.

sexual abuse: Coercing or attempting to coerce any sexual contact or behavior without consent.

sleep disorder: Sleep disorders are clinical conditions that are a consequence of a disturbance in the ability to initiate or maintain the quantity and quality of sleep needed for optimal health, performance and well being.

social phobia: Social phobia is a strong fear of being judged by others and of being embarrassed. This fear can be so strong that it gets in the way of going to work or school or doing other everyday things.

stimulants: A class of drugs that enhances the activity of monamines (such as dopamine) in the brain, increasing arousal, heart rate, blood pressure, and respiration, and decreasing appetite; includes some medications used to treat attention-deficit hyperactivity disorder (e.g., methylphenidate and amphetamines), as well as cocaine and methamphetamine.

tai chi: A mind-body practice that originated in China as a martial art. Individuals doing tai chi move their bodies slowly and gently, while breathing deeply and meditating (tai chi is sometimes called moving meditation).

tolerance: A condition in which higher doses of a drug are required to produce the same effect achieved during initial use; often associated with physical dependence.

trauma: A life-threatening event, such as military combat, natural disasters, terrorist incidents, serious accidents, or physical or sexual assault in adult or childhood.

yoga: A combination of breathing exercises, physical postures, and meditation used to calm the nervous system and balance the body, mind, and spirit.

Chapter 54

Statewide Mental Health Resources

Alabama

Division of Mental Health & Substance Abuse Services
Alabama Department of Mental Health
P.O. Box 301410
Montgomery, AL 36130-1410
Toll-Free: 800-367-0955
Phone: 334-242-3454
Fax: 334-242-0725
Website: www.mh.alabama.gov/UT/ContactUs.aspx
E-mail: webmaster@mh.alabama.gov

Alaska

Division of Behavioral Health
Alaska Department of Health and Social Services
P.O. Box 110620
Juneau, AK 99811-0620
Phone: 907-465-4994
Fax: 907-465-2185
Website: www.dhss.alaska.gov

Resources in this chapter were compiled from several sources deemed reliable; all contact information was verified and updated in September 2017.

Arizona

Behavioral Health Services
Arizona Department of Health
Services
150 N. 18th Ave.
Ste. 200
Phoenix, AZ 85007
Phone: 602-364-2536
Fax: 602-364-4808
Website: www.azdhs.gov/
licensing/index.php#contact-us

Arkansas

**Division of Behavioral
Health Services**
Donaghey Plaza
P.O. Box 1437
Little Rock, AR 72203
Phone: 501-682-1001
TDD: 501-682-8820
Toll-Free TTY: 800-285-1131
Website: www.arkansas.gov

Colorado

**Colorado Department of
Human Services**
1575 Sherman St.
Eighth Fl.
Denver, CO 80203-1714
Phone: 303-866-5700
Fax: 303-866-5563
Website: www.colorado.gov/
pacific/cdhs/contact-us-5
E-mail: cdhs_communications@
state.co.us

Connecticut

**Department of Mental Health
and Addiction Services**
410 Capitol Ave.
P.O. Box 341431
Hartford, CT 06134
Toll-Free: 800-446-7348
Phone: 860-418-7000
TDD: 860-418-6707
Website: www.ct.gov/dmhas/cwp/
view.asp?a=2899&q=334084

Delaware

**Division of Substance Abuse
and Mental Health**
Community Mental Health and
Addiction Services
1901 N. Du Pont Hwy
Main Bldg.
New Castle, DE 19720
Toll-Free: 800-652-2929
Phone: 302-255-9040
Fax: 302-255-4429
Website: www.dhss.delaware.
gov/dhss/contact.html

District of Columbia

**Department of Behavioral
Health**
64 New York Ave. N.E.
Third Fl.
Washington, DC 20002
Phone: 202-673-2200
TTY: 202-673-7500
Fax: 202-673-3433
Website: www.dbh.dc.gov
E-mail: dbh@dc.gov

Florida

ACCESS Central Mail Center
P.O. Box 1770
Ocala, FL 34478-1770
Toll-Free: 866-762-2237
Toll-Free TTY: 800-955-8771
Toll-Free Fax: 866-886-4342
Website: www.myflfamilies.com/
contact-us

Georgia

Department of Behavioral Health & Developmental Disabilities
Two Peachtree St. N.W.
24th Fl.
Atlanta, GA 30303
Toll-Free: 800-436-7442
Phone: 404-657-2252
Website: www.dbhdd.georgia.
gov/contact-us-0

Hawaii

Department of Health
Child and Adolescent Mental
Health Division
3627 Kilauea Ave.
Rm. 101
Honolulu, HI 96816
Phone: 808-733-9333
Fax: 808-733-9357
Website: www.health.hawaii.
gov/camhd

Illinois

Division of Mental Health
Department of Human Services
401 S. Clinton St.
Chicago, IL 60607
Toll-Free: 800-843-6154
Phone: 312-814-5050
Website: www.dhs.state.il.us/
page.aspx?item=36696
E-mail: dhs.mh@illinois.gov

Iowa

Division of Behavioral Health
Department of Public Health
Lucas State Office Bldg.
321 E. 12th St.
Des Moines, IA 50319-0075
Toll-Free: 866-834-9671
Phone: 515-281-7689
Website: www.idph.iowa.gov/
Contact-Us/Address-Phone-
Hours-of-Operation

Kansas

Department for Children and Families
Office of the Secretary
555 S. Kansas Ave.
Topeka, KS 66603
Phone: 785-296-3271
Website: www.dcf.ks.gov/
DCFContacts/Pages/default.aspx

Kentucky

Cabinet for Health and Family Services
Department for Behavioral
Health, Developmental and
Intellectual Disabilities
275 E. Main St.
Frankfort, KY 40621
Phone: 502-564-5497
Fax: 502-564-9523
Website: www.chfs.ky.gov/
contact

Louisiana

Office of Behavioral Health
Department of Health and
Hospitals
628 N. Fourth St.
P.O. Box 629
Baton Rouge, LA 70802
Toll-Free: 888-342-6207
Phone: 225-342-9500
Fax: 225-342-5568
Website: www.dhh.louisiana.
gov/index.cfm/subhome/10/n/6

Maine

Substance Abuse and Mental Health Services
Department of Health and
Human Services
41 Anthony Ave.
Ste. 11 State House Stn
Augusta, ME 04333-0011
Phone: 207-287-2595
Fax: 207-287-9152
Website: www.maine.gov/dhhs/
samhs/about/contacts.htm

Michigan

Department of Health and Human Services
333 S. Grand Ave.
P.O. Box 30195
Lansing, MI 48909
Phone: 517-373-3740
Website: www.michigan.gov/
mdhhs/0,5885,7-339--352302--
,00.html

Minnesota

Department of Human Services
Mental Health Division
P.O. Box 64981
St. Paul, MN 55164-0981
Phone: 651-431-2225
Fax: 651-431-7418
Website: www.mn.gov/dhs/
general-public/about-dhs/
contact-us/division-addresses.jsp

Mississippi

Mississippi Department of Mental Health
1101 Robert E. Lee Bldg.
239 N. Lamar St.
Jackson, MS 39201
Toll-Free: 877-210-8513
Phone: 601-359-1288
TDD: 601-359-6230
Fax: 601-359-6295
Website: www.dmh.ms.gov

Missouri

Division of Behavioral Health
Missouri Department of Mental Health
1706 E. Elm St.
Jefferson City, MO 65101
Toll-Free: 800-575-7480
Phone: 573-751-4942
Fax: 573-751-7814
Website: www.dmh.mo.gov/contactus.html
E-mail: dbhmail@dmh.mo.gov

Montana

Addictive and Mental Disorders Division
Department of Public Health and Human Services
P.O. Box 202905
Ste. 300
Helena, MT 59620-2905
Phone: 406-444-3964
Fax: 406-444-9389
Website: www.dphhs.mt.gov/Portals/85/amdd/ADA%20Compliant%20Docs%20(NEW)/Left%20Panel/AMDDPhoneListSept2017-ADAOK.pdf?ver=2017-09-11-090359-230

Nebraska

Division of Behavioral Health
Department of Health and Human Services
P.O. Box 95026
Lincoln, NE 68509-5026
Phone: 402-471-3121
Website: www.dhhs.ne.gov/Pages/contact.aspx
E-mail: DHHS.Webmaster@Nebraska.gov

New Hampshire

Department of Health and Human Services
129 Pleasant St.
Concord, NH 03301-3852
Toll-Free: 844-ASK-DHHS (844-275-3447)
Phone: 603-271-6738
Fax: 603-271-6105
Website: www.dhhs.nh.gov/contactus/index.htm

New Mexico

Behavioral Health Services Division
Human Services Department
P.O. Box 2348
Santa Fe, NM 87504-2348
Toll-Free: 888-997-2583
Phone: 505-476-9266
Fax: 505-476-9277
Website: www.hsd.state.nm.us/Contact_Us.aspx

New York

Office of Mental Health
44 Holland Ave.
Albany, NY 12229
Toll-Free: 800-597-8481
Website: www.omh.ny.gov

North Dakota

Behavioral Health Services
Department of Human Services
600 E. Blvd. Ave. Dept 325
Bismarck, ND 58505-0250
Toll-Free: 800-472-2622
Phone: 701-328-2310
TTY: 800-366-6888
Fax: 701-328-2359
Website: www.nd.gov/dhs/about/
contact.html
E-mail: dhseo@nd.gov

Ohio

*Ohio Association of
County Behavioral Health
Authorities*
175 S. Third St.
Ste. 900
Columbus, OH 43215
Phone: 614-224-1111
Website: www.oacbha.org

Oklahoma

*Department of Mental
Health and Substance Abuse
Services*
2000 N. Classen Blvd.
Ste. E600
Oklahoma City, OK 73106
Phone: 405-522-3908
Fax: 405-248-9321
Website: www.ok.gov/triton/
contact.php?ac=193&id=169

Oregon

*Addictions and Mental
Health Services*
Oregon Health Authority
500 Summer St. N.E.
Salem, OR 97301-1079
Phone: 503-945-5772
TTY: 800-375-2863
Fax: 503-378-8467
Website: www.oregon.gov/oha/
HSD/AMH/Pages/Contact-Us.
aspx
E-mail: amh.web@state.or.us

Rhode Island

*Department of Behavioral
Healthcare*
Developmental Disabilities and
Hospitals
14 Harrington Rd.
Cranston, RI 02920-3080
Phone: 401-462-3201
Website: www.bhddh.ri.gov
E-mail: BHDDH.AskDD@bhddh.
ri.gov

South Carolina

Department of Mental Health
Administration Building
2414 Bull St.
P.O. Box 485
Columbia, SC 29202
Phone: 803- 898-8581
TTY: 864-297-5130
Website: www.state.sc.us/dmh/
comments.htm

Tennessee

*Department of Mental Health
and Substance Abuse Services*
Andrew Jackson Building
500 Deaderick St.
Sixth Fl.
Nashville, TN 37243
Toll-Free: 800-560-5767
Phone: 615-532-6580
Website: www.tn.gov/
behavioral-health/article/
contact-us
E-mail: OCA.TDMHSAS@tn.gov

Texas

*Mental Health and
Substance Abuse Division*
Department of State Health
Services
P.O. Box 149347
Austin, TX 78714-9347
Toll-Free: 888-963-7111
Phone: 512-776-2150
Toll-Free TDD: 800-735-2989
Website: www.dshs.state.tx.us/
MHSA
E-mail: customer.service@dshs.
texas.gov

Vermont

Department of Mental Health
280 State Dr. NOB 2 N.
Waterbury, VT 05671-2010
Phone: 802-241-0090
Fax: 802-241-0100
Website: www.mentalhealth.
vermont.gov/contact

Virginia

*Department of Behavioral
Health and Developmental
Services*
P.O. Box 1797
Richmond, VA 23218-1797
Phone: 804-786-3921
TDD: 804-371-8977
Fax: 804-371-6638
Website: www.dbhds.virginia.
gov/contact/contactus

West Virginia

*Bureau for Behavioral
Health and Health Facilities*
Department of Health and
Human Resources
350 Capitol St.
Rm. 350
Charleston, WV 25301
Phone: 304-356-4811
Fax: 304-558-1008
Website: www.dhhr.wv.gov/bhhf/
Pages/Contact-Us.aspx

Wisconsin

Department of Health Services
1 W. Wilson St.
Madison, WI 53703
Phone: 608-266-1865
TTY: 800-947-3529
Website: www.dhs.wisconsin.
gov/contacts.htm
E-mail: DHSwebmaster@dhs.
wisconsin.gov

Wyoming

Behavioral Health Division
Mental Health and Substance
Abuse Services
6101 Yellowstone Rd.
Ste. 220
Cheyenne, WY 82002
Toll-Free: 800-535-4006
Phone: 307-777-6494
Fax: 307-777-5849
Website: www.health.wyo.gov/
behavioralhealth

Chapter 55

Directory of Organizations That Help People with Anxiety Disorders and Other Mental Health Concerns

Government Agencies That Provide Information about Mental Health

Agency for Healthcare Research and Quality (AHRQ)
Office of Communications and Knowledge Transfer
5600 Fishers Ln.
Seventh Fl.
Rockville, MD 20857
Phone: 301-427-1364
Website: www.ahrq.gov

Centers for Disease Control and Prevention (CDC)
1600 Clifton Rd.
Atlanta, GA 30329-4027
Toll-Free: 800-CDC-INFO
(800-232-4636)
Phone: 404-639-3311
Toll-Free TTY: 888-232-6348
Website: www.cdc.gov

Resources in this chapter were compiled from several sources deemed reliable; all contact information was verified and updated in September 2017.

Eldercare.gov
Toll-Free: 800-677-1116
TTY: 800-677-1116
Website: www.eldercare.gov/
Eldercare.NET/Public/About/
Contact_Info/Index.aspx
E-mail: eldercarelocator@n4a.
org

Healthfinder®
National Health Information
Center (NHIC)
1101 Wootton Pkwy
Rockville, MD 20852
Website: www.healthfinder.gov
E-mail: healthfinder@hhs.gov

National Cancer Institute (NCI)
Public Inquiries Office
9609 Medical Center Dr.
Bethesda, MD 20892-9760
Toll-Free: 800-4-CANCER
(800-422-6237)
Website: www.cancer.gov
E-mail: cancergovstaff@mail.nih.
gov

National Center for Complementary and Integrative Health (NCCIH)
9000 Rockville Pike
Bethesda, MD 20892
Toll-Free: 888-644-6226
TTY: 866-464-3615
Website: www.nccih.nih.gov/
tools/contact.htm
E-mail: info@nccih.nih.gov

National Institute of Diabetes and Digestive and Kidney Diseases (NIDDK)
31 Center Dr. MSC 2560
Bldg. 31 Rm. 9A06
Bethesda, MD 20892-2560
Phone: 301-496-3583
Website: www.niddk.nih.gov

National Institute of Mental Health (NIMH)
6001 Executive Blvd.
Rm. 6200 MSC 9663
Bethesda, MD 20892-9663
Toll-Free: 866-615-6464
Phone: 301-443-4513
TTY: 301-443-8431/Toll-Free
TTY: 866-415-8051
Fax: 301-443-4279
Website: www.nimh.nih.gov
E-mail: nimhinfo@nih.gov

National Institute of Neurological Disorders and Stroke (NINDS)
P.O. Box 5801
Bethesda, MD 20824
Toll-Free: 800-352-9424
Phone: 301-496-5751
Website: www.ninds.nih.gov

National Institute on Aging (NIA)
31 Center Dr. MSC 2292
Bldg. 31 Rm. 5C27
Bethesda, MD 20892
Toll-Free: 800-222-2225
Phone: 301-496-1752
Toll-Free TTY: 800-222-4225
Website: www.nia.nih.gov
E-mail: niaic@nia.nih.gov

National Institute on Drug Abuse (NIDA)
6001 Executive Blvd.
Rm. 5213 MSC 9561
Bethesda, MD 20892-9561
Website: www.drugabuse.gov
E-mail: media@nida.nih.gov

National Institutes of Health (NIH)
9000 Rockville Pike
Bethesda, MD 20892
Phone: 301-496-4000
Website: www.nih.gov
E-mail: NIHinfo@od.nih.gov

National Science Foundation (NSF)
4201 Wilson Blvd.
Arlington, VA 22230
Toll-Free: 800-877-8339
Phone: 703-292-5111
TDD: 703-292-5090
Website: www.nsf.gov/help/contact.jsp
E-mail: info@nsf.gov

Office on Women's Health (OWH)
200 Independence Ave. S.W.
Rm. 712E
Washington, DC 20201
Toll-Free: 800-994-9662
Phone: 202-690-7650
Toll-Free TDD: 888-220-5446
Fax: 202-205-2631
Website: www.womenshealth.gov
E-mail: info@minorityhealth.hhs.gov

Substance Abuse and Mental Health Services Administration (SAMHSA)
5600 Fishers Ln.
Rockville, MD 20857
Toll-Free: 877-SAMHSA-7 (877-726-4727)
Toll-Free TDD: 800-487-4889
Website: www.samhsa.gov

U.S. Department of Education (ED)
400 Maryland Ave. S.W.
Washington, DC 20202
Toll-Free: 800-USA-LEARN (800-872-5327)
Website: www2.ed.gov/about/contacts/gen/index.html?src=ft

U.S. Department of Health and Human Services (HHS)
200 Independence Ave. S.W.
Washington, DC 20201
Toll-Free: 877-696-6775
Website: www.hhs.gov

U.S. Department of Veterans Affairs (VA)
810 Vermont Ave. N.W.
Washington, DC 20420
Toll-Free: 800-827-1000
Website: www.va.gov

U.S. Food and Drug Administration (FDA)
10903 New Hampshire Ave.
Silver Spring, MD 20993
Toll-Free: 888-INFO-FDA (888-463-6332)
Website: www.fda.gov

Private Agencies That Provide Information about Mental Health

Al-Anon Family Group Headquarters, Inc
1600 Corporate Landing Pkwy
Virginia Beach, VA 23454-5617
Phone: 757-563-1600
Fax: 757-563-1656
Website: www.al-anon.org/
contact-us
Email: wso@al-anon.org

Alzheimer's Association
225 N. Michigan Ave.
17th Fl.
Chicago, IL 60601-7633
Toll-Free: 800-272-3900
Phone: 312-335-8700
TDD: 312-335-5886
Fax: 866-699-1246
Website: www.alz.org/
contact_us.asp

Alzheimer's Foundation of America
322 Eighth Ave.
Seventh Fl.
New York, NY 10001
Toll-Free: 866-232-8484
Website: www.alzfdn.org/
contact-us
E-mail: info@alzfdn.org

American Academy of Child and Adolescent Psychiatry (AACAP)
3615 Wisconsin Ave. N.W.
Washington, DC 20016-3007
Phone: 202-966-7300
Fax: 202-464-0131

Website: www.aacap.org/
AACAP/About_AACAP/Contact.
aspx

American Academy of Family Physicians (AAFP)
11400 Tomahawk Creek Pkwy
Leawood, KS 66211-2680
Toll-Free: 800-274-2237
Phone: 913-906-6000
Fax: 913-906-6075
Website: www.aafp.org
E-mail: aafp@aafp.org

American Academy of Neurology (AAN)
201 Chicago Ave.
Minneapolis, MN 55415
Toll-Free: 800-879-1960
Phone: 612-928-6000
Fax: 612-454-2746
Website: www.aan.com/
contact-aan
E-mail: memberservices@aan.
com

American Academy of Pediatrics (AAP)
141 N.W. Pt. Blvd.
Elk Grove Village, IL
60007-1098
Toll-Free: 800-433-9016
Phone: 847-434-4000
Fax: 847-434-8000
Website: www.aap.org/en-us/
Pages/Contact.aspx
E-mail: kidsdocs@aap.org

American Association for Geriatric Psychiatry (AAGP)
6728 Old McLean Village Dr.
McLean, VA 22101
Phone: 703-556-9222
Fax: 703-556-8729
Website: www.aagponline.org
E-mail: main@aagponline.org

American Association for Marriage and Family Therapy (AAMFT)
112 S. Alfred St.
Alexandria, VA 22314-3061
Phone: 703-838-9808
Fax: 703-838-9805
Website: www.aamft.org/
imis15/aamft/Core/ContactUs/
ContactUs.aspx

American Association of Suicidology (AAS)
5221 Wisconsin Ave. N.W.
Washington, DC 20015
Toll-Free: 800-273-TALK
(800-273-8255)
Phone: 202-237-2280
Fax: 202-237-2282
Website: www.suicidology.org

American Counseling Association (ACA)
6101 Stevenson Ave.
Ste. 600
Alexandria, VA 22304
Toll-Free: 800-347-6647
Phone: 703-823-9800
Toll-Free Fax: 800-473-2329
Website: www.counseling.org/
about-us/contact-us
E-mail: webmaster@counseling.
org

American Foundation for Suicide Prevention (AFSP)
120 Wall St.
29th Fl.
New York, NY 10005
Toll-Free: 888-333-AFSP
(888-333-2377)
Phone: 212-363-3500
Fax: 212-363-6237
Website: www.afsp.org/
about-afsp/contact
E-mail: info@afsp.org

American Group Psychotherapy Association (AGPA)
25 E. 21st St.
Sixth Fl.
New York, NY 10010
Phone: 212-477-2677
Fax: 212-979-6627
Website: www.agpa.org/
contact-us
E-mail: info@agpa.org

American Heart Association
7272 Greenville Ave.
Dallas, TX 75231
Toll-Free: 800-AHA-USA
(800-242-8721)
Website: www.heart.org/
HEARTORG

American Medical Association (AMA)
AMA Plaza
330 N. Wabash Ave.
Ste. 39300
Chicago, IL 60611-5885
Toll-Free: 800-621-8335
Website: www.ama-assn.org/
eform/submit/contact-us

American Pain Society
8735 W. Higgins Rd.
Ste. 300
Chicago, IL 60631
Phone: 847-375-4715
Fax: 866-574-2654
Website: www.
americanpainsociety.org
E-mail: iinfo@
americanpainsociety.org

American Parkinson Disease Association (APDA)
135 Parkinson Ave.
Staten Island, NY 10305
Toll-Free: 800-223-2732
Phone: 718-981-8001
Fax: 718-981-4399
Website: www.apdaparkinson.
org/contact
E-mail: apda@apdaparkinson.
org

American Psychiatric Association (APA)
1000 Wilson Blvd.
Ste. 1825
Arlington, VA 22209
Toll-Free: 888-357-7924
Phone: 703-907-7300
Website: www.psych.org
E-mail: apa@psych.org

American Psychological Association (APA)
750 First St. N.E.
Washington, DC 20002-4242
Toll-Free: 800-374-2721
Phone: 202-336-5500
TDD/TTY: 202-336-6123
Website: www.apa.org
E-mail: public.affairs@apa.org

American Society on Aging
575 Market St.
Ste. 2100
San Francisco, CA 94105-2869
Toll-Free: 800-537-9728
Phone: 415-974-9600
Fax: 415-974-0300
Website: www.asaging.org/form/
contact-us
E-mail: info@asaging.org

Anxiety Disorders Association of America (ADAA)
8701 Georgia Ave.
Ste. 412
Silver Spring, MD 20910
Phone: 240-485-1001
Fax: 240-485-1035
Website: www.adaa.org/
contact-adaa
E-mail: information@adaa.org

Association for Applied Psychophysiology and Biofeedback (AAPB)
10200 W. 44th Ave.
Ste. 304
Wheat Ridge, CO 80033
Toll-Free: 800-477-8892
Phone: 303-422-8436
Website: www.aapb.org/i4a/
pages/index.cfm?pageid=3290
E-mail: info@aapb.org

Association for Behavioral and Cognitive Therapies (ABCT)
305 Seventh Ave.
16th Fl.
New York, NY 10001
Phone: 212-647-1890
Fax: 212-647-1865
Website: www.abct.org/
About/?m=mAbout&fa=
ContactUs
E-mail: clinical.dir@abct.org

Brain & Behavior Research Foundation
90 Park Ave.
16th Fl.
New York, NY 10016
Toll-Free: 800-829-8289
Phone: 646-681-4888
Website: www.bbrfoundation.
org/contact
E-mail: info@bbrfoundation.org

Brain Injury Association of America (BIAA)
1608 Spring Hill Rd., Ste. 110
Vienna, VA 22182
Toll-Free: 800-444-6443
Phone: 703-761-0750
Fax: 703-761-0755
Website: www.biausa.org
E-mail: braininjuryinfo@biausa.org

Brain Trauma Foundation
1 Bdwy.
Sixth Fl.
New York, NY 10004
Phone: 212-772-0608
Fax: 212-772-0357
Website: www.braintrauma.org
E-mail: braininjuryinfo@biausa.
org

Caring.com
2600 S. El Camino Real
Ste. 300
San Mateo, CA 94403
Toll-Free: 800-973-1540
Phone: 650-312-7100
Website: www.caring.com/about/
contact

Cleveland Clinic
9500 Euclid Ave.
Cleveland, OH 44195
Toll-Free: 800-223-2273
Website: www.
my.clevelandclinic.org

Creutzfeldt-Jakob Disease Foundation Inc.
P.O. Box 5312
Akron, OH 44334
Toll-Free: 800-659-1991
Fax: 234-466-7077
Website: www.cjdfoundation.org/
contact
E-mail: help@cjdfoundation.org

The Dana Foundation
505 Fifth Ave.
Sixth Fl.
New York, NY 10017
Phone: 212-223-4040
Fax: 212-317-8721
Website: www.dana.org/About/
Contact_Us
E-mail: danainfo@dana.org

Davis Phinney Foundation
4730 Table Mesa Dr.
Ste. J-200
Boulder, CO 80305
Toll-Free: 866-358-0285
Phone: 303-733-3340
Fax: 303-733-3350
Website: www.
davisphinneyfoundation.org/
contact-us
E-mail: contact@dpf.org

Depressed Anonymous (DA)
P.O. Box 17414
Louisville, KY 40214
Phone: 502-569-1989
Website: www.depressedanon.
com
E-mail: depanon@netpenny.net

*Depression and Bipolar
Support Alliance (DBSA)*
55 E. Jackson Blvd.
Ste. 490
Chicago, IL 60604
Toll-Free: 800-826-3632
Fax: 312-642-7243
Website: www.dbsalliance.org
E-mail: info@dbsalliance.org

*Families for Depression
Awareness*
395 Totten Pond Rd.
Ste. 404
Waltham, MA 02451
Phone: 781-890-0220
Fax: 781-890-2411
Website: www.familyaware.org/
contact-us
E-mail: info@familyaware.org

*Family Caregiver Alliance
(FCA)*
235 Montgomery St.
Ste. 950
San Francisco, CA 94104
Toll-Free: 800-445-8106
Phone: 415-434-3388
Website: www.caregiver.org/
contact

*Geriatric Mental Health
Foundation (GMHF)*
6728 Old McLean Village Dr.
McLean, VA 22101
Phone: 703-556-9222
Fax: 703-556-8729
Website: www.gmhfonline.org
E-mail: web@GMHFonline.org

*Hospice Foundation of
America*
1707 L St. N.W.
Ste. 220
Washington, DC 20036
Toll-Free: 800-854-3402
Phone: 202-457-5811
Fax: 202-457-5815
Website: www.
hospicefoundation.org/
Contact-HFA
E-mail: info@hospicefoundation.
org

*International Foundation for
Research and Education on
Depression*
P.O. Box 17598
Baltimore, MD 21297-1598
Fax: 443-782-0739
Website: www.ifred.org
E-mail: info@ifred.org

*International OCD
Foundation, Inc.*
P.O. Box 961029
Boston, MA 02196
Phone: 617-973-5801
Fax: 617-973-5803
Website: www.iocdf.org/about/
contact-us
E-mail: info@iocdf.org

*International Society for
Traumatic Stress Studies*
111 Deer Lake Rd.
Ste. 100
Deerfield, IL 60015
Phone: 847-480-9028
Fax: 847-480-9282
Website: www.istss.org
E-mail: istss@istss.org

*Lewy Body Dementia
Association (LBDA)*
912 Killian Hill Rd. S.W.
Lilburn, GA 30047
Toll-Free: 800-539-9767
Phone: 404-975-2322
Fax: 480-422-5434
Website: www.lbda.org/contact
E-mail: lbda@lbda.org

Meals on Wheels America
1550 Crystal Dr.
Ste. 1004
Arlington, VA 22202
Toll-Free: 888-998-6325
Fax: 703-548-5274
Website: www.
mealsonwheelsamerica.org

*Mental Health America
(MHA)*
500 Montgomery St.
Ste. 820
Alexandria, VA 22314
Toll-Free: 800-969-6642
Phone: 703-684-7722
Fax: 703-684-5968
Website: www.
mentalhealthamerica.net/
contact-us

Mental Health Minute
Website: www.
mentalhealthminute.info

*National Academy of Elder
Law Attorneys (NAELA)*
1577 Spring Hill Rd.
Ste. 310
Vienna, VA 22182
Phone: 703-942-5711
Fax: 703-563-9504
Website: www.naela.org/
Web/About/ImportTemp/
About_NAELA_New.
aspx?hkey=feb0efd3-bd62-4508-
9ca4-20de373d4784
E-mail: naela@naela.org

*National Alliance for
Caregiving (NAC)*
4720 Montgomery Ln.
Ste. 205
Bethesda, MD 20814
Phone: 301-718-8444
Fax: 301-951-9067
Website: www.caregiving.org
E-mail: info@caregiving.org

National Alliance on Mental Illness (NAMI)
3803 N. Fairfax Dr., Ste. 100
Arlington, VA 22203
Toll-Free: 800-950-6264
Phone: 703-524-7600
Fax: 703-524-9094
Website: www.nami.org

National Association of Anorexia Nervosa and Associated Disorders (ANAD)
220 N. Green St.
Chicago, IL 60607
Phone: 630-577-1330
Fax: 630-577-1333
Website: www.anad.org
E-mail: hello@anad.org

National Association of School Psychologists (NASP)
4340 E. West Hwy
Ste. 402
Bethesda, MD 20814
Toll-Free: 866-331-NASP
(866-331-6277)
Phone: 301-657-0270
Fax: 301-657-0275
Website: www.apps.nasponline.org/about-nasp/contact-us.aspx

National Center for Victims of Crime
2000 M St. N.W.
Ste. 480
Washington, DC 20036
Phone: 202-467-8700
Fax: 202-467-8701
Website: www.ncvc.org
E-mail: webmaster@ncvc.org

National Council on Problem Gambling
730 11th St. N.W.
Ste. 601
Washington, DC 20001
Toll-Free: 800-522-4700
Phone: 202-547-9204
Fax: 202-547-9206
Website: www.ncpgambling.org
E-mail: ncpg@ncpgambling.org

National Eating Disorders Association (NEDA)
165 W. 46th St., Ste. 402
New York, NY 10036
Toll-Free: 800-931-2237
Phone: 212-575-6200
Fax: 212-575-1650
Website: www.nationaleatingdisorders.org
E-mail: info@NationalEatingDisorders.org

National Federation of Families for Children's Mental Health
9605 Medical Center Dr.
Ste. 280
Rockville, MD 20850
Phone: 240-403-1901
Fax: 240-403-1909
Website: www.ffcmh.org
E-mail: ffcmh@ffcmh.org

National Gerontological Nursing Association (NGNA)
121 W. State St.
Geneva, IL 60134
Phone: 630-748-4616
Website: www.ngna.org
E-mail: ngna@affinity-strategies.com

National Hospice and Palliative Care Organization (NHPCO)
1731 King St., Ste. 100
Alexandria, VA 22314
Toll-Free: 800-646-6460
Phone: 703-837-1500
Fax: 703-837-1233
Website: www.nhpco.org
E-mail: nhpco_info@nhpco.org

National Rehabilitation Information Center (NARIC)
8400 Corporate Dr., Ste. 500
Landover, MD 20785
Toll-Free: 800-346-2742
TTY: 301-459-5984
Fax: 301-459-5984
Website: www.naric.com

National Stroke Association
9707 E. Easter Ln.
Ste. B
Centennial, CO 80112
Toll-Free: 800-STROKES
(800-787-6537)
Phone: 303-649-9299
Website: www.stroke.org/
webform/contact-us
E-mail: info@stroke.org

Parkinson's Institute and Clinical Center
675 Almanor Ave.
Sunnyvale, CA 94085-2934
Toll-Free: 800-655-2273
Phone: 408-734-2800
Fax: 408-734-8455
Website: www.thepi.org/contact-the-parkinsons-institute-and-clinical-center
E-mail: info@thepi.org

Parkinson's Disease Foundation (PDF)
1359 Bdwy., Ste. 1509
New York, NY 10018
Toll-Free: 800-457-6676
Phone: 212-923-4700
Fax: 212-923-4778
Website: www.pdf.org/contact_us
E-mail: info@pdf.org

Postpartum Support International (PSI)
6706 S.W. 54th Ave.
Portland, OR 97219
Toll-Free: 800-944-4PPD
(800-944-4773)
Phone: 503-894-9453
Fax: 503-894-9452
Website: www.postpartum.net/
contact-us
E-mail: support@postpartum.net

Psych Central
55 Pleasant St.
Ste. 207
Newburyport, MA 01950
Website: www.psychcentral.com/
about/feedback
E-mail: talkback@psychcentral.
com

Society of Certified Senior Advisors
720 S. Colorado Blvd.
Ste. 750 N.
Denver, CO 80246
Toll-Free: 800-653-1785
Website: www.csa.us/page/
Contact
E-mail: Society@csa.us

Suicide Awareness Voices of Education (SAVE)
8120 Penn Ave. S.
Ste. 470
Bloomington, MN 55431
Toll-Free: 800-273-8255
Phone: 952-946-7998
Website: www.save.org/contact

Suicide Prevention Resource Center (SPRC)
Education Development Center, Inc.
43 Foundry Ave.
Waltham, MA 02453-8313
Toll-Free: 877-GET-SPRC
(877-438-7772)
TTY: 617-964-5448
Website: www.sprc.org/
contact-us
E-mail: info@sprc.org

Visiting Nurses Associations of America (VNAA)
2121 Crystal Dr.
Ste. 750
Arlington, VA 22202
Toll-Free: 888-866-8773
Phone: 571-527-1520
Fax: 571-527-1521
Website: www.vnaa.org/
contact-us
E-mail: vnaa@vnaa.org

Well Spouse Association
63 W. Main St.,Ste. H
Freehold, NJ 07728
Toll-Free: 800-838-0879
Phone: 732-577-8899
Fax: 732-577-8644
Website: www.wellspouse.org
E-mail: info@wellspouse.org

Index

Index

Page numbers followed by 'n' indicate a footnote. Page numbers in *italics* indicate a table or illustration.